Clostridioides difficile Infection, 2nd Edition

Clostridioides difficile Infection, 2nd Edition

Editor

Guido Granata

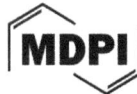

Basel • Beijing • Wuhan • Barcelona • Belgrade • Novi Sad • Cluj • Manchester

Guido Granata
Clinical and Research Department
for Infectious Diseases
National Institute for Infectious
Diseases L. Spallanzani, IRCCS
Rome
Italy

Editorial Office
MDPI AG
Grosspeteranlage 5
4052 Basel, Switzerland

This is a reprint of articles from the Special Issue published online in the open access journal *Antibiotics* (ISSN 2079-6382) (available at: www.mdpi.com/journal/antibiotics/special_issues/Clostridioides_2nd).

For citation purposes, cite each article independently as indicated on the article page online and using the guide below:

Lastname, A.A.; Lastname, B.B. Article Title. *Journal Name* **Year**, *Volume Number*, Page Range.

ISBN 978-3-7258-1642-2 (Hbk)
ISBN 978-3-7258-1641-5 (PDF)
https://doi.org/10.3390/books978-3-7258-1641-5

© 2024 by the authors. Articles in this book are Open Access and distributed under the Creative Commons Attribution (CC BY) license. The book as a whole is distributed by MDPI under the terms and conditions of the Creative Commons Attribution-NonCommercial-NoDerivs (CC BY-NC-ND) license (https://creativecommons.org/licenses/by-nc-nd/4.0/).

Contents

About the Editor vii

Preface ix

Guido Granata
Introduction to the Special Issue on *Clostridioides difficile* Infection, Second Edition
Reprinted from: *Antibiotics* 2024, 13, 607, doi:10.3390/antibiotics13070607 1

Mircea Stoian, Adina Andone, Alina Boeriu, Sergio Rareș Bândilă, Daniela Dobru and Sergiu Ștefan Laszlo et al.
COVID-19 and *Clostridioides difficile* Coinfection Analysis in the Intensive Care Unit
Reprinted from: *Antibiotics* 2024, 13, 367, doi:10.3390/antibiotics13040367 3

Bogdan Ioan Vintila, Anca Maria Arseniu, Claudiu Morgovan, Anca Butuca, Victoria Bîrluțiu and Carmen Maximiliana Dobrea et al.
A Real-World Study on the Clinical Characteristics, Outcomes, and Relationship between Antibiotic Exposure and *Clostridioides difficile* Infection
Reprinted from: *Antibiotics* 2024, 13, 144, doi:10.3390/antibiotics13020144 16

Dongxuan Li, Yi Song, Zhanfeng Bai, Xin Xi, Feng Liu and Yang Zhang et al.
Real-World Data in Pharmacovigilance Database Provides a New Perspective for Understanding the Risk of *Clostridium difficile* Infection Associated with Antibacterial Drug Exposure
Reprinted from: *Antibiotics* 2023, 12, 1109, doi:10.3390/antibiotics12071109 37

Łukasz Lis, Andrzej Konieczny, Michał Sroka, Anna Ciszewska, Kornelia Krakowska and Tomasz Gołębiowski et al.
Clinical Determinants Predicting *Clostridioides difficile* Infection among Patients with Chronic Kidney Disease
Reprinted from: *Antibiotics* 2022, 11, 785, doi:10.3390/antibiotics11060785 50

Nobuaki Mori, Jun Hirai, Wataru Ohashi, Nobuhiro Asai, Yuichi Shibata and Hiroshige Mikamo
Clinical Efficacy of Fidaxomicin and Oral Metronidazole for Treating *Clostridioides difficile* Infection and the Associated Recurrence Rate: A Retrospective Cohort Study
Reprinted from: *Antibiotics* 2023, 12, 1323, doi:10.3390/antibiotics12081323 57

Artsiom Klimko, Cristian George Tieranu, Ana-Maria Curte, Carmen Monica Preda, Ioana Tieranu and Andrei Ovidiu Olteanu et al.
Clostridioides Difficile Enteritis: Case Report and Literature Review
Reprinted from: *Antibiotics* 2022, 11, 206, doi:10.3390/antibiotics11020206 66

Tri-Hanh-Dung Doan, Marie-Françoise Bernet-Camard, Sandra Hoÿs, Claire Janoir and Séverine Péchiné
Impact of Subinhibitory Concentrations of Metronidazole on Morphology, Motility, Biofilm Formation and Colonization of *Clostridioides difficile*
Reprinted from: *Antibiotics* 2022, 11, 624, doi:10.3390/antibiotics11050624 77

Sean Lee, Neha Nanda, Kenichiro Yamaguchi, Yelim Lee and Rosemary C. She
Clostridioides difficile Toxin B PCR Cycle Threshold as a Predictor of Toxin Testing in Stool Specimens from Hospitalized Adults
Reprinted from: *Antibiotics* 2022, 11, 576, doi:10.3390/antibiotics11050576 93

Daniele Roberto Giacobbe, Antonio Vena, Marco Falcone, Francesco Menichetti and Matteo Bassetti
Fidaxomicin for the Treatment of *Clostridioides difficile* Infection in Adult Patients: An Update on Results from Randomized Controlled Trials
Reprinted from: *Antibiotics* **2022**, *11*, 1365, doi:10.3390/antibiotics11101365 . . . . **102**

Guido Granata, Francesco Schiavone and Giuseppe Pipitone
Bezlotoxumab in Patients with a Primary *Clostridioides difficile* Infection: A Literature Review
Reprinted from: *Antibiotics* **2022**, *11*, 1495, doi:10.3390/antibiotics11111495 . . . . **118**

Maria Chiara de Stefano, Benedetta Mazzanti, Francesca Vespasiano, Letizia Lombardini and Massimo Cardillo
The Regulatory Approach for Faecal Microbiota Transplantation as Treatment for *Clostridioides difficile* Infection in Italy
Reprinted from: *Antibiotics* **2022**, *11*, 480, doi:10.3390/antibiotics11040480 . . . . **125**

About the Editor

Guido Granata

Guido Granata, M.D., Ph.D., Infectious disease specialist, allergology and clinical immunology specialist, and consultant in infectious diseases.

In 2010, medical degree, Sapienza University of Rome, Italy. In 2016, Board Certification in Allergology and Clinical Immunology, Sapienza University of Rome, Italy. In 2016, visiting research fellow at the Rheumatology Research Group, Institute of Infection, Inflammation and Ageing, University of Birmingham, UK. In 2017, research fellow at the Italian National Institute for Infectious Diseases "L. Spallanzani", Rome, Italy. In 2017, collaborator, "CCM 2016" project: "Clostridium difficile: good practices for the diagnosis, surveillance, communication and the infection control", funded by the Italian Ministry of Health. In 2018, consultant in infectious diseases, Severe and Immunocompromised Host Infections Unit, National Institute for Infectious Diseases "L. Spallanzani", Rome, Italy. In 2019, principal investigator in the project "ReCloDi–Real Incidence of Clostridioides difficile infection in Italy" and winner of the Italian Society of Anti-Infective Therapy 2019 Young Investigator Grant. In 2020, Doctor of Philosophy degree "Monocytes surface expression of FFA4, a G Protein coupled, free fatty acid sensing receptor in HIV infected subjects", Department of Clinical Medicine, Sapienza University of Rome. In 2021, principal investigator of the study: "A prospective study on incidence, risk factors and outcome of recurrent Clostridioides difficile infection: the ReCloDi study" and winner of the 31s European Society of Clinical Microbiology and Infectious Diseases ECCMID 2021 Travel Grant.

Research activities: infection control, *Clostridioides difficile* infection, antimicrobial treatment, and antimicrobial resistance. Clinical and Research Department, National Institute for Infectious Diseases "L. Spallanzani" IRCCS, Rome, Italy.

Preface

Clostridioides difficile is a Gram-positive, anaerobic bacterium that is one of the most common causes of healthcare-associated infections worldwide.

Despite research efforts and progress made regarding the epidemiology and clinical management of *Clostridioides difficile* infection in the last decade, several critical aspects of this complex disease remain unclear.

This reprint collects multidisciplinary research articles focusing on *Clostridioides difficile* infection. The contributions collected here shed light on grey areas of our knowledge about *Clostridioides difficile*, including the identification of *Clostridioides difficile* carriers at high risk of developing infection or infection recurrence, the intra-hospital and community spread of *Clostridioides difficile* the rate of *Clostridioides difficile* infection during the SARS-CoV-2 pandemic, and the current treatment approach.

I would like to thank the scientific community for their interest in this collection and for submitting manuscripts. I am grateful to the editor-in-chief of *Antibiotics*, Professor Nicholas Dixon, and the managing editor, Ms. Monica He, for their invaluable support.

Special thanks go to my mentor, Professor Nicola Petrosillo, who introduced me to my career and research interests and always supported me, and to my beloved family, Patricia, Meletta-Flaminia, and Maritozza-Cecilia.

Guido Granata
Editor

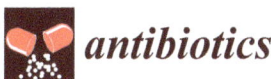

Editorial

Introduction to the Special Issue on *Clostridioides difficile* Infection, Second Edition

Guido Granata

Clinical and Research Department for Infectious Diseases, National Institute for Infectious Diseases L. Spallanzani, IRCCS, 00149 Rome, Italy; guido.granata@inmi.it

Clostridioides difficile (CD) is a Gram-positive, anaerobic bacterium that is one of the most common causes of infective diarrhoea worldwide [1].

Among hospitalized patients, *Clostridioides difficile* infection (CDI) leads to increased morbidity, mortality, and extended hospital stays. Despite research efforts and progress made regarding the epidemiology and clinical management of CDI in the last decade, several critical aspects of this complex disease remain unclear. Firstly, the clinical spectrum of CDI is wide-ranging, from asymptomatic carriage and mild diarrhoea to severe colitis, toxic megacolon, and fatality [1,2]. The mortality rates associated with CDI vary considerably across studies, ranging from less than 2% to 17% [2].

The identification of CD carriers at high risk of developing infection and CDI patients at high risk of developing severe CDI and experiencing recurrence remains a significant challenge [3].

Another concern is the intra-hospital and community spread of CD [4]. Understanding the transmission routes is crucial for the development of targeted interventions to reduce the spread of CDI. Antimicrobial stewardship and infection control programmes may help to prevent CDI, even during the ongoing SARS-CoV-2 pandemic [4].

The molecular pathogenesis of CDI remains uncertain. Further research is required to elucidate the interactions between CD, the gut microbiota, host immunity, and the specific roles of CD toxin A, toxin B, and binary toxin [5,6].

Finally, CDI recurrences present a significant challenge, increasing hospitalization costs and morbidity and mortality rates [3]. While oral vancomycin or fidaxomicin represent the recommended first-line antimicrobial therapies, further study is required to confirm the efficacy and safety of innovative non-antimicrobial approaches, including monoclonal anti-toxin antibodies, fecal microbiota transplantation, vaccines, and phage therapy [1,7].

The Second Edition of the Special Issue *Clostridioides difficile* Infection includes seven full research articles, two review articles, and one perspective and one communication article. These contributions aim to add clarity on the open issues surrounding this topic.

Among the contributions, the work by Stoian, M. et al. examined the correlation between COVID-19 and CDI in the intensive care unit [8]. Of interest, the authors identified immuno-modulator or steroid treatment, antibiotic administration, and proton pump inhibitor treatment as significant risk factors for CDI coinfection among COVID-19 patients admitted to intensive care, and reported an increased mortality rate among these patients [8].

The study by Lis L. et al. aimed to identify the clinical determinants predicting CDI among the subgroup of hospitalized patients with chronic kidney disease [9]. The results confirmed that serum albumin has a protective effect against CDI severity. The multivariate analysis showed that the stage of chronic kidney disease and the length of antibiotic use increased the risk of CDI, whereas a lower Norton scale score had a protective impact [9].

Regarding CDI treatment in specific subgroups of high-risk patients, Giacobbe, D. R. et al. discussed the updated evidence on the efficacy of fidaxomicin for the treatment of either the first CDI episode or recurrent CDI. The authors reported evidence supporting the

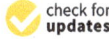

Citation: Granata, G. Introduction to the Special Issue on *Clostridioides difficile* Infection, Second Edition. *Antibiotics* 2024, 13, 607. https://doi.org/10.3390/antibiotics13070607

Received: 14 June 2024
Accepted: 24 June 2024
Published: 29 June 2024

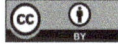

Copyright: © 2024 by the author. Licensee MDPI, Basel, Switzerland. This article is an open access article distributed under the terms and conditions of the Creative Commons Attribution (CC BY) license (https://creativecommons.org/licenses/by/4.0/).

use of fidaxomicin despite its high cost. According to the authors, risk models for recurrent CDI should be used to select patients for fidaxomicin treatment [10].

Future studies should focus on identifying high-risk groups for recurrent CDI. At present, bezlotoxumab may be considered in specific, high-risk patients with immunosuppression. Granata, G. et al. collected the available evidence on bezlotoxumab for preventing recurrent CDI during a first CDI episode [11]. Their findings support the administration of bezlotoxumab in patients with a primary CDI episode, despite the high cost. According to the authors, it is likely that the future guidance may change from "administer bezlotoxumab only in high-risk patients" to "consider bezlotoxumab even for a primary CDI episode, in view of the patient benefits and the cost-effectiveness of reducing expensive recurrent CDI episodes" [11].

This Special Issue presents a compendium of multidisciplinary research on CDI. The collected works serve as a comprehensive resource for scholars engaged in the field of CDI, and the Guest Editor is grateful for the interest and contributions that have been received.

Funding: This research received no external funding.

Conflicts of Interest: The author declares no conflicts of interest.

References

1. Di Bella, S.; Sanson, G.; Monticelli, J.; Zerbato, V.; Principe, L.; Giuffrè, M.; Pipitone, G.; Luzzati, R. Clostridioides difficile infection: History, epidemiology, risk factors, prevention, clinical manifestations, treatment, and future options. *Clin. Microbiol. Rev.* **2024**, *37*, e0013523. [CrossRef] [PubMed]
2. Czepiel, J.; Krutova, M.; Mizrahi, A.; Khanafer, N.; Enoch, D.A.; Patyi, M.; Deptuła, A.; Agodi, A.; Nuvials, X.; Pituch, H.; et al. Mortality Following Clostridioides difficile Infection in Europe: A Retrospective Multicenter Case-Control Study. *Antibiotics* **2021**, *10*, 299. [CrossRef] [PubMed]
3. Granata, G.; Petrosillo, N.; Adamoli, L.; Bartoletti, M.; Bartoloni, A.; Basile, G.; Bassetti, M.; Bonfanti, P.; Borromeo, R.; Ceccarelli, G.; et al. Prospective Study on Incidence, Risk Factors and Outcome of Recurrent Clostridioides difficile Infections. *J. Clin. Med.* **2021**, *10*, 1127. [CrossRef] [PubMed]
4. Viprey, V.F.; Granata, G.; Vendrik, K.E.W.; Davis, G.L.; Petrosillo, N.; Kuijper, E.J.; Vilken, T.; Lammens, C.; Schotsman, J.J.; Benson, A.D.; et al. European survey on the current surveillance practices, management guidelines, treatment pathways and heterogeneity of testing of Clostridioides difficile, 2018–2019: Results from The Combatting Bacterial Resistance in Europe CDI (COMBACTE-CDI). *J. Hosp. Infect.* **2023**, *131*, 213–220. [CrossRef] [PubMed]
5. Kordus, S.L.; Thomas, A.K.; Lacy, D.B. Clostridioides difficile toxins: Mechanisms of action and antitoxin therapeutics. *Nat. Rev. Microbiol.* **2022**, *20*, 285–298. [CrossRef] [PubMed]
6. Granata, G.; Mariotti, D.; Ascenzi, P.; Petrosillo, N.; di Masi, A. High Serum Levels of Toxin A Correlate with Disease Severity in Patients with Clostridioides difficile Infection. *Antibiotics* **2021**, *10*, 1093. [CrossRef] [PubMed]
7. van Prehn, J.; Reigadas, E.; Vogelzang, E.H.; Bouza, E.; Hristea, A.; Guery, B.; Krutova, M.; Norén, T.; Allerberger, F.; Coia, J.E.; et al. European Society of Clinical Microbiology and Infectious Diseases: 2021 update on the treatment guidance document for Clostridioides difficile infection in adults. *Clin. Microbiol. Infect.* **2021**, *27* (Suppl. 2), S1–S21. [CrossRef] [PubMed]
8. Stoian, M.; Andone, A.; Boeriu, A.; Bândilă, S.R.; Dobru, D.; Laszlo, S.Ș.; Corău, D.; Arbănași, E.M.; Russu, E.; Stoian, A. COVID-19 and Clostridioides difficile Coinfection Analysis in the Intensive Care Unit. *Antibiotics* **2024**, *13*, 367. [CrossRef] [PubMed]
9. Lis, Ł.; Konieczny, A.; Sroka, M.; Ciszewska, A.; Krakowska, K.; Gołębiowski, T.; Hruby, Z. Clinical Determinants Predicting Clostridioides difficile Infection among Patients with Chronic Kidney Disease. *Antibiotics* **2022**, *11*, 785. [CrossRef] [PubMed]
10. Giacobbe, D.R.; Vena, A.; Falcone, M.; Menichetti, F.; Bassetti, M. Fidaxomicin for the Treatment of Clostridioides difficile Infection in Adult Patients: An Update on Results from Randomized Controlled Trials. *Antibiotics* **2022**, *11*, 1365. [CrossRef] [PubMed]
11. Granata, G.; Schiavone, F.; Pipitone, G. Bezlotoxumab in Patients with a Primary Clostridioides difficile Infection: A Literature Review. *Antibiotics* **2022**, *11*, 1495. [CrossRef] [PubMed]

Disclaimer/Publisher's Note: The statements, opinions and data contained in all publications are solely those of the individual author(s) and contributor(s) and not of MDPI and/or the editor(s). MDPI and/or the editor(s) disclaim responsibility for any injury to people or property resulting from any ideas, methods, instructions or products referred to in the content.

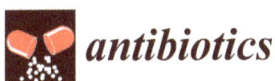

Article

COVID-19 and *Clostridioides difficile* Coinfection Analysis in the Intensive Care Unit

Mircea Stoian [1], Adina Andone [2,*], Alina Boeriu [2], Sergio Rareș Bândilă [3], Daniela Dobru [2], Sergiu Ștefan Laszlo [4], Dragoș Corău [4], Emil Marian Arbănași [5,6,7], Eliza Russu [6,7] and Adina Stoian [8]

1. Department of Anesthesiology and Intensive Care, George Emil Palade University of Medicine, Pharmacy, Sciences and Technology of Targu Mures, 540139 Targu Mures, Romania; mircea.stoian@umfst.ro
2. Gastroenterology Department, George Emil Palade University of Medicine, Pharmacy, Sciences and Technology of Targu Mures, 540142 Targu Mures, Romania; aboeriu@gmail.com (A.B.); daniela.dobru@umfst.ro (D.D.)
3. Orthopedic Surgery and Traumatology Service, Marina Baixa Hospital, Av. Alcade En Jaume Botella Mayor, 03570 Villajoyosa, Spain; sergiob1976@gmail.com
4. Intensive Care Unit, Mures, County Hospital, Street Gheorghe Marinescu No 1, 540136 Targu Mures, Romania; laszlo.sergiu.stefan@gmail.com (S.Ș.L.); dragos.corau@gmail.com (D.C.)
5. Department of Vascular Surgery, George Emil Palade University of Medicine, Pharmacy, Science and Technology of Targu Mures, 540139 Targu Mures, Romania; emilarbanasi1@gmail.com
6. Clinic of Vascular Surgery, Mures County Emergency Hospital, 540136 Targu Mures, Romania; eliza.russu@umfst.ro
7. Doctoral School of Medicine and Pharmacy, George Emil Palade University of Medicine, Pharmacy, Sciences and Technology of Targu Mures, 540142 Targu Mures, Romania
8. Department of Pathophysiology, George Emil Palade University of Medicine, Pharmacy, Sciences and Technology of Targu Mures, 540136 Targu Mures, Romania; adina.stoian@umfst.ro
* Correspondence: adina.roman91@gmail.com

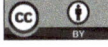

Citation: Stoian, M.; Andone, A.; Boeriu, A.; Bândilă, S.R.; Dobru, D.; Laszlo, S.Ș.; Corău, D.; Arbănași, E.M.; Russu, E.; Stoian, A. COVID-19 and *Clostridioides difficile* Coinfection Analysis in the Intensive Care Unit. *Antibiotics* **2024**, *13*, 367. https://doi.org/10.3390/antibiotics13040367

Academic Editor: Guido Granata

Received: 25 March 2024
Revised: 14 April 2024
Accepted: 16 April 2024
Published: 17 April 2024

Copyright: © 2024 by the authors. Licensee MDPI, Basel, Switzerland. This article is an open access article distributed under the terms and conditions of the Creative Commons Attribution (CC BY) license (https://creativecommons.org/licenses/by/4.0/).

Abstract: Since the emergence of SARS-CoV-2 in late 2019, the global mortality attributable to COVID-19 has reached 6,972,152 deaths according to the World Health Organization (WHO). The association between coinfection with *Clostridioides difficile* (CDI) and SARS-CoV-2 has limited data in the literature. This retrospective study, conducted at Mureș County Clinical Hospital in Romania, involved 3002 ICU patients. Following stringent inclusion and exclusion criteria, 63 patients were enrolled, with a division into two subgroups—SARS-CoV-2 + CDI patients and CDI patients. Throughout their hospitalization, the patients were closely monitored. Analysis revealed no significant correlation between comorbidities and invasive mechanical ventilation (IMV) or non-invasive mechanical ventilation (NIMV). However, statistically significant associations were noted between renal and hepatic comorbidties ($p = 0.009$), death and CDI-SARS-CoV-2 coinfection ($p = 0.09$), flourochinolone treatment and CDI-SARS-CoV-2 infection ($p = 0.03$), and an association between diabetes mellitus and SARS-CoV-2-CDI infection ($p = 0.04$), as well as the need for invasive mechanical ventilation ($p = 0.04$). The patients with CDI treatment were significantly younger and received immuno-modulator or corticotherapy treatment, which was a risk factor for opportunistic agents. Antibiotic and PPI (proton pump inhibitor) treatment were significant risk factors for CDI coinfection, as well as for death, with PPI treatment in combination with antibiotic treatment being a more significant risk factor.

Keywords: *Clostridioides difficile*; SARS-CoV-2; antibiotic therapy; corticosteroid therapy; intensive care unit

1. Introduction

The literature has limited data regarding the association between coinfection with *Clostridioides difficile* and SARS-CoV-2 in Intensive Care Units. Most of the publications have assessed the characteristics of *C. difficile* comparatively between the COVID-19 pandemic and the pre-pandemic period. Starting from this comparison, our goal was to analyze the data of critical patients admitted to the Intensive Care Unit (ICU) with SARS-CoV-2 infection and compare them with critical patients with CDI admitted to the ICU.

Since the end of 2019, global healthcare has been affected by the COVID-19 pandemic and its consequences. At the end of October 2023, nearly 4 years after the onset of the pandemic, 771,408,825 confirmed COVID-19 cases were declared, with a total number of 6,972,152 cumulative deaths. There are still reports of new-onset cases, without an epidemiological risk of a new pandemic [1]. In Romania, the first case of COVID-19 was identified on the 15 February 2020, and since then, more than 3,485,792 COVID-19 cases were reported, with a cumulative 68,455 death cases.

COVID-19 can present with various associated symptoms, varying from loss of smell to nasal obstruction, fever, or difficulty breathing. Interestingly, diarrhea was reported with an incidence of 19% [2]. Most of the COVID-19 cases had a mild or moderate severity and did not require hospitalization or advanced medical care [3]. Severe forms of COVID-19 manifested with pneumonia and difficulty breathing, with associated pulmonary infiltrations evidenced by thoracic imagistic scans. Pneumonia can be complicated by respiratory insufficiency, which requires oxygen supplementations or mechanical ventilation (invasive or non-invasive) [4,5]. Other severe complications of COVID-19 include thromboembolic events (pulmonary embolism or stroke), circulatory shock, myocardial lesions, arrhythmias and encephalopathies [6,7], loss of taste and smell [8], generalized headache [9], dizziness with vertigo [10], seizures [11], encephalitis [12], and Guillain–Barré syndrome [13]. Nevertheless, the exact mechanisms of these changes are still being studied. Several digestive symptoms, such as nausea, vomiting, diarrhea, and acute abdominal pain, were observed in COVID-19 cases [14].

The severe form of COVID-19 usually appears one week after the first symptoms, and the clinical manifestations can become catastrophic. Observational studies emphasized the role of dysbiosis in acute and post-acute COVID-19 and its connection to the severity of the disease [15]. The COVID-19 pandemic placed a significant burden on worldwide healthcare through the economic challenges related to increasing medical healthcare costs and the incidence of medical-system-associated infections (nosocomial infections). One of the most frequently associated infections is *C. difficile* infection (CDI). The incidence of CDI has been reported with an increasing pattern since the onset of the COVID-19 pandemic [16,17]. Multiple mechanisms have been proposed to explain the association between COVID-19 and CDI, from which we mention intestinal dysbiosis, the lack of adherence to proper hand hygiene, and excessive empiric antibiotic treatment [18–20]. The increasing use of antibiotics during the COVID-19 pandemic, especially for treating bacterial coinfections and as a prophylactic measure, could have contributed to a higher incidence of CDI and the development of resistant strains of *C. difficile*. Excessive use of antibiotics modifies the normal intestinal flora, which can lead to an increased risk of CDI [18]. CDI is easily transmitted through spores and appears in medical healthcare and the community [21]. The associated symptoms vary from mild diarrhea to toxic megacolon, which can become life-threatening.

While a part of the literature data available show an increased incidence of CDI during the COVID-19 pandemic, other studies show a weak association between the two types of infection [22]. Comparisons between the pre-COVID-19 incidence of CDI and the COVID-19 pandemic CDI infection levels showed a positive correlation between the two disorders, nevertheless showing uncertain significance [23].

This study aimed to assess whether the incidence of CDI and the severity of the clinical and microbiological forms of CDI are different between COVID-19 patients and non-COVID-19 patients during the pandemic.

It is essential to acknowledge the mechanism by which concomitant infection with CDI affects patients and their medical care.

2. Results

2.1. Hospital Characteristics

Mures County Clinical Hospital has 1182 beds, and it is the second hospital for number of beds in Romania, with a total of 44 beds assigned to the ICU (23 beds for the General (Polyvalent) Intensive Care Unit and 21 beds for the Postanesthesia Care Unit Intermediate Intensive Therapy (PACU). In February 2020, the hospital was assigned to the care of COVID-19 patients exclusively, as per the order of the Ministry of Health nr. 444; therefore, the admissions were open only for COVID-19 patients or other medical or surgical emergencies related to these patients. This led to a decrease of 50% in the number of admissions in comparison to previous years.

2.2. CDI Patient Characteristics

In the two years, between 30 March 2020 and 31 March 2022, a total of 19,414 patients were admitted in Mures County Clinical Hospital (HCM), from which 6340 patients were admitted with different forms of COVID-19 and 368 patients were diagnosed with CDI. In the ICU, without PACU, a total of 3002 critical patients were admitted: 1691 with SARS-CoV-2 infection; 1311 non-COVID-19 patients, of which 62 presented with CDI; and 38 had a coinfection with CDI and SARS-CoV-2.

All patients included are presented in Figure 1.

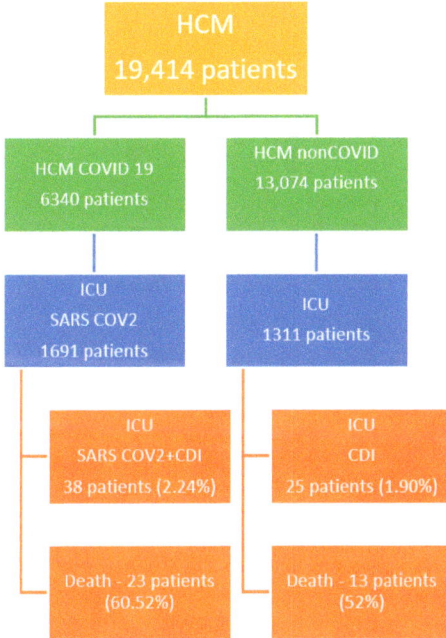

Figure 1. CDI patients' characteristics.

Thirty-six critical patients died during the ICU admission. Twenty-one patients from Group 1 came from an urban environment (55.26%).

The presence of a positive toxin A + B *C. difficile* infection was seen in 58 of the studied patients, and in 5 patients, we saw only toxin A *C. difficile*-positive tests.

The annual incidence of CDI in Mures County Clinical Hospital is seen in Figure 2.

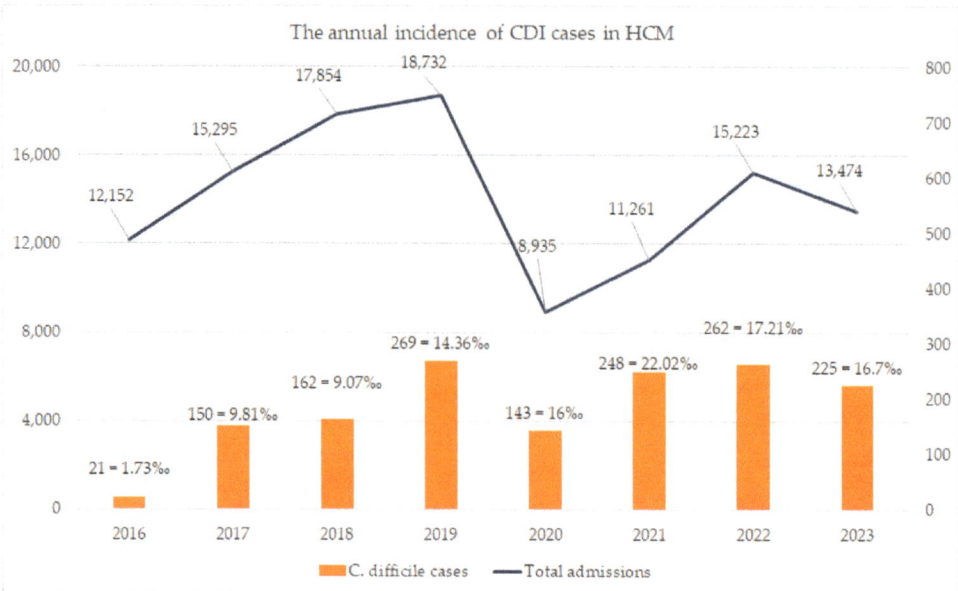

Figure 2. The annual incidence of CDI in HCM.

We can see in Figure 2 an annual increase in the CDI infections starting from 2020 (pandemic period) compared to the pre-pandemic period. In 2020 and 2021, our hospital admitted only COVID-19 cases to the ICU department at a proportion of 80%, showing a direct correlation of the increase in the incidence of CDI with COVID-19 cases, an incidence which dropped in the 2022 and 2023 periods, when our admission pool was mixed (COVID-19 and non-COVID-19 cases). In the remaining 20% of non-COVID-19 admissions, the percentage of CDI infection was very low (1.2 per 1000 cases).

2.3. Incidence Analysis

The total number of admissions is described in Figure 2. We see an increase in CDI incidence in the pre-pandemic period, which varies from 0.8 up to 5.29 per 1000 patients, which increased during the pandemic period, varying from 6.02 per 1000 patients, when we admitted only COVID-19 cases in the HCM. This represents the total number gathered from our electronic databases of nosocomial infections. The patients were not admitted with a diagnosis of CDI before their admission.

In the ICU department, we found 51 cases during 2020–2021 (COVID-19 group), with an incidence of 5.6/1000 cases discharged, and 99 cases during 2017–2018 (pre-COVID-19 group), with an incidence of 6.1/1000 cases discharged ($p = 0.6$). Although the incidence in our selected patients was not statistically different, the annual incidence as seen in Figure 2 has risen, taking into consideration there were only COVID-19 patients admitted in the ICU department.

We found 38 cases of CDI in the COVID-19 group, with an incidence reported for all admitted patients in the ICU of 2.24%, and 25 cases in the non-COVID-19 group, with an incidence of 1.83%. The mean age of the COVID-19 group was 68.79 ± 16.24 years, whereas in the non-COVID-19 group, it was 68.83 ± 12.83 years during the 2-year period of analysis.

The mean duration of ICU admissions in the COVID-19 group was 13.57 ± 8.34 days, whereas in the non-COVID-19 group it was 9.21 ± 9.02 days.

Comparing the mean results, we have a significant statistical difference between the two groups (CDI + COVID-19 group and CDI group) regarding Carmeli score ($p < 0.01$), leukocyte count both at admission and at discharge ($p = 0.01$, $p = 0.04$), neutrophil count at admission and at discharge ($p = 0.03$, $p = 0.01$), creatinine level ($p = 0.001$), ALT ($p = 0.05$), LDH ($p = 0.025$), and platelet count ($p < 0.01$). The paraclinical evolution of patients is seen in Table 1.

Table 1. Paraclinical examinations performed on admission and on discharge.

	Group	Admission	Discharge	Unpaired t-Test p
CRP (mg/dL)	1	36.32 ± 49.6	10.50 ± 11.80	0.731
	2	41.83 ± 72.76	12.95 ± 15.90	0.507
Fibrinogen (mg/dL)	1	475.88 ± 214.02	426.06 ± 187.94	0.374
	2	428.28 ± 184.23	439.59 ± 160.63	0.773
Ferritin (ng/mL)	1	1332.99 ± 901.43	2008.032 ± 2320.15	0.139
	2	838.05 ± 1176.75	724.33 ± 1120.29	0.07
LDH (U/L)	1	480.49 ± 231.26	510.43 ± 342.53	**0.02**
	2	319.00 ± 289.69	249.30 ± 101.82	**0.002**
Leucocytes (/mm^3)	1	10.25 ± 5.06	16.51 ± 8.48	**0.01**
	2	13.67 ± 5.83	12.40 ± 5.66	**0.04**
AST (U/L)	1	57.89 ± 62.36	104.73 ± 268.58	0.08
	2	33.88 ± 28.20	34.46 ± 30.62	0.20
ALT (U/L)	1	74.43 ± 90.98	128.70 ± 235.63	**0.05**
	2	35.83 ± 30.47	32.17 ± 25.25	**0.05**
Creatinine (mg/dL)	1	1.07 ± 0.58	1.34 ± 1.28	**0.001**
	2	2.65 ± 2.73	1.95 ± 2.18	0.17
Urea (mg/dL)	1	70.52 ± 37.85	111.38 ± 93.41	0.06
	2	94.15 ± 60.59	83.90 ± 59.43	0.20

Group 1—COVID-19 + CDI; Group 2—CDI.

Regarding the antibiotic treatment administered, we had a number of patients on cephalosporin treatment (n = 21), carbapenems (n = 11), fluoroquinolones (n = 5), beta-lactamines (n = 6), and aminoglycosides (n = 5). All antibiotic treatments were administered before the hospital admission, there were no patients with previous antibiotic therapy, and not all patients with SARS-CoV-2 infection received antibiotic treatment.

Fluoroquinolone treatment was statistically associated with cephalosporine treatment ($p = 0.03$, Chi-Square test), beta-lactamine, and cephalosporine treatment ($p = 0.001$, Chi-Square test).

Death and CDI-SARS-CoV-2 coinfection were statistically significantly associated with PPI treatment ($p = 0.01$, Chi-Square test; $p = 0.03$, Chi-Square test).

From all patients included in this study who died during ICU admission, 75% of deaths occurred in CDI-SARS-CoV-2 coinfection patients ($p = 0.09$, Chi-Square test).

2.4. Comorbidities Analysis

We found no statistical differences by performing the analysis between the two groups regarding hepatic comorbities, diabetes mellitus, renal comorbidities, cardiovascular comorbidities, antibiotic treatment administered, and sex.

There was a statistically significant association between renal and hepatic comorbidities ($p = 0.009$, Chi-Square test).

CDI + SARS-CoV-2 coinfection was statistically associated with death ($p = 0.01$, Chi-Square test) as well as the status of ventilation ($p = 0.02$, Chi-Square test).

As far as comorbidities, the only comorbidity that was associated with death was diabetes mellitus ($p = 0.05$, Chi-Square test) in the CDI + SARS-CoV-2 group.

There was an association between the need for invasive ventilation and CDI + SARS-CoV-2 coinfection ($p = 0.00$, Chi-Square test), and diabetes mellitus was statistically associated with CDI + SARS-CoV-2 infection ($p = 0.04$, Chi-Square test) and the need for invasive ventilation ($p = 0.04$, Chi-Square test).

Gastrointestinal symptoms such as anorexia, nausea, vomiting, and abdominal pain were reported in 5 patients in the SARS-CoV-2 group (20%) and 16 patients in the SARS-CoV-2-CDI group (42.1%). There were no associated gastrointestinal disorders in either of the two groups studied.

2.5. Severity Score Analysis

The Carmeli score calculated at admission was 1.79 + 0.74 in the COVID-19/-CDI coinfection patients and 2.46 ± 0.5 in patients with CDI ($p = 0.001$, Student t-test). The APACHE score in CDI + COVID-19 coinfection patients was 18.08 ± 4.68 and 25 ± 8.54 in the CDI group ($p = 0.06$, Student t-test). The SOFA median score was 8.96 ± 2.05 in CDI + COVID-19 coinfection patients, and 9 ± 3.5 in CDI patients ($p = 0.965$, Student, t-test).

3. Discussion

The COVID-19 pandemic represented an unprecedented health crisis, bringing about radical changes in medical practice in a very short time. The implementation and strong adherence to infection prevention protocols, wearing protective equipment, and improving hand hygiene are considered changes that have influenced the decrease in the incidence of hospital-acquired infections, including CDI [24–26]. Analyzing the incidence of CDI from 2016 to 2023 at our hospital, we observe a progressive increase in the number of diagnosed cases of CDI rather than a decrease as expected. If in 2016 the number of cases was 1.73‰, it progressively increased to 9.81‰ in 2017, 14.36‰ in 2019, 16‰ in 2020, reaching the highest incidence of 22.02‰ in 2021, followed by a slight decline to 17.21‰ in 2022, and then 16.7‰. An increase in CDI incidence is reported in other studies, explaining that this rise is because of increased use of antibiotics and/or steroids, or even the modification of the patient population profile admitted during the pandemic [18,27–29]. In another study, Markovic-Denic L reported that the incidence density rate was three times higher when the hospital was a dedicated COVID-19 hospital, meaning only COVID-19-positive patients were admitted, compared to the period when it was a non-COVID-19 hospital, before and during the COVID-19 pandemic [30]. Kuijper EJ et al. show that CDI incidence increased in the mid-first decade of the 21st century due to highly virulent new strains of C. difficile, such as ribotype (RT) 027 [31]. Following these findings, measures have been introduced for rational antibiotic use, infection prevention, and control, factors considered essential in CDI prevention, thus becoming a major national priority in many states [32].

Analyzing the incidence of CDI from 30 March 2020 to 31 March 2021 in critically ill patients in the ICU, we found a higher incidence of CDI in the COVID-19 group at 2.24%, compared to the non-COVID-19 group, with an incidence of 1.83%. The average age of the COVID-19 group was 68.79 ± 16.24 years, while in the non-COVID-19 group it was 68.83 ± 12.83 years over a period of 2 years of analysis. Boeriu et al. show an average age of 69.56 ± 12.389 in the COVID-19 group and 64.84 ± 15.78 in the non-COVID-19 group, with a higher incidence of CDI at older age ($p = 0.025$) [33]. In our study group, there were no significant differences in the incidence regarding the age of patients with CDI. The average length of stay in the ICU for the COVID-19 group was 13.57 ± 8.34 days, while for the non-COVID-19 group it was 9.21 ± 9.02 days, indicating the severity of COVID-19-CDI coinfection. These data highlight the prolonged hospitalization period and increased mortality of patients with dual infection. Gavrielatou et al. show that the average length of stay in the ICU for patients with COVID-19-CDI coinfection was 12 days (range 1–59 days), and the mortality of this group of patients increased to 7/11 (63%) [34]. Buetti N et al., using prospectively collected multicenter data, showed that the risk of COVID-19 patients admitted to the ICU developing BSI (blood stream infection) was higher than that for patients without COVID-19 after seven days of ICU stay. Clinicians should be particularly attentive to late ICU-BSI in patients with COVID-19 [35]. The literature data have focused on the evolution of patients with CDI and COVID-19 coinfection. Negative outcomes are associated with prolonged hospitalization of COVID-19 and CDI patients, as well as CDI recurrence after hospital discharge [36]. The incidence of mortality during ICU hospitalization of patients with CDI-SARS-CoV-2 coinfection was 75% ($p = 0.09$, Chi-Square test). Allegreti et al. showed a significantly higher mortality incidence in patients with associated infections (80% in COVID-19 with CDI versus 12.2% in patients with only COVID-19, $p < 0.0001$) [37], while Sandhu A et al. showed that four out of nine patients with COVID-19 and CDI coinfection died during hospitalization [38]. Awan RU et al. found that in-hospital mortality was significantly higher among patients with COVID-19 with CDI compared to patients with COVID-19 without CDI (23% vs. 13.4%, OR: 1.3, 95% CI: 1.2–1.5, $p = 0.01$) [16]. Carmeli score evaluation showed a significant statistical difference between the two groups ($p < 0.01$), highlighting once again the role of repeated hospitalizations and antibiotic therapy in triggering CDI infection. Van Rossen TM et al. identified the only risk factors associated with CDI recurrence as older age, healthcare-associated CDI, previous hospitalization (<3 months), PPI initiated during/after CDI diagnosis, and CDI recurrence, while for severe forms of CDI, only older age was identified as a risk factor [39].

The most prescribed antibiotics for the patients included in this study were cephalosporins (33.33%), carbapenems (17.46%), beta-lactams (9.52%), fluoroquinolones (7.93%), and aminoglycosides (7.93%). The association of antibiotic treatment with fluoroquinolone–cephalosporin ($p = 0.03$, Chi-Square test) and beta-lactams–cephalosporin ($p = 0.001$, Chi-Square test) in patients with coinfection is associated with an unfavorable outcome for them.

The statistical analysis in our study showed the association between comorbidities in our selected patients and the intense use of antibiotic treatment; together with PPI treatment, it was a high-risk factor for CDI infection, which led to a higher fatality, even though the patients had respiratory distress and lung failure.

We observed a high percentage of patients with COVID-19-CDI coinfection who received antibiotic treatment with one or more class of antibiotics. This is one of the most important result in our study, as antibiotic use should be limited in patients at risk of developing CDI, and treatment guidelines in COVID-19 were modified at a late stage after SARS-CoV-2 detection with caution rules regarding antibiotic treatment. Despotović A et al. show that the most frequently used antibiotics in COVID-19 patients were macrolides (32.4%), cephalosporins (29.6%), and fluoroquinolones (28.2%). A third of patients (34.5%) reported using more than one antibiotic [40]. We found no statistical differences between hepatic comorbidities, diabetes mellitus, renal comorbidities, cardiovascular comorbidities, antibiotic treatment administered, and the sex of patients between the two studied groups. Diabetes is frequently observed in hospitalized patients with COVID-19, with a reported prevalence between 7 and 30%. It can lead to chronic inflammation and an exaggerated immune response, as observed in COVID-19 infection [41]. Chronic liver disease is known as an independent risk factor for CDI infection, as well as for COVID-19 infection, due to frequent hospitalizations and reduced immunity [16,42]. It has also been noted that patients with concurrent COVID-19 and CDI have a higher prevalence of essential hypertension (HTN), coronary artery disease (CAD), and congestive heart failure (CHF) [43]. A meta-analysis showed that pre-existing coronary artery disease (CAD) is present in about one-tenth of hospitalized patients with COVID-19 [44].

In our analysis, the only comorbidity associated with the death of patients with COVID-19-CDI coinfection was diabetes mellitus ($p = 0.05$, Chi-Square test). Diabetics have a higher antibiotic consumption due to frequent infections, thus increasing their predisposition to CDI due to intestinal dysbiosis [41,45,46], thereby triggering increased morbidity and mortality when combined. This could indicate the possibility of a genetic background being involved in the intestinal dysbiosis, and a possible genetic susceptibility to develop autoimmune gastrointestinal disorders even after this episode of CDI or CDI and SARS-CoV-2 coinfection. Also, the association with fatality of COVID-19 + CDI coinfection in patients with diabetes mellitus was proven in our study, compared to other comorbidities.

Even though it is well known that diabetes mellitus is an important risk factor for fatality in COVID-19 cases, the role of CDI infection in these selected patients is significant.

Ghosdal et al. related in their study the incidence and significance of gastrointestinal symptoms in COVID-19 infection and concluded that a percentage as high as 25% of patients had gastrointestinal symptoms as the only manifestation, in relation to the disease severity and having high clinical implications [47].

In our study, the percentage was higher in the SARS-CoV-2 and CDI group, even though we excluded from the analysis diarrhea as a gastrointestinal symptom, showing the clinical implication of gastrointestinal symptoms even before the diagnosis of CDI. Taking this into consideration, we could conclude that SARS-CoV-2 infection facilitates CDI, and CDI does not worsen the gastrointestinal symptoms associated with SARS-CoV-2.

Yibirin et al., in their systematic review of the literature, presented the adverse effects associated with PPI use, signaling the risk of acquiring CDI, alongside respiratory infections, kidney disease, gastrointestinal malignancies, liver disease, and fracture risk [48].

In our study, the relation to death and PPI use was demonstrated only in the CDI-SARS-CoV-2 group, showing in fact the risk of PPI and CDI acquirement, which associated a higher risk of complications and fatality with these associated conditions.

CDI + SARS-CoV-2 coinfection is an independent factor of severity and is statistically associated with the death of patients ($p = 0.01$, Chi-Square test). The association of mechanical ventilation in patients with coinfection is associated with increased morbidity and mortality ($p = 0.02$, Chi-Square test).

Micek S.T et al. reported a mortality rate of 25.1% in patients with CDI requiring mechanical ventilation [44]

Through the analysis of the Carmeli score, calculated upon admission to the ICU for both groups, we obtained a value of 1.79 + 0.74 for COVID-19-CDI coinfection and 2.46 ± 0.5 in patients with CDI alone ($p = 0.001$, Student's t-test). This score is used in Romania for screening patients susceptible to colonization with multidrug-resistant bacteria. In this study, the score emphasizes the risk of developing *C. difficile* infection, in addition to the risk of colonization with MDR germs.

The APACHE score in the group with CDI + COVID-19 coinfection was 18.08 ± 4.68 and, respectively 25 ± 8.54 in the CDI group ($p = 0.06$, Student's t-test). Even in this severity score, calculated upon admission to the ICU, patients in the group with CDI infection without COVID-19 presented a higher risk of mortality. APACHE II is a predictive instrument that assesses the extent of a patient's illness and predicts the prognosis of the disease, usually in terms of mortality, for patients admitted to the ICU [49]. Thus, we observe that although the group has an unfavorable prognosis, it has a better survival rate in the case of *C. difficile* mono-infection.

Another score evaluated upon admission to the ICU was the SOFA score, which had a value of 8.96 ± 2.05 in patients with concomitant infection with CDI + COVID-19 and 9 ± 3.5 in patients with CDI ($p = 0.965$, Student's t-test). The differences between the two groups are practically statistically insignificant, so its use does not bring additional data for patients with COVID-19 infection. This was also observed by Moisa et al. in their study, where they proposed a new mortality predictability score at 28 days for patients admitted to the ICU [50].

Stoian et al. showed in a case presentation and literature review the significant number of patients which require ICU services due to severe respiratory, thrombotic, and septic complications and who require long-term hospitalization, by presenting a case of a 54-year-old woman with severe COVID-19 infection and an associated critical illness: polyneuropathy [51]. Although in our study we did not have cases with the critical illness polyneuropathy, the likelihood of them developing this condition was increased due to the association of both COVID-19 and *C. difficile* infection. The case presented was treated with high-dose intravenous immunoglobulins, which needs to be taken in to consideration if this pathology is suspected.

In other study by Stoian et al., the significance and large spectrum of the disease COVID-19 is presented by the study of the occurrence of acute disseminated encephalomyelitis in SARS-CoV-2 infection/vaccination [52]. We did not have cases of encephalomyelitis, but the rate of SARS-CoV-2 vaccination in our studied patients was extremely low, and neurological complications may have appeared in the long course of the disease, which was limited due to the *C. difficile*-associated infection.

In our previous study, published by Stoian et al., we followed up patients in the ICU, with a focus on long-term radiological pulmonary changes in mechanically ventilated patients with respiratory failure due to SARS-CoV-2 infection [5].

The radiological pulmonary changes were also recorded in our patients, but we did not follow them up radiologically, due to the increased mortality rate due to the association of these two separate conditions: SARS-CoV-2 infection and *C. difficile* infection.

In their study regarding the evolution and incidence of COVID-19 and CDI in a Romanian institution, Marinescu et al. showed that CDI has complicated the outcome of COVID-19 patients, especially for those with comorbidities or previously exposed to the healthcare system, and addressed the same need for vigilance for the extensive use of antibiotics, similar to our study [53].

Study Limitations

Since only critically ill patients are admitted to the ICU, this study included a limited number of patients, leading to a small sample size. Additionally, this study was conducted in a single medical unit and was not a multicenter study. The number of patients admitted during that period to our unit was limited to medical emergencies and COVID-19-positive patients.

The evaluation of severity scores such as APACHE II and SOFA is limited to patients with COVID-19-CDI coinfection; thus, more comprehensive studies or meta-analyses of these predictability scores are needed.

4. Materials and Methods

4.1. Data Collection and Analysis

We performed a retrospective observational study using the data offered by the informatic system of Mures County Clinical Hospital and the analysis of the observational charts and the surveillance charts of CDI patients with COVID-19 infection admitted to the ICU. The follow-up period was 2 years, from the moment of admission of the first COVID-19 patient in the ICU on 31 March 2020 up until 31 March 2022.

We collected and analyzed the following data: age, environment, sex, comorbidities, incidence of CDI in the pre-COVID19 period and COVID-19 period, APACHE score, SOFA score, duration of treatment in the ICU, the status of mechanical ventilation, treatment administered (H2 blockers, PPI, empirical antibiotic treatment, the class of antibiotics administered), the identified pathogen, and documented infections. The following paraclinical examinations were followed up: leukocyte count, neutrophil count, lymphocyte count, monocyte count, platelet count, seric urea, creatinine, ALT, AST, GGT, LDH, ferritin, albumin, total proteins, glycemia, potassium, sodium, detection of toxin A + B *C. difficile*, and RT PCR SARS-CoV-2 status.

All the paraclinical examinations were conducted in the Mures County Clinical Hospital laboratory through spectrophotometry, flow cytometry, impedance testing, turbidimetry (PCR), molecular diagnosis, and immunochromatography for toxin A + B *C. difficile*.

We created 2 subgroups of patients: the first group—patients with SARS-CoV-2 and CDI coinfection—and the second group—patients with mono-infection with CDI.

Inclusion criteria:

- Critical patients admitted to the ICU department;
- SARS-CoV-2 infection, confirmed by RT-PCR SARS-CoV-2;
- Diagnosis of CDI, confirmed by toxin A + B *C. difficile*.

Statistical analysis was performed using software applications such as IBM SPSS Statistics v26 and Microsoft Excel 2019. We assessed parametric variables (ANOVA test), describing the data as continuous (mean, standard deviation [SD], median, min/max) depending on their distribution. We used correlations for quantitative variables with Pearson's correlation coefficient (rho), with alpha set at 0.05. A p-value ≤ 0.05 was considered significant. Contingency tables and the Chi-Squared test were used to assess the correlation between the distributions of the categorical variables.

We analyzed two types of data: the incidence of CDI for Mures County Clinical Hospital in the 2016–2023 period and the comparative analysis of the two groups, coinfection with SARS-CoV-2 and CDI group and CDI group, during the two-year period.

4.2. Ethics Statement

For this study, we used data from the hospital's informatic system and the observation charts and surveillance charts during the admissions. We did not collect supplementary data or materials or require any supplementary data from the patients included in this study.

The data do not include data regarding personal identity. We obtained the Ethics Committee of Mures County Clinical Hospital's approval; 6077 from 7 April 2023.

5. Conclusions

The incidence of CDI infection in both COVID-19 and non-COVID-19 groups is practically similar. All patients underwent curative antibiotic treatment for a documented infection with at least one pathogen agent. The patients with CDI treatment were significantly younger and received immunomodulator or corticotherapy treatment, which was a risk factor for opportunistic agents.

Antibiotic and PPI treatment were significant risk factors for CDI coinfection, as well as for death, with PPI treatment associated with antibiotic treatment being a more significant risk factor. This was one of the most important aspects of our study, as COVID-19 treatment guidelines included, for a long period of time, recommendations for antibiotic treatment. Diabetes mellitus was a significant comorbidity associated with CDI-COVID-19 coinfections as well as death.

Most patients received empiric antibiotic treatment from the initial days of hospitalization.

For all patients admitted in the intensive care unit in a critical condition, the association of CDI with SARS-CoV-2 infection was associated with a worse prognosis and an increased risk of fatality.

Author Contributions: Conceptualization, methodology, writing—original draft preparation, M.S., A.S., A.A. and S.Ș.L.; software, A.A., S.Ș.L. and D.C.; formal analysis, investigation, D.D., M.S., S.R.B. and A.B.; resources, A.S., S.R.B., E.M.A., E.R. and D.D.; writing—review and editing, A.S., M.S., A.A. and S.Ș.L.; project administration, visualization, supervision, M.S., A.S., A.A. and A.B.; validation, all authors. All authors have read and agreed to the published version of the manuscript.

Funding: This work was supported by the George Emil Palade University of Medicine, Pharmacy, Science, and Technology of Târgu Mureș. Research grant number 170/1/09.01.2024.

Institutional Review Board Statement: This study was conducted in accordance with the Declaration of Helsinki, and approved in Institutional Review 6077 from 7 April 2023.

Data Availability Statement: Data are available based on request from the corresponding author.

Conflicts of Interest: The authors declare no conflicts of interest.

Abbreviations

ALT	alanine aminotransferase
APACHE II	Acute Physiology and Chronic Health Evaluation II
AST	aspartate aminotransferase
CAD	coronary artery disease
CDI	Clostridioides Difficile Infection

CHF	cardiac heart failure
GGT	gamma-glutamyl transferase
HCM	Hospital County Mures
HTN	hypertension
GDH	glutamate dehydrogenase
ICU	intensive care units
LDH	lactate dehydrogenase
MDR	multidrug resistance
RT PCR SARS-CoV-2	Real-Time Polymerase Chain Reaction SARS-CoV-2
PPI	proton-pump inhibitors
PACU	Post-Anesthesia Care Unit
PCR	polymerase chain reaction
PCT	procalcitonin
SOFA	Sequential Organ Failure Assessment
VSH (ESR)	Erythrocyte Sedimentation Rate

References

1. World Health Organization. Available online: https://www.who.int/emergencies/diseases/novel-coronavirus-2019 (accessed on 19 December 2023).
2. European Centre for Disease Prevention and Control. Clinical Characteristics of COVID-19. 7 September 2021. Available online: https://www.ecdc.europa.eu/en/covid-19/latest-evidence/clinical (accessed on 12 June 2023).
3. Long, B.; Carius, B.M.; Chavez, S.; Liang, S.Y.; Brady, W.J.; Koyfman, A.; Gottlieb, M. Clinical update on COVID-19 for the emergency clinician: Presentation and evaluation. Am. J. Emerg. Med. 2022, 54, 46–57. [CrossRef]
4. Wang, D.; Hu, B.; Hu, C.; Zhu, F.; Liu, X.; Zhang, J.; Wang, B.; Xiang, H.; Cheng, Z.; Xiong, Y.; et al. Clinical Characteristics of 138 Hospitalized Patients with 2019 Novel Coronavirus-Infected Pneumonia in Wuhan, China. JAMA 2020, 323, 1061–1069. [CrossRef]
5. Stoian, M.; Roman, A.; Boeriu, A.; Onișor, D.; Bandila, S.R.; Babă, D.F.; Cocuz, I.; Niculescu, R.; Costan, A.; Laszlo, S.Ș.; et al. Long-Term Radiological Pulmonary Changes in Mechanically Ventilated Patients with Respiratory Failure due to SARS-CoV-2 Infection. Biomedicines 2023, 11, 2637. [CrossRef] [PubMed]
6. Klok, F.A.; Kruip, M.J.H.A.; van der Meer, N.J.M.; Arbous, M.S.; Gommers, D.A.M.P.J.; Kant, K.M.; Kaptein, F.H.J.; van Paassen, J.; Stals, M.A.M.; Huisman, M.V.; et al. Incidence of thrombotic complications in critically ill ICU patients with COVID-19. Thromb. Res. 2020, 191, 145–147. [CrossRef]
7. Xie, Y.; Xu, E.; Bowe, B.; Al-Aly, Z. Long-term cardiovascular outcomes of COVID-19. Nat. Med. 2022, 28, 583–590. [CrossRef]
8. Javed, N.; Ijaz, Z.; Khair, A.H.; Dar, A.A.; Lopez, E.D.; Abbas, R.; Sheikh, A.B. COVID-19 loss of taste and smell: Potential psychological repercussions. Pan Afr. Med. J. 2022, 43, 38. [CrossRef]
9. Tana, C.; Bentivegna, E.; Cho, S.-J.; Harriott, A.M.; García-Azorín, D.; Labastida-Ramirez, A.; Ornello, R.; Raffaelli, B.; Beltrán, E.R.; Ruscheweyh, R.; et al. Long COVID headache. J. Headache Pain 2022, 23, 93. [CrossRef] [PubMed]
10. Korres, G.; Kitsos, D.K.; Kaski, D.; Tsogka, A.; Giannopoulos, S.; Giannopapas, V.; Sideris, G.; Tyrellis, G.; Voumvourakis, K. The Prevalence of Dizziness and Vertigo in COVID-19 Patients: A Systematic Review. Brain Sci. 2022, 12, 948. [CrossRef] [PubMed]
11. Nikbakht, F.; Mohammadkhanizadeh, A.; Mohammadi, E. How does the COVID-19 cause seizure and epilepsy in patients? The potential mechanisms. Mult. Scler. Relat. Disord. 2023, 46, 102535. [CrossRef] [PubMed]
12. Siow, I.; Lee, K.S.; Zhang, J.J.Y.; Saffari, S.E.; Ng, A. Encephalitis as a neurological complication of COVID-19: A systematic review and meta-analysis of incidence, outcomes, and predictors. Eur. J. Neurol. 2023, 28, 3491–3502. [CrossRef]
13. Khan, F.; Sharma, P.; Pandey, S.; Sharma, D.; Vijayavarman, V.; Kumar, N.; Shukla, S.; Dandu, H.; Jain, A.; Garg, R.K.; et al. COVID-19-associated Guillain-Barre syndrome: Postinfectious alone or neuroinvasive too? J. Med. Virol. 2023, 93, 6045–6049. [CrossRef] [PubMed]
14. Groff, A.; Kavanaugh, M.; Ramgobin, D.; McClafferty, B.; Aggarwal, C.S.; Golamari, R.; Jain, R. Gastrointestinal Manifestations of COVID-19: A Review of What We Know. Ochsner J. 2021, 21, 177–180. [CrossRef] [PubMed]
15. Akter, S.; Tasnim, S.; Barua, R.; Choubey, M.; Arbee, S.; Mohib, M.M.; Minhaz, N.; Choudhury, A.; Sarker, P.; Mohiuddin, M.S. The Effect of COVID-19 on Gut Microbiota: Exploring the Complex Interplay and Implications for Human Health. Gastrointest. Disord. 2023, 5, 340–355. [CrossRef]
16. Awan, R.U.; Gangu, K.; Nguyen, A.; Chourasia, P.; Borja Montes, O.F.; Butt, M.A.; Muzammil, T.S.; Afzal, R.M.; Nabeel, A.; Shekhar, R.; et al. COVID-19 and Clostridioides difficile Coinfection Outcomes among Hospitalized Patients in the United States: An Insight from National Inpatient Database. Infect. Dis. Rep. 2023, 15, 279–291. [CrossRef] [PubMed]
17. Bentivegna, E.; Alessio, G.; Spuntarelli, V.; Luciani, M.; Santino, I.; Simmaco, M.; Martelletti, P. Impact of COVID-19 prevention measures on risk of health care-associated Clostridium difficile infection. Am. J. Infect. Control 2021, 49, 640–642. [CrossRef] [PubMed]
18. Granata, G.; Petrosillo, N.; Al Moghazi, S.; Caraffa, E.; Puro, V.; Tillotson, G.; Cataldo, M.A. The burden of Clostridioides difficile infection in COVID-19 patients: A systematic review and meta-analysis. Anaerobe 2022, 74, 102484. [CrossRef] [PubMed]

19. Langford, B.J.; So, M.; Raybardhan, S.; Leung, V.; Soucy, J.-P.R.; Westwood, D.; Daneman, N.; MacFadden, D.R. Antibiotic prescribing in patients with COVID-19: Rapid review and meta-analysis. *Clin. Microbiol. Infect.* **2021**, *27*, 520–531. [CrossRef] [PubMed]
20. Linares-García, L.; Cárdenas-Barragán, M.E.; Hernández-Ceballos, W.; Pérez-Solano, C.S.; Morales-Guzmán, A.S.; Miller, D.S.; Schmulson, M. Bacterial and Fungal Gut Dysbiosis and Clostridium difficile in COVID-19: A Review. *J. Clin. Gastroenterol.* **2022**, *56*, 285–298. [CrossRef] [PubMed]
21. Rupnik, M.; Wilcox, M.H.; Gerding, D.N. Clostridium difficile infection: New developments in epidemiology and pathogenesis. *Nat. Rev. Microbiol.* **2009**, *7*, 526–536. [CrossRef]
22. Laszkowska, M.; Kim, J.; Faye, A.S.; Joelson, A.M.; Ingram, M.; Truong, H.; Silver, E.R.; May, B.; Greendyke, W.G.; Zucker, J.; et al. Prevalence of Clostridioides difficile and Other Gastrointestinal Pathogens in Patients with COVID-19. *Dig. Dis. Sci.* **2021**, *66*, 4398–4405. [CrossRef]
23. Lewandowski, K.; Rosołowski, M.; Kaniewska, M.; Kucha, P.; Meler, A.; Wierzba, W.; Rydzewska, G. Clostridioides difficile infection in coronavirus disease 2019 (COVID-19): An underestimated problem? *Pol. Arch. Intern. Med.* **2021**, *131*, 121–127.
24. Israel, S.; Harpaz, K.; Radvogin, E.; Schwartz, C.; Gross, I.; Mazeh, H.; Cohen, M.J.; Benenson, S. Dramatically improved hand hygiene performance rates at time of coronavirus pandemic. *Clin. Microbiol. Infect.* **2020**, *26*, 1566–1568. [CrossRef] [PubMed]
25. Kakiuchi, S.; Livorsi, D.J.; Perencevich, E.N.; Diekema, D.J.; Ince, D.; Prasidthrathsint, K.; Kinn, P.; Percival, K.; Heintz, B.H.; Goto, M. Days of Antibiotic Spectrum Coverage: A Novel Metric for Inpatient Antibiotic Consumption. *Clin. Infect. Dis.* **2022**, *75*, 567–576. [CrossRef] [PubMed]
26. Dieringer, T.D.; Furukawa, D.; Graber, C.J.; Stevens, V.W.; Jones, M.M.; Rubin, M.A.; Goetz, M.B. Inpatient antibiotic utilization in the Veterans' Health Administration during the coronavirus disease 2019 (COVID-19) pandemic. *Infect. Control Hosp. Epidemiol.* **2021**, *42*, 751–753. [CrossRef] [PubMed]
27. Sipos, S.; Vlad, C.; Prejbeanu, R.; Haragus, H.; Vlad, D.; Cristian, H.; Dumitrascu, C.; Popescu, R.; Dumitrascu, V.; Predescu, V. Impact of COVID-19 prevention measures on Clostridioides difficile infections in a regional acute care hospital. *Exp. Ther. Med.* **2021**, *22*, 1215. [CrossRef] [PubMed]
28. Zouridis, S.; Sangha, M.; Feustel, P.; Richter, S. Clostridium difficile Infection Rates during the Pandemic in New York Capital Area: A Single-Center Study. *Cureus* **2023**, *15*, e37576. [CrossRef] [PubMed]
29. Cojocariu, C.; Girleanu, I.; Trifan, A.; Olteanu, A.; Muzica, C.M.; Huiban, L.; Chiriac, S.; Singeap, A.M.; Cuciureanu, T.; Sfarti, C.; et al. Did the severe acute respiratory syndrome-coronavirus 2 pandemic cause an endemic Clostridium difficile infection? *World J. Clin. Cases* **2021**, *9*, 10180–10188. [CrossRef] [PubMed]
30. Markovic-Denic, L.; Nikolic, V.; Toskovic, B.; Brankovic, M.; Crnokrak, B.; Popadic, V.; Radojevic, A.; Radovanovic, D.; Zdravkovic, M. Incidence and Risk Factors for Clostridioides difficile Infections in Non-COVID and COVID-19 Patients: Experience from a Tertiary Care Hospital. *Microorganisms* **2023**, *11*, 435. [CrossRef] [PubMed]
31. Kuijper, E.J.; Coignard, B.; Tüll, P.; ESCMID Study Group for Clostridium difficile; EU Member States; European Centre for Disease Prevention and Control. Emergence of Clostridium difficile-associated disease in North America and Europe. *Clin. Microbiol. Infect.* **2006**, *12* (Suppl. 6), 2–18. [CrossRef]
32. Mu, Y.; Dudeck, M.; Jones, K.; Li, Q.; Soe, M.; Nkwata, A.; Edwards, J. Trends in Hospital Onset Clostridioides difficile Infection Incidence, National Healthcare Safety Network, 2010–2018. *Infect. Control Hosp. Epidemiol.* **2020**, *41*, S53–S54. [CrossRef]
33. Boeriu, A.; Roman, A.; Dobru, D.; Stoian, M.; Voidăzan, S.; Fofiu, C. The Impact of Clostridioides Difficile Infection in Hospitalized Patients: What Changed during the Pandemic? *Diagnostics* **2022**, *12*, 3196. [CrossRef] [PubMed]
34. Gavrielatou, E.; Tsimaras, M. 707. Hospital-Onset Clostridioides difficile Infection Rates during COVID-19 Pandemic in the ICU Patients. *Open Forum Infect. Dis.* **2021**, *8* (Suppl. 1), S453. [CrossRef] [PubMed Central]
35. Buetti, N.; Ruckly, S.; de Montmollin, E.; Reignier, J.; Terzi, N.; Cohen, Y.; Siami, S.; Dupuis, C.; Timsit, J.F. COVID-19 increased the risk of ICU-acquired bloodstream infections: A case-cohort study from the multicentric OUTCOMEREA network. *Intensive Care Med.* **2021**, *47*, 180–187. [CrossRef] [PubMed]
36. Granata, G.; Bartoloni, A.; Codeluppi, M.; Contadini, I.; Cristini, F.; Fantoni, M.; Ferraresi, A.; Fornabaio, C.; Grasselli, S.; Lagi, F.; et al. The Burden of Clostridioides Difficile Infection during the COVID-19 Pandemic: A Retrospective Case-Control Study in Italian Hospitals (CloVid). *J. Clin. Med.* **2020**, *9*, 3855. [CrossRef]
37. Allegretti, J.R.; Nije, C.; McClure, E.; Redd, W.D.; Wong, D.; Zhou, J.C.; Bazarbashi, A.N.; McCarty, T.R.; Hathorn, K.E.; Shen, L.; et al. Prevalence and Impact of Clostridioides difficile Infection among Hospitalized Patients with Coranavirus Disease 2019. *JGH Open* **2021**, *5*, 622–625. [CrossRef] [PubMed]
38. Sandhu, A.; Tillotson, G.; Polistico, J.; Salimnia, H.; Cranis, M.; Moshos, J.; Cullen, L.; Jabbo, L.; Diebel, L.; Chopra, T. Clostridioides Difficile in COVID-19 Patients, Detroit, Michigan, USA, March–April 2020. *Emerg. Infect. Dis.* **2020**, *26*, 2272–2274. [CrossRef] [PubMed]
39. van Rossen, T.M.; Ooijevaar, R.E.; Vandenbroucke-Grauls, C.M.J.E.; Dekkers, O.M.; Kuijper, E.J.; Keller, J.J.; van Prehn, J. Prognostic factors for severe and recurrent Clostridioides difficile infection: A systematic review. *Clin. Microbiol. Infect.* **2022**, *28*, 321–331. [CrossRef] [PubMed]
40. Despotović, A.; Barać, A.; Cucanić, T.; Cucanić, K.; Stevanović, G. Antibiotic (Mis)Use in COVID-19 Patients before and after Admission to a Tertiary Hospital in Serbia. *Antibiotics* **2022**, *11*, 847. [CrossRef]

41. Lima-Martínez, M.M.; Carrera Boada, C.; Madera-Silva, M.D.; Marín, W.; Contreras, M. COVID-19 and diabetes: A bidirectional relationship. *Clínica Investig. Arterioscler. (Engl. Ed.)* **2021**, *33*, 151–157. [CrossRef]
42. Marjot, T.; Webb, G.J.; Barritt, A.S.; Moon, A.M.; Stamataki, Z.; Wong, V.W.; Barnes, E. COVID-19 and liver disease: Mechanistic and clinical perspectives. *Nat. Rev. Gastroenterol. Hepatol.* **2021**, *18*, 348–364. [CrossRef]
43. Zuin, M.; Rigatelli, G.; Bilato, C.; Rigatelli, A.; Roncon, L.; Ribichini, F. Preexisting coronary artery disease among coronavirus disease 2019 patients: A systematic review and meta-analysis. *J. Cardiovasc. Med.* **2022**, *23*, 535–545. [CrossRef] [PubMed]
44. Micek, S.T.; Schramm, G.; Morrow, L.; Frazee, E.; Personett, H.; Doherty, J.A.; Hampton, N.; Hoban, A.; Lieu, A.; McKenzie, M.; et al. Clostridium difficile infection: A multicenter study of epidemiology and outcomes in mechanically ventilated patients. *Crit. Care Med.* **2013**, *41*, 1968–1975. [CrossRef] [PubMed]
45. Qu, H.Q.; Jiang, Z.D. Clostridium difficile infection in diabetes. *Diabetes Res. Clin. Pract.* **2014**, *105*, 285–294. [CrossRef] [PubMed]
46. Slavcovici, A.; Streinu-Cercel, A.; Țățulescu, D.; Radulescu, A.; Mera, S.; Marcu, C.; Vesbianu, D.; Topan, A. The role of risk factors 'carmeli score' and infective endocarditis classification in the assessment of appropriate empirical therapy. *Ther. Pharmacol. Clin. Toxicol.* **2009**, *XIII*, 52–56.
47. Ghoshal, U.C.; Ghosal, U.; Mathur, A.; Singh, R.; Nath, A.; Garg, A.; Singh, D.; Singh, S.; Singh, J.; Pandey, A.; et al. The spectrum of gastrointestinal symptoms in patients with coronavirus disease-19: Predictors, relationship with disease severity, and outcome. *Clin. Transl. Gastroenterol.* **2020**, *11*, e00259. [CrossRef] [PubMed]
48. Yibirin, M.; De Oliveira, D.; Valera, R.; Plitt, A.E.; Lutgen, S. Adverse effects associated with proton pump inhibitor use. *Cureus* **2021**, *13*, e12759. [CrossRef] [PubMed]
49. Knaus, W.A.; Draper, E.A.; Wagner, D.P.; Zimmerman, J.E. APACHE II: A severity of disease classification system. *Crit. Care Med.* **1985**, *13*, 818–829. [CrossRef] [PubMed]
50. Moisa, E.; Corneci, D.; Negutu, M.I.; Filimon, C.R.; Serbu, A.; Popescu, M.; Negoita, S.; Grintescu, I.M. Development and Internal Validation of a New Prognostic Model Powered to Predict 28-Day All-Cause Mortality in ICU COVID-19 Patients-The COVID-SOFA Score. *J. Clin. Med.* **2022**, *11*, 4160. [CrossRef]
51. Stoian, A.; Bajko, Z.; Maier, S.; Cioflinc, R.A.; Grigorescu, B.; Moțățăianu, A.; Bărcuțean, L.; Balașa, R.; Stoian, M. High-dose intravenous immunoglobulins as a therapeutic option in critical illness polyneuropathy accompanying SARS-CoV-2 infection: A case-based review of the literature (Review). *Exp. Ther. Med.* **2021**, *22*, 1182. [CrossRef]
52. Stoian, A.; Bajko, Z.; Stoian, M.; Cioflinc, R.A.; Niculescu, R.; Arbănași, E.M.; Russu, E.; Botoncea, M.; Bălașa, R. The Occurrence of Acute Disseminated Encephalomyelitis in SARS-CoV-2 Infection/Vaccination: Our Experience and a Systematic Review of the Literature. *Vaccines* **2023**, *11*, 1225. [CrossRef]
53. Marinescu, A.R.; Laza, R.; Musta, V.F.; Cut, T.G.; Dumache, R.; Tudor, A.; Porosnicu, M.; Lazureanu, V.E.; Licker, M. Clostridium Difficile and COVID-19: General Data, Ribotype, Clinical Form, Treatment-Our Experience from the Largest Infectious Diseases Hospital in Western Romania. *Medicina* **2021**, *57*, 1099. [CrossRef] [PubMed]

Disclaimer/Publisher's Note: The statements, opinions and data contained in all publications are solely those of the individual author(s) and contributor(s) and not of MDPI and/or the editor(s). MDPI and/or the editor(s) disclaim responsibility for any injury to people or property resulting from any ideas, methods, instructions or products referred to in the content.

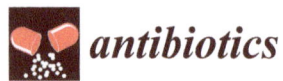

Article

A Real-World Study on the Clinical Characteristics, Outcomes, and Relationship between Antibiotic Exposure and *Clostridioides difficile* Infection

Bogdan Ioan Vintila [1,2], Anca Maria Arseniu [3,*], Claudiu Morgovan [3], Anca Butuca [3], Victoria Bîrluțiu [2,4], Carmen Maximiliana Dobrea [3], Luca Liviu Rus [3], Steliana Ghibu [5], Alina Simona Bereanu [1,2,*], Rares Arseniu [6], Ioana Roxana Codru [1,2], Mihai Sava [1,2,†] and Felicia Gabriela Gligor [3,†]

1. Clinical Surgical Department, Faculty of Medicine, "Lucian Blaga" University of Sibiu, 550169 Sibiu, Romania; bogdan.vintila@ulbsibiu.ro (B.I.V.); ioanaroxana.bera@ulbsibiu.ro (I.R.C.); mihai.sava@ulbsibiu.ro (M.S.)
2. County Clinical Emergency Hospital, 550245 Sibiu, Romania; victoria.birlutiu@ulbsibiu.ro
3. Preclinical Department, Faculty of Medicine, "Lucian Blaga" University of Sibiu, 550169 Sibiu, Romania; claudiu.morgovan@ulbsibiu.ro (C.M.); anca.butuca@ulbsibiu.ro (A.B.); carmen.dobrea@ulbsibiu.ro (C.M.D.); liviu.rus@ulbsibiu.ro (L.L.R.); felicia.gligor@ulbsibiu.ro (F.G.G.)
4. Clinical Medical Department, Faculty of Medicine, "Lucian Blaga" University of Sibiu, 550169 Sibiu, Romania
5. Department of Pharmacology, Physiology and Pathophysiology, Faculty of Pharmacy, "Iuliu Hatieganu" University of Medicine and Pharmacy, 400012 Cluj-Napoca, Romania; steliana.ghibu@umfcluj.ro
6. County Emergency Clinical Hospital "Pius Brînzeu", 300723 Timișoara, Romania; arseniurares@gmail.com

* Correspondence: anca.arseniu@ulbsibiu.ro (A.M.A.); alina.bereanu@ulbsibiu.ro (A.S.B.)
† These authors contributed equally to this work.

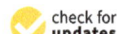

Citation: Vintila, B.I.; Arseniu, A.M.; Morgovan, C.; Butuca, A.; Bîrluțiu, V.; Dobrea, C.M.; Rus, L.L.; Ghibu, S.; Bereanu, A.S.; Arseniu, R.; et al. A Real-World Study on the Clinical Characteristics, Outcomes, and Relationship between Antibiotic Exposure and *Clostridioides difficile* Infection. *Antibiotics* **2024**, *13*, 144. https://doi.org/10.3390/antibiotics13020144

Academic Editor: Guido Granata

Received: 23 December 2023
Revised: 24 January 2024
Accepted: 30 January 2024
Published: 1 February 2024

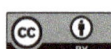

Copyright: © 2024 by the authors. Licensee MDPI, Basel, Switzerland. This article is an open access article distributed under the terms and conditions of the Creative Commons Attribution (CC BY) license (https://creativecommons.org/licenses/by/4.0/).

Abstract: *Clostridioides difficile* is a Gram-positive bacteria that causes nosocomial infections, significantly impacting public health. In the present study, we aimed to describe the clinical characteristics, outcomes, and relationship between antibiotic exposure and *Clostridioides difficile* infection (CDI) in patients based on reports from two databases. Thus, we conducted a retrospective study of patients diagnosed with CDI from Sibiu County Clinical Emergency Hospital (SCCEH), Romania, followed by a descriptive analysis based on spontaneous reports submitted to the EudraVigilance (EV) database. From 1 January to 31 December 2022, we included 111 hospitalized patients with CDI from SCCEH. Moreover, 249 individual case safety reports (ICSRs) from EVs were analyzed. According to the data collected from SCCEH, CDI was most frequently reported in patients aged 65–85 years (66.7%) and in females (55%). In total, 71.2% of all patients showed positive medical progress. Most cases were reported in the internal medicine (n = 30, 27%), general surgery (n = 26, 23.4%), and infectious disease (n = 22, 19.8%) departments. Patients were most frequently exposed to ceftriaxone (CFT) and meropenem (MER). Also, in the EV database, most CDI-related ADRs were reported for CFT, PIP/TAZ (piperacillin/tazobactam), MER, and CPX (ciprofloxacin). Understanding the association between previous antibiotic exposure and the risk of CDI may help update antibiotic stewardship protocols and reduce the incidence of CDI by lowering exposure to high-risk antibiotics.

Keywords: *Clostridioides difficile*; *Clostridioides difficile* infections; CDI; antibiotic exposure; EudraVigilance; single-center retrospective study; healthcare-associated infections

1. Introduction

Clostridioides difficile (CD) is a bacterium characterized by its Gram-positive nature, spore-forming ability, and anaerobic properties [1,2]. The microorganism commonly occurs in the human gastrointestinal tract, which harbors a variety of bacteria, mainly anaerobic, but it can also occur in animals and various environments [3].

CD infection (CDI) is a highly prevalent hospital-acquired infection [4] that has increased in frequency and severity over the past decade. CD most often causes healthcare-associated infections. They are one of the top three threats to public health, according to the Centers for Disease Control and Prevention [5,6]. On the other hand, a recent population-based study found that as much as 41% of CDI cases are actually contracted in the community. Interestingly, the study also revealed that while community-acquired CDI generally has a milder clinical course than the hospital-acquired form, it is still a significant concern. It is essential to be aware of the prevalence of CDI in community settings to identify high-risk individuals early on [7].

CDI is frequently linked to a set of risk factors. Many factors contribute to CDI, including antimicrobial use, advanced age, hospitalization, and a compromised immune system. Advanced age is strongly associated with complications and death, especially in patients with co-infections and high comorbidity scores [8].

It is a well-known fact that patients who receive antibiotics during their hospital stay are at a higher risk of developing CDI [9,10]. Carbapenems are a class of broad-spectrum antibiotics that are highly effective against many bacteria, including Gram-positive and Gram-negative bacteria. They are considered last-resort antibiotics typically used to treat severe and often life-threatening infections resistant to other antibiotics [11]. However, their increasing use is a matter of concern for several reasons, and one is the imbalances produced in the microbiota, with a high risk of CDI [12]. A member of the oxazolidinone antibiotic family, linezolid (LIN) stands out as the first representative of its class [13]. The drug has been approved for treating infections caused by *Enterococcus faecium*, which is resistant to vancomycin; *Staphylococcus aureus* pneumonia, which occurs in hospitals; and complex skin and skin structure infections. Furthermore, LIN is well known for its effectiveness as an antibiotic in treating infections in the ICU [13]. In recent years, there has been renewed attention on polymyxins due to the emergence of Gram-negative bacteria resistant to multiple antibiotics, leaving few alternative treatment options available [14]. It is common for healthcare professionals to administer antibiotics, including piperacillin and tazobactam (PIP/TAZ), ceftriaxone (CFT), ciprofloxacin (CPX), and gentamicin (GEN), in intensive care settings. PIP/TAZ is recognized for its β-lactam/β-lactamase solid-inhibiting properties [15,16]. Upon conducting a thorough examination of the medical records of 640 patients treated in an ICU, it was discovered that a significant majority of 73.4% of patients had received CFT. Interestingly, it was noted that CPX and GEN were administered to fewer than 3% of patients who were admitted to the ICU [17]. One notable benefit of using CPX and GEN to treat patients who are critically ill is that they can effectively treat pathogens that are not as responsive to the typical antibiotics administered in intensive care scenarios, particularly in the context of urinary tract infections [18,19].

Healthcare providers can improve patient care in managing CDI by using a range of therapeutic techniques and expanding their knowledge of the unique characteristics of individuals at higher risks of acquiring infections during their hospital stay [20]. This information allows for tailoring antibiotic therapies and decreasing the probability of contracting hospital-acquired infections, such as CDI [21,22].

In the present study, we aimed to describe the clinical characteristics, outcomes, and relationship between previous antibiotic exposure and *Clostridioides difficile* infection in patients based on reports from two databases. We conducted a retrospective analysis of medical records and data for patients diagnosed with healthcare-associated CDI at the Sibiu County Clinical Emergency Hospital (SCCEH) in 2022. We analyzed patient demographics, comorbidity scores, antibiotic prescriptions, the duration of hospitalization, the need for intensive care admission, and clinical outcomes related to *Clostridioides difficile* infection. The antibiotics of interest for our study were PIP/TAZ, CFT, CPX, GEN, meropenem (MER), colistimethate or colistin (COL), and LIN. Moreover, in the present study, we examined each antibiotic's independent potential contribution to the development of CDI. Consecutively, we evaluated data reported in EudraVigilance (EV), an extensive database for reporting adverse drug reactions (ADRs), as individual case safety reports (ICSRs). To evaluate the real-world situation, we compared the reports regarding CDI from both databases and related to patients' exposure to all seven antibiotics.

2. Results

2.1. Descriptive Analysis of Reports from Sibiu County Clinical Emergency Hospital (SCCEH)

2.1.1. Baseline Patients' Characteristics

The patients' characteristics are represented in Table 1. The average age of patients was 72.1 years. The most frequent cases were registered in the 65–85 years category (66.7%) and in the female group (55%). A favorable evolution was observed in 71.2% of patients. For surgical patients, favorable outcomes were registered for a high proportion of patients (86.8%) compared to non-surgical patients (63.0%). Regarding the detection mode, 57.7% of the cases were active, and 42.3% were passive.

Table 1. *Clostridium difficile* infection patients' characteristics.

	Patient Characteristic	Cases n (%)
Age Mean (Minimum–Maximum)	72.1 years (18.3–94.8 years)	111
Age category * Mean (Minimum–Maximum)	18–64 years 54.7 years (18.3–63.9 years)	25 (22.5)
	65–85 years 75.1 years (65.3–84.3 years)	74 (66.7)
	>85 years 89.7 years (85.8–94.8 years)	12 (10.8)
Gender	Female	61 (55.0)
	Male	50 (45.0)
Patients' category	Surgical favorable outcome unfavorable outcome	38 (34.2) 33 (86.8) 5 (13.2)
	Non-surgical favorable outcome unfavorable outcome	73 (65.8) 46 (63.0) 27 (37.0)
Evolution	Favorable resolved/recovered	79 (71.2) 79 (100)
	Unfavorable aggravated condition Death not resolved/not recovered	32 (28.8) 3 (9.0) 28 (88.0) 1 (3.0)
Detection mode	Active	64 (57.7)
	Passive	47 (42.3)

* $p < 0.001$.

2.1.2. Hospital Length of Stay

In the studied group, the total hospital length of stay (T-HLS) was 20.18 days. The media of hospital length of stay until the detection (HLS-UD) was 9.2 days (minimum 0–maximum 34 days). A longer period was observed for the duration of hospitalization after CDI detection (11.03 days, minimum 0–maximum 31 days). The average hospital length of stay in ICU (HL-ICU) was 3.45 days (minimum 0–maximum 45 days) (Figure 1).

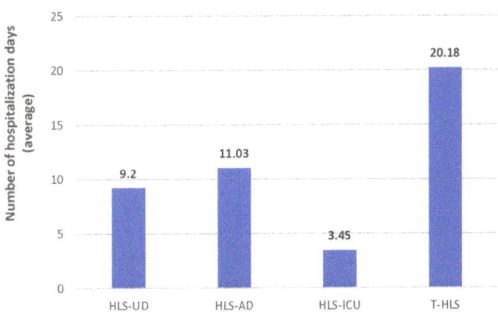

Figure 1. Hospital length of stay. HLS-AD—hospital length of stay after detection (days); HLS-ICU—hospital length of stay in ICU (days); HLS-UD—hospital length of stay until detection (days); T-HLS—total hospital length of stay (days).

According to the data presented in Table 2, no statistical difference regarding the outcomes could be observed in the four categories (HLS-UD, HLS-AD, HLS-ICU, T-HLS).

Table 2. The relationship between the number of hospitalization days and patients' outcomes. HLS-AD—hospital length of stay after detection (days); HLS-ICU—hospital length of stay in ICU (days); HLS-UD—hospital length of stay until detection (days); T-HLS—total hospital length of stay (days).

	Outcome	Average Duration of Hospitalization (Days)	p-Value
HLS-UD	favorable	9.78	$p > 0.05$
	unfavorable	7.75	
HLS-AD	favorable	11.08	$p > 0.05$
	unfavorable	10.91	
HLS-ICU	favorable	2.57	$p > 0.05$
	unfavorable	5.63	
T-HLS	favorable	20.80	$p > 0.05$
	unfavorable	18.66	

2.1.3. Influence of Age on the Patients' Outcome

According to the data presented in Table 3, a favorable outcome was obtained in the first two subgroups (18–64 years and 65–85 years). As observed, the unfavorable outcome resulted in a proportion of 12% in the 18–64 years group, over 29.7% in the 65–85 years group, and 58.3% in people aged more than 85 years old.

Table 3. The distribution of the outcome by age category. n—number of patients.

Age Category	Favorable n (%)	Unfavorable n (%)
18–64 years	22 (88.0)	3 (12.0)
65–85 years	52 (70.3)	22 (29.7)
>85 years	5 (41.7)	7 (58.3)

2.1.4. Wards

The highest number of cases was reported in internal medicine (n = 30, 27.0%), general surgery (n = 26, 23.4%), and infectious disease (n = 22, 19.8%). The rest of the wards reported fewer than four cases, except neurology (n = 7, 6.3%). In seven wards, the favorable outcomes represented 100% of total cases, and only in two wards, the favorable outcome represented 0%. It can be noticed that a higher percentage of favorable outcomes was reported in the wards with the most cases, such as general surgery (92.3%) and internal medicine (70.0%) (Figure 2).

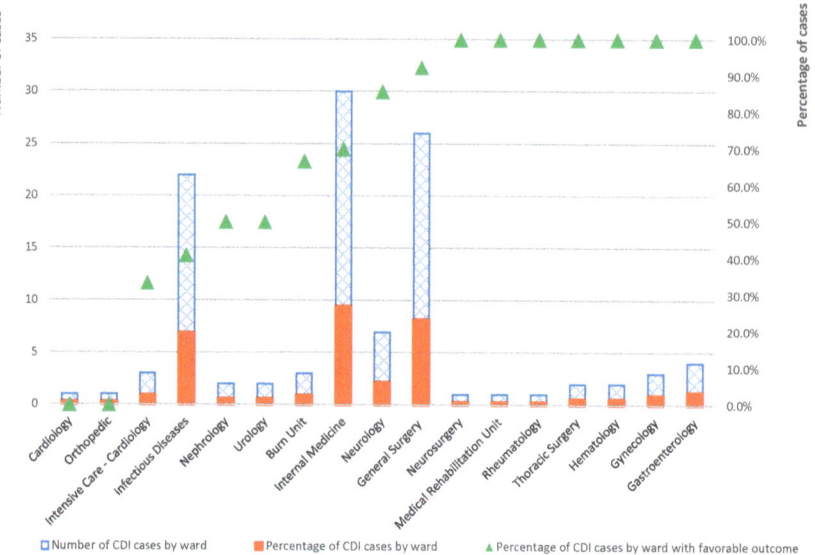

Figure 2. The distribution of cases by ward.

2.1.5. Admission Diagnosis

According to the results presented in Figure 3, we observed that among the cases diagnosed with CDI in SCCEH, the majority of them were found in patients with an admission diagnosis of oncological pathology (n = 17, 15.3%; favorable outcome = 94.1%), SARS-COV2 (n = 13, 11.7%; favorable outcome = 38.5%), chronic liver disease (n = 13, 11.7%; favorable outcome = 84.6%), stroke (n = 7, 6.3%; favorable outcome = 85.7%), and urinary tract infection (n = 6, 5.4%; favorable outcome = 50%).

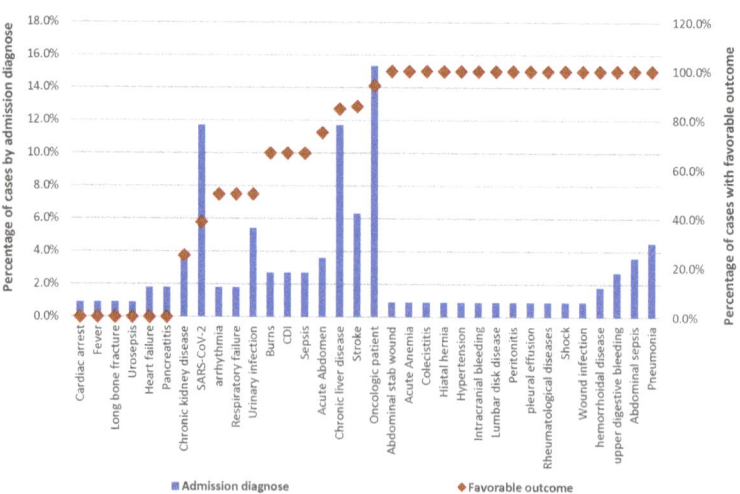

Figure 3. The distribution of cases by admission diagnoses. CDI—*Clostridioides difficile* infection.

2.1.6. Charlson Comorbidity Index

Table 4 presented the Charlson comorbidity index (CCI) for patients with CDI from SCCEH (average CCI: 7.6). No significant differences could be observed in females compared to males. Still, significant differences could be observed between age categories and evolution groups (favorable compared to unfavorable).

Table 4. Charlson comorbidity index for patients with *Clostridoides difficile* infection.

Variables		Charlson Comorbidity Index		p-Value
		Average	Range	
All patients		7.6	(0–16 points)	
Gender	Female	8.04	(4–15 points)	$p > 0.05$
	Male	7.14	(0–16 points)	
Category of age	18–64 years	6	(4–16 points)	$p < 0.01$
	65–85 years	8.1	(0–15 points)	
	>85 years	8.2	(6–11 points)	
Outcome	Favorable	7.2	(0–15 points)	$p < 0.01$
	resolved/recovered	7.2	(0–15 points)	
	Unfavorable	8.8	(4–16 points)	
	aggravated condition	8.3	(7–11 points)	
	death	8.8	(4–16 points)	
	not resolved/not recovered	11	(11 points)	

2.1.7. Antibiotic Exposure

The mean of antibiotics used by all patients is 1.50 ± 1.09. In subgroup 1, the mean has a higher value (1.68 ± 1.22) than the other two subgroups (1.5 ± 1.11 for 65–85 years and 1.17 ± 0.39 for > 85 years subgroup). The median of the antibiotics used by all patients is 1. Except for subgroup 1 (median = 2), the other subgroups have a median equal to 1. The value of the mode (maximum repeated value) is 1 for the entire group and subgroups 2 and 3. For subgroup 1, the mode is 3 (Table 5).

Table 5. The exposure of patients to antibiotics.

	All Group	Subgroup 1 18–64 Years	Subgroup 2 65–85 Years	Subgroup 3 >85 Years
Mean	1.504505	1.68	1.5	1.166667
Standard Error	0.103084	0.243036	0.129434	0.112367
Median	1	2	1	1
Mode	1	3	1	1
Standard Deviation	1.086059	1.215182	1.11343	0.389249
Sample Variance	1.179525	1.476667	1.239726	0.151515
Kurtosis	0.202974	−1.16656	0.517144	2.64
Skewness	0.66032	0.07172	0.734379	2.055237
Range	5	4	5	1
Minimum	0	0	0	1
Maximum	5	4	5	2
Sum	167	42	111	14
Count	111	25	74	12

Although there is no statistical difference regarding the outcomes, it can still be observed that the cases with favorable outcomes were exposed to a more significant number of antibiotics (1.53 ± 1.07) compared to the unfavorable ones (1.44 ± 1.13). The median of the antibiotics used by patients is 1 in both subgroups. (Table 6).

Table 6. Distribution of cases by number of antibiotics and outcome.

	Favorable	Unfavorable
Mean	1.531646	1.4375
Standard Error	0.120633	0.200491
Median	1	1
Mode	1	1
Standard Deviation	1.072206	1.134147
Sample Variance	1.149627	1.28629
Kurtosis	0.439452	−0.07617
Skewness	0.652101	0.730805
Range	5	4
Minimum	0	0
Maximum	5	4
Sum	121	46
Count	79	32

Regarding previous antibiotic exposure, the patients in the analyzed group were most frequently exposed to CFT (n = 32) and MER (n = 20) and the least to COL (n = 3). Exposure to the other four antibiotics was as follows: LIN (n = 11), GEN (n = 10), PIP/TAZ (n = 8), and CPX (n = 7).

According to Figure 4, the proportion of the recovered/resolved cases from the total cases was higher for GEN (100%, n = 10), PIP/TAZ (88%, n = 7), and CFT (75%, n = 24). Also, a lower proportion of recovered/resolved cases was registered in patients treated with COL (0%, n = 0), LIN (45%, n = 5), and MER (55%, n = 11). The highest proportion of fatal cases was registered for MER (45%, n = 9), LIN (45%, n = 5), and COL (100%, n = 3).

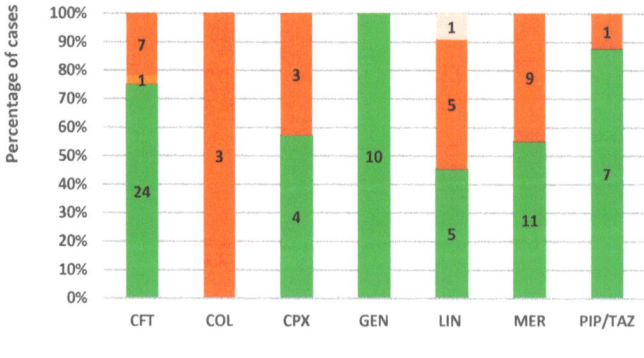

Figure 4. The percentage of cases by outcome in total reports. CFT—ceftriaxone; COL—colistin; CPX—ciprofloxacin; GEN—gentamicin; LIN—linezolid; MER—meropenem; PIP/TAZ—piperacillin and tazobactam.

2.2. Analysis of Spontaneous Reports from EudraVigilance

2.2.1. Descriptive Analysis of ICSRs Uploaded in 2022

In 2022, the EV database registered 249 ICSRs for all antibiotics analyzed in the present study, most of them being reported for CFT (n = 85), PIP/TAZ (n = 78), MER (n = 36), and CPX (n = 36). For all seven drugs analyzed, health professionals uploaded the majority of reports, but only for COL, GEN, and LIN, the majority of ICSRs were reported from the European Economic Area (EEA).

It can also be noted that CDI was most frequently reported for patients in the following age groups: 65–85 years (n = 107, 43.0%), more than 85 years (n = 67, 26.9%), and 18–64 years (n = 61, 24.5%).

The proportion of reports between the two genders was similar (male—122, female—124), but for males, CDI associated with the consumption of MER (72.2%), CFT (55.3%), and GEN (50%) were reported more frequently (Table 7).

Table 7. Characteristics of ICSR related to CDI recorded in EudraVigilance (1 January–31 December 2022). EEA—European Economic Area, non-EEA—non-European Economic Area; HP—healthcare professionals, N-HPs—non-healthcare professionals; n—number of reports.

			CFT	COL	CPX	GEN	LIN	MER	PIP/TAZ
	Total ICSRs, n		85	2	36	6	6	36	78
Reporter Group	HPs	n	85	2	30	6	6	34	76
		(%)	(100)	(100)	(85.7)	(100)	(100)	(94.4)	(97.4)
	N-HPs	n	0	0	5	0	0	2	2
		(%)	(0.0)	(0.0)	(14.3)	(0.0)	(0.0)	(5.6)	(2.6)
Countries	EEA	n	27	2	7	6	5	10	14
		(%)	(31.8)	(100.0)	(20.0)	(100.0)	(83.3)	(27.8)	(17.9)
	Non-EEA	n	58	0	28	0	1	26	64
		(%)	(68.2)	(0.0)	(80.0)	(0.0)	(16.7)	(72.2)	(82.1)
Age Category	2 months–2 years	n	0	0	0	0	0	0	2
		(%)	(0.0)	(0.0)	(0.0)	(0.0)	(0.0)	(0.0)	(2.6)
	3–11 years	n	1	0	0	0	0	0	1
		(%)	(1.2)	(0.0)	(0.0)	(0.0)	(0.0)	(0.0)	(1.3)
	18–64 years	n	17	2	13	1	2	13	13
		(%)	(20.0)	(100.)	(36.1)	(16.7)	(33.3)	(36.1)	(16.7)
	65–85 years	n	34	0	17	3	4	18	31
		(%)	(40.0)	(0.0)	(47.2)	(50.0)	(66.7)	(50.0)	(39.7)
	>85 years	n	31	0	4	1	0	4	27
		(%)	(36.5)	(0.0)	(11.1)	(16.7)	(0.0)	(11.1)	(34.6)
	Not specified	n	2	0	2	1	0	1	4
		(%)	(2.4)	(0.0)	(5.6)	(16.7)	(0.0)	(2.8)	(5.1)
Gender	Male	n	47	0	14	3	2	26	30
		(%)	(55.3)	(0.0)	(38.9)	(50.0)	(33.3)	(72.2)	(38.5)
	Female	n	38	2	22	3	4	9	46.00
		(%)	(44.7)	(100.0)	(61.1)	(50.0)	(66.7)	(25.0)	(59.0)
	Not specified	n	0.00	0.00	0.00	0.00	0.00	1.00	2.00
		(%)	(0.0)	(0.0)	(0.0)	(0.0)	(0.0)	(2.8)	(2.6)

2.2.2. Outcomes

Figure 5 presents the outcomes included in ICSRs for all seven drugs analyzed. More than 61.1% of total reports are related to a favorable outcome (recovered/resolved—38.2% and recovering/resolving—22.9%). Death was reported in 18 ICSRs (7.2%), and not recovered/not resolved outcome was reported in 7 ICSRs (2.8%).

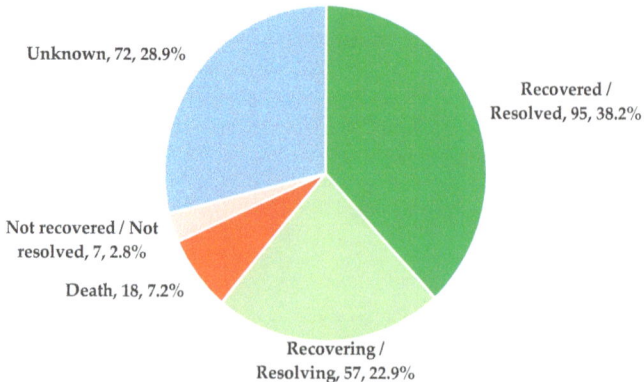

Figure 5. Outcomes presented in ICSRs reported in EV in 2022.

Although favorable results were reported for most antibiotics, unfavorable results were recorded in some reports for LIN (16.7%), CPX (11.1%), CFT (10.6%), and PIP/TAZ (10.3%) (Figure 6).

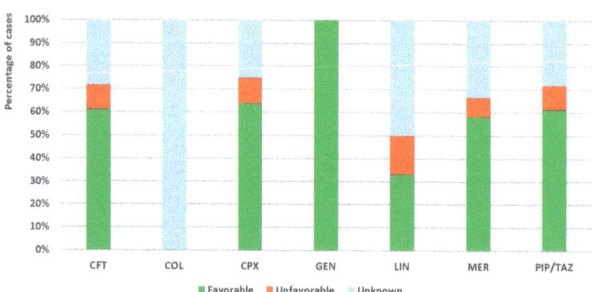

Figure 6. Distribution of ICSR by category of outcomes and antibiotic. CFT—ceftriaxone; COL—colistin; CPX—ciprofloxacin; GEN—gentamicin; LIN—linezolid; MER—meropenem; PIP/TAZ—piperacillin and tazobactam.

Figure 7 showed that all analyzed antibiotics caused/prolonged hospitalization in percentages between 66.7% (GEN and LIN) and 100% (COL).

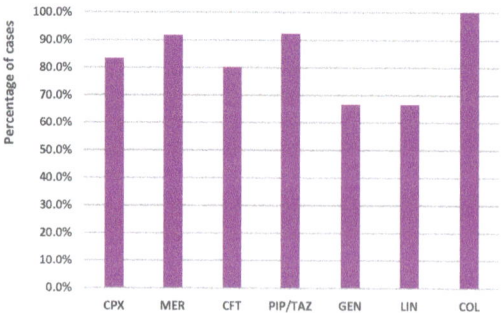

Figure 7. Distribution of cases associated with caused/prolonged hospitalization reported in EV in 2022. CFT—ceftriaxone; COL—colistin; CPX—ciprofloxacin; GEN—gentamicin; LIN—linezolid; MER—meropenem; PIP/TAZ—piperacillin and tazobactam.

2.3. Comparison between the Reports from Sibiu County Clinical Emergency Hospital (SCCEH) and the Spontaneous Reports from EudraVigilance (EV)

2.3.1. Exposure to Analyzed Drugs as a Single Suspected Antibiotic

Figure 8 showed a similar situation in SCCEH and EV, referring to the proportion of cases associated with COL (0%—SCCEH, 0%—EV) and MER (11.11%—EV, 10%—SCCEH) as a single suspected antibiotic for CDI. A large difference was noticed regarding the CPX (0%—SCCEH, 31.43%—EV), CFT (62.5%—SCCEH, 31.76%—EV), and GEN (0%—SCCEH, 16.67%—EV) as being the only suspected antibiotics.

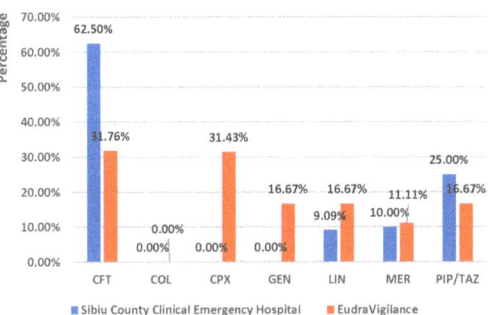

Figure 8. Comparison of the proportion of reports associated with each drug as the only suspected antibiotic in all reports associated with the analyzed drug in SCCEH vs. EudraVigilance (2022). CFT—ceftriaxone; COL—colistin; CPX—ciprofloxacin; GEN—gentamicin; LIN—linezolid; MER—meropenem; PIP/TAZ—piperacillin and tazobactam.

2.3.2. Frequency of Exposure to Other Antibiotics in Cases Where the Analyzed Drug Was Not the Only Suspected Antibiotic

The frequency of exposure to other antibiotics in cases where the analyzed drug was not the only suspected antibiotic in EV database reports (A_{Ev}) and in hospital database reports (A_H), respectively, are presented in Figure 9. Similar values could be observed for CFT (A_{Ev} = 0.8 and A_H = 0.5) and PIP/TAZ (A_{Ev} = 0.5 and A_H = 0.9) (Figure 9).

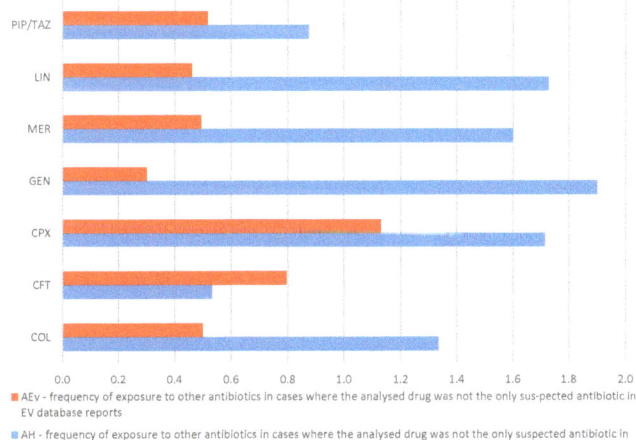

Figure 9. Frequency of exposure to other antibiotics in cases where the analyzed drug was not the only suspected antibiotic—comparison between A_{Ev} and A_H reports. CFT—ceftriaxone; COL—colistin; CPX—ciprofloxacin; GEN—gentamicin; LIN—linezolid; MER—meropenem; PIP/TAZ—piperacillin and tazobactam.

Subsequently, we identified the other suspected antibiotics associated with the analyzed drug. The frequency of exposure (R) to each suspected antibiotic, in the total number of exposures for each of the seven studied antibiotics, was compared between the two databases. Thus, in Figure 10, it can be observed that amoxicillin/clavulanic acid was most frequently reported as a suspected drug in CDI cases associated with GEN and PIP/TAZ in the EV database but not found in any SCCEH reports. The proportion of reports showing ampicillin as a suspected drug in CDI cases associated with GEN is similar in both databases (SCCEH: R = 0.10 and EV: R = 0.11). The same observation is available for MER in CDI cases associated with COL (SCCEH: R = 0.50 and EV: R = 0.50), CFT in CDI cases associated with PIP/TAZ (SCCEH: R = 0.14 and EV: R = 0.13), and PIP/TAZ in CDI cases associated with CPX (SCCEH: R = 0.17 and EV: R = 0.13).

	EUDRAVIGILANCE DATABASE							HOSPITAL DATABASE						
	CFT	CPX	COL	GEN	LIN	MER	PIP/TAZ		CFT	CPX	COL	GEN	LIN	MER	PIP/TAZ
Common antibiotics between the two databases															
AMI				0.10				AMI	0.12			0.05			0.14
AMP				0.10	0.08			AMP				0.11			
CLX							0.07	CLX				0.05			
CFT		0.39		0.08	0.22		0.13	CFT		0.25	0.16				0.14
CPX	0.11			0.08	0.08			CPX					0.11	0.16	0.29
LIN			0.50					LIN		0.17	0.25			0.22	0.29
MER	0.14	0.19	0.50		0.23		0.07	MER		0.42	0.50	0.16	0.37		
PIP/TAZ	0.18	0.13		0.20		0.15		PIP/TAZ		0.17			0.11		
SFX/TMT					0.08			SFX/TMT				0.05			
Non common antibiotics															
AMO / CLA				0.15			0.19	CFD	0.24	0.25		0.05	0.32	0.19	
CTX				0.15				CFR	0.12			0.11			0.14
CLR				0.10				FOS				0.05			
CLI					0.08			GEN	0.18						
COL					0.15			OXA				0.11			
ERT							0.07	PEN				0.05			
IMI					0.15			RFM				0.05			
LEV						0.13									
RFX					0.08										

Figure 10. Comparison between the most frequently reported antibiotics as suspected drugs in CDI cases associated with the analyzed antibiotics in EudraVigilance and SCCEH database in 2022. The numbers represent the frequency of exposure (R) to each suspected antibiotic, in the total number of exposures for each of the seven studied antibiotics. AMI—amikacin; AMO/CLA—amoxicillin + clavulanic acid; AMP—ampicillin; CFD—ceftazidime; CFR—cefuroxime; CFT—ceftriaxone; CLR—clarithromycin; CLX—cephalexin; COL—colistin; CPX—ciprofloxacin; CTX—cefotaxime; ERT—ertapenem; FOS—fosfomycin; GEN—gentamicin; IMI—imipenem + cilastatin; LEV—levofloxacin; LIN—linezolid; MER—meropenem; MOX—moxifloxacin; OXA—oxacillin; PEN—penicillin G; RFM—rifampicin; PIP/TAZ—piperacillin and tazobactam; RFX—rifaximin. The red cells include results with similar R values; the blue cells include results with non-similar R values; and the grey cells include results that can not be compared.

3. Discussion

CDI is a frequently occurring disease that affects patients previously exposed to antibiotics. This infection is an essential concern for healthcare professionals, as it can lead to significant morbidity and mortality worldwide [23].

From 30,608 patients admitted to SCCEH in 2022, 111 patients were diagnosed with CDI, representing an incidence rate of 3.63 per 1000 admissions. A study performed in another hospital in Romania revealed a high incidence of CDI (20.57/15.70 to 1000 discharged patients in 2013/2014) [24]. A meta-analysis that included 229 publications with data from 41 countries identified a yearly incidence of up to 35.15 CDI per 1000 admissions [25]. A retrospective, multicenter cohort study performed in 43 hospitals in the United States of America between 1 January 2013 and 31 December 2017 showed that the median total incidence has increased from 7.9 CDIs per 1000 admissions to 9.3 CDIs per 1000 admissions [26]. Also, a study by Kuntz et al. reported a higher incidence (13.3 CDIs per 1000 patient admissions) [27] than that observed in SCCEH. On the other hand, a teaching hospital from Okayama City (Japan) reported a low incidence rate, between 1.71 cases per 1000 admissions in an old hospital and 0.46 cases per 1000 admissions in a new hospital [28]. Also, a low incidence of CDI was recorded in a Portuguese hospital (20.7 per 10,000 admissions) [29]. The mortality rate from SCCEH was 252.3 deaths/1000 cases/year (25%). Mortality rates due to CDI vary widely between studies. A systematic review of HA-CDI in Europe based on studies published between 2000 and 2010 estimated in-hospital mortality ranging between 0% (Latvia) and 44% (Austria) [30]. A retrospective study of patients diagnosed with CDI in a healthcare facility in Taiwan reported an in-hospital mortality of 28.7% [31]. Another multicenter cohort study from the Netherlands found a 2.5-fold increase in 30-day mortality due to CDI [32]. Age and the presence of comorbidities were found to be among the most reported risk factors for mortality in CDI patients [33].

A significant proportion (77.5%) of all patients admitted to SCCEH and affected by CDI are represented by the elderly population ($\geq$65 years). Also, in the three age subgroups, the proportion of unfavorable outcomes doubles from one group to another. Thus, elderly people who are over 85 years old are exposed to a higher risk of unfavorable outcomes associated with CDI. Also, in the descriptive analysis of the spontaneous reports recorded in EV during 2022 and associated with the use of CFT, COL, CPX, GEN, LIN, MER, and PIP/TAZ, it was observed that CDI was most frequently reported in patients aged 65–85 years, followed by individuals over 85 years. According to other studies, the elderly have a weakened immune response, which makes them more vulnerable to infections, including CDI, especially when they have other illnesses [34,35]. The elderly population is often exposed to long-term medical care and interventions, and frequent drugs used by this patient population (e.g., antibiotics and proton pump inhibitors) can disrupt the microbial balance, creating an environment for CD proliferation [35–38]. Moreover, according to the literature, the mortality rate within 30 days is higher in individuals over the age of 60. This risk increases substantially in those aged 80 and above. This highlights the increased susceptibility of older populations, particularly those over 80, to the negative consequences of CDI [39].

In total, 55% of all patients admitted to SCCEH and affected by CDI were females. Regarding the occurrence of CDI-related ADRs recorded in EV, no major difference was observed between females (50.4%) and males (49.6%). Previous studies have shown that females have higher rates of CDI compared to males [40,41]. This suggests that sex-specific dynamics, particularly concerning the gut microbiome, may be at play. Research has revealed that differences in the gut microbiome between males and females are closely linked to hormonal variations. Hormone levels have been identified as mediators influencing the distinct microbial composition observed in both sexes [42,43].

Out of all the cases of CDI from SCCEH, only 34.2% were surgical cases. However, we observed that 86.8% of these cases had favorable outcomes, suggesting good antibiotic stewardship in terms of antibiotic prophylaxis. On the other hand, non-surgical patients had favorable outcomes in only 63% of cases. This indicates a significant difference in the clinical paths and ultimate prognosis between these two groups of patients. Several studies and reports have shown a strong link between the occurrence of CDI in individuals who undergo surgical procedures [44,45]. This correlation is mainly attributed to the widespread use of broad-spectrum antibiotics in surgical care. Moreover, the increasing incidence of CDI in surgical patients is closely related to the rising number of elderly individuals and those with weakened immune systems who undergo various surgical interventions [44]. A recent study found that patients undergoing surgical procedures are more likely to develop severe CDI [46]. Although these patients tend to have a more challenging clinical course with CDI, their overall outcomes are better than those of medical patients [46]. On the other hand, medical patients experience a shorter hospital stay, an earlier onset of CDI, and higher rates of 30-day and overall mortality, with deaths occurring earlier after the onset of CDI [46].

The results of our study showed that, on average, it takes around 9.2 days from the time of admission until the detection of CDI in hospitalized patients from SCCEH. Additionally, once CDI is identified, the average hospital stay significantly increases to 11.03 days. However, the reports from EV showed that COL, PIP/TAZ, MER, CFT, and CPX were associated with caused/prolonged hospitalization in a high proportion (100%, 92.3%, 91.7%, 80%, and 83.3%, respectively). A recent study found that CDI adds an average of three days to hospital stays, significantly impacting hospital discharge rates [47]. For example, in the context of the United Kingdom, CDI was linked to a considerable reduction in the daily discharge rate, specifically by about 28% [48]. On the other hand, a prospective study has reported a relatively short duration of hospitalization, with a median stay of only five days and a range spanning from 3 to 11 days [49]. The difference in hospitalization duration highlights the variability across different studies and the importance of considering contextual factors and study design when interpreting such results.

The highest incidence of cases reported across various medical and surgical wards from SCCEH was found in infectious disease (n = 22, 19.8%), general surgery (n = 26, 23.4%), and internal medicine (n = 30, 27.0%). A noteworthy trend emerged when examining outcomes. In seven wards, favorable outcomes represented 100% of total cases, highlighting a notable success in patient management. On the other hand, out of all the wards, only two (cardiology and orthopedics) had a 0% rate of favorable outcomes, indicating difficulties in achieving positive patient results in those particular contexts. However, it is essential to consider that the patients in those wards were of advanced age and had severe underlying medical conditions and a high comorbidity index. According to a recent study, the ICU and internal medicine wards have a higher prevalence of CDI cases. The analysis revealed that the median number of CDI cases per admission was consistently higher in these wards and had the highest incidence rate and density [25]. Another recent study showed a notable number of CDI cases in general medicine wards. The study further suggests that patients admitted to general medicine wards tend to be older and may have pre-existing medical conditions that make them more susceptible to acquiring the infection [50].

The Charlson comorbidity index (CCI) is reliable for assessing critical outcomes such as mortality, hospital stay, functional disability, and healthcare utilization [51]. Patients with a high CCI score, mainly those exceeding 7, are more likely to experience recurrent condition occurrences [52,53]. In our study, we analyzed the application of the CCI for patients from SCCEH diagnosed with CDI. The average CCI of the patients was calculated at 7.6. This indicates a significant burden of comorbidities that the studied patient population had. While analyzing the data by gender, we observed no significant differences between men and women regarding the CCI scores. However, a pattern could be observed when exploring the correlation between CCI, age categories, and the evolution of CDI outcomes. Some significant differences were identified, particularly when comparing different age groups within the favorable and unfavorable evolution categories. These differences underscore the importance of considering demographic and comorbidity factors in managing CDI.

Specific diagnoses have a high incidence of unfavorable outcomes, as shown in our analysis. In some instances, the gravity of concurrent diagnoses leads to 100% unfavorable outcomes. This includes specific conditions such as cardiac arrest (n = 1), fever (n = 1), long bone fracture (n = 1), urosepsis (n = 1), heart failure (n = 2), and pancreatitis (n = 2), underlining the critical nature of these medical situations. In total, 75% of cases with chronic kidney disease (n = 4) had unfavorable outcomes. This substantial proportion emphasizes the challenging clinical trajectory associated with chronic kidney disease. The impact of SARS-CoV-2 is particularly noteworthy, with 61.5% of cases (n = 13) leading to unfavorable outcomes. This underscores the complex and often unpredictable nature of outcomes associated with COVID-19. Additionally, diagnoses such as arrhythmia (n = 2), respiratory failure (n = 2), and urinary infection (n = 3) exhibit a 50% frequency of unfavorable outcomes.

Regarding the exposure of patients to antibiotics, it was observed that in SCCEH, the mean of antibiotics used by all patients is 1.50. According to the United States Centers for Disease and Control Prevention, exposure to antibiotics increases the risk of CDI by 7 to 10 times by killing the good germs from saprophytic flora capable of fighting against opportunistic bacteria like CD [54,55]. A recent study examined the effect of prior antibiotic use on the risk of developing CDI. The study found that the amount of antibiotics used before hospitalization is the most significant factor contributing to the risk of developing CDI [56]. Additionally, the study suggests that while all types of antibiotics carry some risks, the level of risk varies depending on the specific drug and method of administration [56]. The results are consistent with previous studies, indicating that the risk of developing CDI is higher in individuals exposed to antibiotics. The risk of developing CDI is cumulative and increases with each day of antibiotic exposure [57]. The most significant risk occurs within the first 60 days after taking antibiotics. In the dataset analyzed, the odds of developing CDI increased by 12.8% per day of individual antibiotic exposure [58,59].

Moreover, the elderly people (>85 years) were exposed only to 1.17 antibiotics compared to all groups (1.50). Statistical analysis shows that the coefficient of skewness has positive values for the entire group (0.66) and subgroups 2 (0.73) and 3 (2.06). For subgroup 1, a symmetrical distribution of values (skewness = 0.07) could be observed, and a constant trend in the use of antibiotics could be implicitly observed. Additionally, a leptokurtic distribution (kurtosis > 0) could be noticed in all group, subgroups 2, and 3, showing a small range, variance, and standard deviation with most data points near the mean. The opposite of subgroup 1 could be observed as a platykurtic distribution (kurtosis < 0), which shows an extensive range, variance, and standard deviation [60,61]. Moreover, patients who had favorable outcomes were exposed to a slightly higher number of antibiotics (1.53) compared to those who had unfavorable outcomes (1.44). Skewness has positive values for both subgroups (0.65 and 0.73). These values indicate asymmetry [60,61] and could suggest a mildly increasing tendency to use antibiotics. Additionally, a leptokurtic distribution (kurtosis > 0) could be noticed in patients from the subgroup with favorable outcomes (kurtosis = 0.439452) that shows a small range, variance, and standard deviation with the majority of data points near the mean. In subgroups with unfavorable outcomes, a normal distribution (kurtosis = −0.07617) [60,61] is observed.

Of the seven studied antibiotics, patients from SCCEH were most frequently exposed to CFT and MER. In the EV database, most CDI-related ADRs were reported for CFT, PIP/TAZ, MER, and CPX. Moreover, our results indicated that there are some similarities between cases associated with COL and MER between the two databases regarding the patient exposure to each analyzed drug as a single suspected antibiotic, while there were large differences between cases associated with CFT and CPX. Furthermore, for all analyzed antibiotics except CFT, exposure to other antibiotics was increased in SCCEH reports compared to EV. Some antibiotics were frequently reported as suspected drugs only in the EV database: (i) AMO/CLA, CTX, and CLR in CDI cases associated with GEN; (ii) CLI, COL, IMI, and RFX in CDI cases associated with LIN; (iii) AMO/CLA, ERT, and LEV CDI cases associated with PIP/TAZ. Only in the reports from SCCEH, it was observed that (i) CFD was frequently reported as a suspected drug in CDI cases associated with CFT, CPX, GEN, LIN, and MER; (ii) CFR in CDI cases associated with CFT, GEN, and PIP/TAZ; and (iii) FOS, OXA, PEN, RFM in CDI cases associated with GEN. A recent study compared the risk of CDI associated with 27 antibiotics. The results showed that clindamycin has a high risk of causing CDI. The fluoroquinolones, such as ciprofloxacin and moxifloxacin, as well as later-generation cephalosporin like cefaclor, have odds ratios ranging from 4.16 to 6.83. Meanwhile, linezolid, cefprozil, cephalexin, cefadroxil, ampicillin, levofloxacin, and sulfamethoxazole/trimethoprim have odds ratios between 2.15 and 3.58 [62]. A hospital-acquired CDI meta-analysis found that certain antibiotics are more strongly associated with CDI than others. The order of association from strongest to weakest is third-generation cephalosporins, clindamycin, second-generation cephalosporins, fourth-generation cephalosporins, carbapenems, trimethoprim-sulfonamides, fluoroquinolones, and penicillin combinations [63].

To ensure the safety of patients in hospitals, it is important to implement strict infection control measures and sanitation protocols to address bacterial contamination. The issue of CD contamination in hospitals can be effectively tackled through a comprehensive approach that includes multiple strategies. These strategies may include promoting the responsible use of antibiotics, implementing effective infection control practices, enhancing environmental cleaning, providing education and training on infection prevention, using probiotics, adopting early detection methods, and isolating affected patients [64].

Limitations

As this is a retrospective observational study, it has some limitations. The level of evidence is low, and this study's representativeness is limited due to inconsistent data reporting, uneven use of terminology, etc. This study's small representation in the general population is due to data being reported in a year and collected only from a single center. The lack of clinical and laboratory information can cause a possible alteration in the identification of the first symptoms to establish the onset of the disease and the identification of all cases of CDI, which could lead to an under-reporting of these cases. Not all risk factors have been identified, so causality cannot be established. The outcomes could be potentially influenced by differences between the specialists' vigilance in detecting non-severe cases of CDI. It should be noted that this study did not include all of the cumulative risk factors for CDI. Some factors that were not considered include using proton pump inhibitors or anti-inflammatory medications, prolonged hospitalization exceeding 20 days, surgical interventions on the digestive tract, the presence of a nasogastric tube, or parenteral nutrition. The patients' follow-up could be considered another study limitation due to the lack of information regarding their evolution after discharge, especially in patients with improved or aggravated status.

Although our study has significant advantages based on the EV database data extraction technology, there are also limitations that we need to consider. First of all, the EV database is a spontaneous reporting system. This means the reporting may be selective, incomplete, inaccurate, and unverified. Thus, it is not easy to take into account certain factors such as dose, duration of use, comorbidities, drug combinations, and other factors that may influence the occurrence of CDI. Secondly, the EV database only contains cases with adverse events, and the incidence rate cannot be calculated due to the lack of the total number of patients receiving antibiotic treatment. In other words, we do not have the denominator of drug exposure. Finally, disproportionality analysis based on EV did not quantify risk or causality but only assessed signal strength. Therefore, it is essential to remember that the analysis only indicates a signal that needs further investigation but does not provide conclusive evidence.

One issue with spontaneous reporting is the occurrence of duplicate reports, where multiple sources submit the same report (a patient and a medical professional). Additionally, there may be various reports where the reporter modifies an existing case follow-up report with additional information. To address this, EV periodically identifies and merges these duplicate reports during quality review. Furthermore, in this study, we used a deduplication procedure to identify and eliminate these reports based on the unique EU local number code, making the reporting process more efficient and accurate. The two databases can only be compared in a few aspects due to the differing levels and information types. The case reports in the two databases differ, making it difficult to compare the results.

4. Materials and Methods

4.1. Study Design

A retrospective pharmacovigilance study referring to CDI was performed. The real-world data reported in 2022 from SCCEH were analyzed. All cases investigated (n = 111) from the hospital's database were classified as nosocomial infections associated with medical procedures, with none attributed to community transmission. The infections observed in SCCEH are classified by the hospital's infection surveillance department as nosocomial infections. Nosocomial CDI was defined as the development of new-onset diarrhea either at admission in patients with recent hospitalization within twelve weeks or $\geq$48 h from admission in patients without recent prior hospitalization, plus a confirmed CDI [65]. Institutional review board approval was obtained before the initiation of this study.

Subsequently, another study, including a descriptive analysis, was performed based on the spontaneous reports registered in the EV database (n = 249) between 1 January and 31 December 2022 at https://www.adrreports.eu (accessed on 11 October 2023) [66]. The ICSRs refer to the EEA or non-EEA and could be reported by healthcare professionals or non-healthcare professionals (e.g., patients, lawyers, etc.) [67]. For this study, no ethics committee approval is required because ICSRs do not include any patients' personal information [68].

4.2. Materials

Seven antibiotics that are frequently used in hospital settings were chosen: CFT, COL, CPX, GEN, LIN, MER, and PIP/TAZ. The analyzed data were reported in EV between 1 January and 31 December 2022. Preferred terms related to CDI were as follows: "Clostridial infection", "Clostridial sepsis", "*Clostridium* bacteremia", "*Clostridium* colitis", "*Clostridium difficile* colitis", "*Clostridium difficile* infection", and "Gastroenteritis clostridial".

4.3. Data Analysis

4.3.1. Descriptive Analysis of Reports from Sibiu County Clinical Emergency Hospital

A descriptive analysis of data registered in 2022 in SCCEH was realized. Many criteria were considered to evaluate the baseline patients' characteristics:

- Demographic data: age, gender, patient's category (surgical or non-surgical patient). The data collected from SCCEH referred to adult patients, and the age categories were chosen according to European Medicines Agency regulations regarding pharmacovigilance activity. This is to enable better comparison between the two datasets.
- Evolution: resolved/recovered, aggravated conditions, not resolved/not recovered (transfers), or death. The resolved/recovered cases represented the favorable evolution, and unfavorable evolution included aggravated conditions, not resolved/not recovered (transfers included), or death.
- Type of detection: active or passive. The active or passive detection mode indicates how the infection was reported to the infection surveillance department from SCCEH. Active detection means that the patient's attending physician reported the infection, while passive detection means that the infection surveillance department detected the infection.

The descriptive analysis presents (i) the influence of age on the outcome (favorable or unfavorable), (ii) the distribution of cases by wards (cases, percentage of total cases, proportion of favorable outcomes), (iii) the distribution of cases by medical diagnoses (cases, percentage of total cases, proportion of favorable outcomes), (iv) CCI (for the group, by sex, by age category, by outcome), (v) hospital length of stay (HLS-AD—hospital length of stay after the detection, HLS-ICU—hospital length of stay in ICU, HLS-UD—hospital length of stay until the detection, and T-HLS—total hospital length of stay), and (vi) exposure to antibiotics (analysis regarding the antibiotics' exposure, distribution of cases by the number of antibiotics used and outcome, the proportion of cases by outcome in relation with the total number of cases). All administered antibiotics in the last month were considered suspected except those specific for treating CDI (vancomycin, metronidazole, tigecycline, and rifaximin). The value of CCI was used to predict the 10-year survival in patients with multiple comorbidities. This indicator was calculated with MDcalc [69], and the values took into account comorbidities such as diabetes, cancers, cardiovascular diseases, renal failure, AIDS, etc. [70].

4.3.2. Analysis of Spontaneous Reports from EudraVigilance

A descriptive analysis of CDI reported as a spontaneous adverse reaction related to using CFT, COL, CPX, GEN, LIN, MER, and PIP/TAZ was performed. Many criteria were used to carry out this analysis: age category, gender, reporter group, and outcomes. The resolved/recovered cases and resolving/recovering were considered with a favorable evolution, and an unfavorable evolution was considered for not resolved/not recovered or death conditions.

4.3.3. Comparison between the Reports from Sibiu County Clinical Emergency Hospital (SCCEH) and the Spontaneous Reports from EudraVigilance (EV)

To carry out a comparison between both databases, the proportion of reports associated with each drug as the only suspected antibiotic in all reports associated with the analyzed drug in SCCEH versus EudraVigilance was determined.

Moreover, the frequency of exposure to other antibiotics in cases where the analyzed drug was not the only suspected antibiotic in EV database reports (A_{Ev}) and in hospital database reports (A_H), respectively, was examined. A_{Ev} was calculated as the ratio of the total number of other antibiotics suspected of CDI reported in association with each analyzed drug (COL, CFT, CPX, GEN, LIN, MER, or PIP/TAZ) to the total number of reports registered for each analyzed drug. A similar ratio was calculated for hospital settings (A_H). Consecutively, both ratios (A_{Ev} and A_H) were compared.

$$A_{Ev} = \frac{N_{SEV}}{N_{EV}} \quad (1)$$

A_{Ev} = frequency of exposure to other antibiotics in cases where the analyzed drug was not the only suspected antibiotic in EV database reports;

N_{SEV} = total number of other antibiotics suspected of CDI reported in association with each analyzed drug in EV database reports;

N_{EV} = total number of reports registered for each analyzed drug in the EV database.

$$A_H = \frac{N_{SH}}{N_H} \quad (2)$$

A_H = frequency of exposure to other antibiotics in cases where the analyzed drug was not the only suspected antibiotic in hospital database reports;

N_{SH} = total number of other antibiotics suspected of CDI reported in association with each analyzed drug in hospital database reports;

N_H = total number of reports registered for each analyzed drug in the hospital database.

Subsequently, we identified the other suspected antibiotics associated with the analyzed drug. The frequency of exposure to each suspected antibiotic, in the total number of exposures for each of the seven studied antibiotics, was compared between the two databases.

A frequency indicator (R) was obtained for both databases (hospital and EudraVigilance) as the ratio of the number of reports for each other suspected antibiotic identified (N_A) and the total number of other suspected antibiotics associated with each studied drug (N_{TA}). The first three frequency values for both databases (hospital and EV) were extracted and used for comparison.

$$R = \frac{N_A}{N_{TA}} \quad (3)$$

where:

R—frequency indicator;

N_A—number of reports for each other suspected antibiotic identified;

N_{TA}—total number of other suspected antibiotics associated with each studied drug.

4.4. Statistical Analysis

The data were analyzed using Microsoft Excel 2010 software—Data Analysis Tools. The variables that describe the characteristics of the population were presented in absolute numbers, frequencies, and percentages, or mean and standard deviation. To evaluate the antibiotics exposure, skewness (a measure of symmetry) and Kurtosis (a measure that quantifies the shape of the probability distribution) were considered. The comparison between subgroups was considered significant if p-value < 0.05.

5. Conclusions

This study stands out by using a unique approach, comparing the results from two different datasets collected from a clinical setting and the European spontaneous reporting system. This methodology helps us to better understand the clinical characteristics and the effects of antibiotic use on CDI, providing a more accurate representation of real-world outcomes. The present study offers valuable insights to the scientific community, emphasizing the crucial need for responsible antibiotic use and effective infection prevention and control measures. Future studies are encouraged to investigate further into the complexities of antibiotic-associated colitis, to enhance our knowledge and improve signal detection in pharmacovigilance practices.

Author Contributions: Conceptualization, B.I.V., A.M.A., A.B., C.M. and F.G.G.; methodology, B.I.V., A.M.A., A.B., C.M.D., L.L.R., S.G, R.A. and F.G.G.; software, B.I.V., A.M.A., A.B., I.R.C. and C.M.; validation, B.I.V., A.M.A., M.S., V.B., S.G., C.M. and F.G.G.; formal analysis, B.I.V., A.M.A., A.B., A.S.B., I.R.C. and C.M.; investigation, B.I.V., A.M.A., A.B., A.S.B., S.G. and C.M.; resources, B.I.V., A.M.A., A.B., C.M. and F.G.G.; writing—original draft preparation, B.I.V., A.M.A., C.M.D., L.L.R., A.B. and C.M.; writing—review and editing, B.I.V., A.M.A., A.B., M.S., V.B., S.G., R.A., C.M. and F.G.G.; visualization, B.I.V., A.M.A., A.B., M.S., V.B., C.M.D., L.L.R., S.G., C.M., R.A. and F.G.G.; supervision, A.M.A., A.B., C.M., M.S. and F.G.G. All authors have read and agreed to the published version of the manuscript.

Funding: This project is financed by Lucian Blaga University of Sibiu through the research grant LBUS-IRG-2022-08/No. 2878, 18 July 2022.

Institutional Review Board Statement: The study protocols are approved by the Institutional Review Board of the Ethics Committee of the Sibiu County Clinical Emergency Hospital, No. 26995/13.11.2023.

Informed Consent Statement: Not applicable.

Data Availability Statement: Data are contained within this article.

Conflicts of Interest: The authors declare no conflicts of interest.

References

1. Popa, D.; Neamtu, B.; Mihalache, M.; Boicean, A.; Banciu, A.; Banciu, D.D.; Moga, D.F.C.; Birlutiu, V. Fecal Microbiota Transplant in Severe and Non-Severe Clostridioides Difficile Infection. Is There a Role of FMT in Primary Severe CDI? *J. Clin. Med.* **2021**, *10*, 5822. [CrossRef] [PubMed]
2. Chiș, A.A.; Rus, L.L.; Morgovan, C.; Arseniu, A.M.; Frum, A.; Vonica-țincu, A.L.; Gligor, F.G.; Mureșan, M.L.; Dobrea, C.M. Microbial Resistance to Antibiotics and Effective Antibiotherapy. *Biomedicines* **2022**, *10*, 1121. [CrossRef] [PubMed]
3. Czepiel, J.; Dróżdż, M.; Pituch, H.; Kuijper, E.J.; Perucki, W.; Mielimonka, A.; Goldman, S.; Wultańska, D.; Garlicki, A.; Biesiada, G. Clostridium Difficile Infection: Review. *Eur. J. Clin. Microbiol. Infect. Dis.* **2019**, *38*, 1211. [CrossRef] [PubMed]
4. Birlutiu, V.; Dobritoiu, E.S.; Lupu, C.D.; Herteliu, C.; Birlutiu, R.M.; Dragomirescu, D.; Vorovenci, A. Our Experience with 80 Cases of SARS-CoV-2-Clostridioides Difficile Co-Infection: An Observational Study. *Medicine* **2022**, *101*, E29823. [CrossRef] [PubMed]
5. Centers for Disease Control and Prevention. *Antibiotic Resistance Threats in the United States*; Centers for Disease Control and Prevention: Atlanta, GA, USA, 2013.
6. Magill, S.S.; Edwards, J.R.; Bamberg, W.; Beldavs, Z.G.; Dumyati, G.; Kainer, M.A.; Lynfield, R.; Maloney, M.; McAllister-Hollod, L.; Nadle, J.; et al. Multistate Point-Prevalence Survey of Health Care-Associated Infections. *N. Engl. J. Med.* **2014**, *370*, 1198–1208. [CrossRef] [PubMed]
7. Kim, G.; Zhu, N.A. Community-Acquired Clostridium Difficile Infection. *Can. Fam. Physician* **2017**, *63*, 131.

8. Boicean, A.; Neamtu, B.; Birsan, S.; Batar, F.; Tanasescu, C.; Dura, H.; Roman, M.D.; Hașegan, A.; Bratu, D.; Mihetiu, A.; et al. Fecal Microbiota Transplantation in Patients Co-Infected with SARS-CoV2 and Clostridioides Difficile. *Biomedicines* **2022**, *11*, 7. [CrossRef]
9. Slimings, C.; Riley, T.V. Antibiotics and Healthcare Facility-Associated Clostridioides Difficile Infection: Systematic Review and Meta-Analysis 2020 Update. *J. Antimicrob. Chemother.* **2021**, *76*, 1676–1688. [CrossRef]
10. Perić, A.; Rančić, N.; Dragojević-Simić, V.; Milenković, B.; Ljubenović, N.; Rakonjac, B.; Begović-Kuprešanin, V.; Šuljagić, V. Association between Antibiotic Use and Hospital-Onset Clostridioides Difficile Infection in University Tertiary Hospital in Serbia, 2011–2021: An Ecological Analysis. *Antibiotics* **2022**, *11*, 1178. [CrossRef]
11. Armstrong, T.; Fenn, S.J.; Hardie, K.R. JMM Profile: Carbapenems: A Broad-Spectrum Antibiotic. *J. Med. Microbiol.* **2021**, *70*, 1462. [CrossRef]
12. Janssen, J.; Kinkade, A.; Man, D. CARBapenem UtilizatiON Evaluation in a Large Community Hospital (CARBON): A Quality Improvement Study. *Can. J. Hosp. Pharm.* **2015**, *68*, 327. [CrossRef]
13. Hashemian, S.M.R.; Farhadi, T.; Ganjparvar, M. Linezolid: A Review of Its Properties, Function, and Use in Critical Care. *Drug Des. Devel. Ther.* **2018**, *12*, 1759–1767. [CrossRef]
14. Moubareck, C.A. Polymyxins and Bacterial Membranes: A Review of Antibacterial Activity and Mechanisms of Resistance. *Membranes* **2020**, *10*, 181. [CrossRef]
15. Khilnani, G.C.; Zirpe, K.; Hadda, V.; Mehta, Y.; Madan, K.; Kulkarni, A.; Mohan, A.; Dixit, S.; Guleria, R.; Bhattacharya, P. Guidelines for Antibiotic Prescription in Intensive Care Unit. *Indian J. Crit. Care Med.* **2019**, *23*, S1. [CrossRef]
16. El-Haffaf, I.; Caissy, J.A.; Marsot, A. Piperacillin-Tazobactam in Intensive Care Units: A Review of Population Pharmacokinetic Analyses. *Clin. Pharmacokinet.* **2021**, *60*, 855–875. [CrossRef]
17. Kayambankadzanja, R.K.; Lihaka, M.; Barratt-Due, A.; Kachingwe, M.; Kumwenda, W.; Lester, R.; Bilima, S.; Eriksen, J.; Baker, T. The Use of Antibiotics in the Intensive Care Unit of a Tertiary Hospital in Malawi. *BMC Infect. Dis.* **2020**, *20*, 776. [CrossRef]
18. Grigore, N.; Totan, M.; Pirvut, V.; Mitariu, S.I.C.; Chicea, R.; Sava, M.; Hasegan, A. A Risk Assessment of Clostridium Difficile Infection after Antibiotherapy for Urinary Tract Infections in the Urology Department for Hospitalized Patients. *Rev. Chim.* **2017**, *68*, 1453–1456. [CrossRef]
19. Gieling, E.M.; Wallenburg, E.; Frenzel, T.; de Lange, D.W.; Schouten, J.A.; ten Oever, J.; Kolwijck, E.; Burger, D.M.; Pickkers, P.; ter Heine, R.; et al. Higher Dosage of Ciprofloxacin Necessary in Critically Ill Patients: A New Dosing Algorithm Based on Renal Function and Pathogen Susceptibility. *Clin. Pharmacol. Ther.* **2020**, *108*, 770–774. [CrossRef]
20. Codru, I.R.; Sava, M.; Vintilă, B.I.; Bereanu, A.S.; Bîrluțiu, V. A Study on the Contributions of Sonication to the Identification of Bacteria Associated with Intubation Cannula Biofilm and the Risk of Ventilator-Associated Pneumonia. *Medicina* **2023**, *59*, 1058. [CrossRef]
21. Vintila, B.I.; Arseniu, A.M.; Morgovan, C.; Butuca, A.; Sava, M.; Bîrluțiu, V.; Rus, L.L.; Ghibu, S.; Bereanu, A.S.; Codru, I.R.; et al. A Pharmacovigilance Study Regarding the Risk of Antibiotic-Associated Clostridioides Difficile Infection Based on Reports from the EudraVigilance Database: Analysis of Some of the Most Used Antibiotics in Intensive Care Units. *Pharmaceuticals* **2023**, *16*, 1585. [CrossRef]
22. Vintila, B.I.; Arseniu, A.M.; Butuca, A.; Sava, M.; Bîrluțiu, V.; Rus, L.L.; Axente, D.D.; Morgovan, C.; Gligor, F.G. Adverse Drug Reactions Relevant to Drug Resistance and Ineffectiveness Associated with Meropenem, Linezolid, and Colistin: An Analysis Based on Spontaneous Reports from the European Pharmacovigilance Database. *Antibiotics* **2023**, *12*, 918. [CrossRef]
23. Mullish, B.H.; Williams, H.R.T. Clostridium Difficile Infection and Antibiotic-Associated Diarrhoea. *Clin. Med. (Northfield. Il)* **2018**, *18*, 237. [CrossRef]
24. Laza, R.; Jurac, R.; Crișan, A.; Lăzureanu, V.; Licker, M.; Popovici, E.D.; Bădițoiu, L.M. Clostridium Difficile in Western Romania: Unfavourable Outcome Predictors in a Hospital for Infectious Diseases. *BMC Infect. Dis.* **2015**, *15*, 1–9. [CrossRef]
25. Balsells, E.; Shi, T.; Leese, C.; Lyell, I.; Burrows, J.; Wiuff, C.; Campbell, H.; Kyaw, M.H.; Nair, H. Global Burden of Clostridium Difficile Infections: A Systematic Review and Meta-Analysis. *J. Glob. Health* **2019**, *9*, 10407. [CrossRef]
26. Turner, N.A.; Grambow, S.C.; Woods, C.W.; Fowler, V.G.; Moehring, R.W.; Anderson, D.J.; Lewis, S.S. Epidemiologic Trends in Clostridioides Difficile Infections in a Regional Community Hospital Network. *JAMA Netw. Open* **2019**, *2*, e1914149. [CrossRef]
27. Kuntz, J.L.; Smith, D.H.; Petrik, A.F.; Yang, X.; Thorp, M.L.; Barton, T.; Barton, K.; Labreche, M.; Spindel, S.J.; Johnson, E.S. Predicting the Risk of Clostridium Difficile Infection upon Admission: A Score to Identify Patients for Antimicrobial Stewardship Efforts. *Perm. J.* **2016**, *20*, 20–25. [CrossRef]
28. Shiode, J.; Fujii, M.; Nasu, J.; Itoh, M.; Ishiyama, S.; Fujiwara, A.; Yoshioka, M. Correlation between Hospital-Onset and Community-Onset Clostridioides Difficile Infection Incidence: Ward-Level Analysis Following Hospital Relocation. *Am. J. Infect. Control* **2022**, *50*, 1240–1245. [CrossRef]
29. Fonseca, F.; Forrester, M.; Advinha, A.M.; Coutinho, A.; Landeira, N.; Pereira, M. Clostridioides Difficile Infection in Hospitalized Patients—A Retrospective Epidemiological Study. *Healthcare* **2024**, *12*, 76. [CrossRef]
30. Wiegand, P.N.; Nathwani, D.; Wilcox, M.H.; Stephens, J.; Shelbaya, A.; Haider, S. Clinical and Economic Burden of Clostridium Difficile Infection in Europe: A Systematic Review of Healthcare-Facility-Acquired Infection. *J. Hosp. Infect.* **2012**, *81*, 1–14. [CrossRef]
31. Chu, Y.; Lee, C.; Chen, H.; Hung, C. Predictors of Mortality in Patients with Clostridium Difficile Infection. *Adv. Dig. Med.* **2020**, *7*, 77–82. [CrossRef]

32. Hensgens, M.P.M.; Goorhuis, A.; Dekkers, O.M.; Van Benthem, B.H.B.; Kuijper, E.J. All-Cause and Disease-Specific Mortality in Hospitalized Patients with Clostridium Difficile Infection: A Multicenter Cohort Study. *Clin. Infect. Dis.* **2013**, *56*, 1108–1116. [CrossRef]
33. Czepiel, J.; Krutova, M.; Mizrahi, A.; Khanafer, N.; Enoch, D.A.; Patyi, M.; Deptuła, A.; Agodi, A.; Nuvials, X.; Pituch, H.; et al. Mortality Following Clostridioides Difficile Infection in Europe: A Retrospective Multicenter Case-Control Study. *Antibiotics* **2021**, *10*, 299. [CrossRef]
34. Tartof, S.Y.; Yu, K.C.; Wei, R.; Tseng, H.F.; Jacobsen, S.J.; Rieg, G.K. Incidence of Polymerase Chain Reaction-Diagnosed Clostridium Difficile in a Large High-Risk Cohort, 2011–2012. *Mayo Clin. Proc.* **2014**, *89*, 1229–1238. [CrossRef]
35. Biagi, E.; Nylund, L.; Candela, M.; Ostan, R.; Bucci, L.; Pini, E.; Nikkïla, J.; Monti, D.; Satokari, R.; Franceschi, C.; et al. Through Ageing, and beyond: Gut Microbiota and Inflammatory Status in Seniors and Centenarians. *PLoS ONE* **2010**, *5*, e10667. [CrossRef]
36. Lee, G.C.; Reveles, K.R.; Attridge, R.T.; Lawson, K.A.; Mansi, I.A.; Lewis, J.S.; Frei, C.R. Outpatient Antibiotic Prescribing in the United States: 2000 to 2010. *BMC Med.* **2014**, *12*, 1–8. [CrossRef]
37. Seto, C.T.; Jeraldo, P.; Orenstein, R.; Chia, N.; DiBaise, J.K. Prolonged Use of a Proton Pump Inhibitor Reduces Microbial Diversity: Implications for Clostridium Difficile Susceptibility. *Microbiome* **2014**, *2*, 42. [CrossRef]
38. Owens, R.C.; Donskey, C.J.; Gaynes, R.P.; Loo, V.G.; Muto, C.A. Antimicrobial-Associated Risk Factors for Clostridium Difficile Infection. *Clin. Infect. Dis.* **2008**, *46* (Suppl. S1), S19–S31. [CrossRef]
39. Shin, J.H.; High, K.P.; Warren, C.A. Older Is Not Wiser, Immunologically Speaking: Effect of Aging on Host Response to Clostridium Difficile Infections. *J. Gerontol. A. Biol. Sci. Med. Sci.* **2016**, *71*, 916–922. [CrossRef]
40. Rogers, M.A.M.; Greene, M.T.; Young, V.B.; Saint, S.; Langa, K.M.; Kao, J.Y.; Aronoff, D.M. Depression, Antidepressant Medications, and Risk of Clostridium Difficile Infection. *BMC Med.* **2013**, *11*, 121. [CrossRef]
41. Rogers, M.A.M.; Greene, M.T.; Saint, S.; Chenoweth, C.E.; Malani, P.N.; Trivedi, I.; Aronoff, D.M. Higher Rates of Clostridium Difficile Infection among Smokers. *PLoS ONE* **2012**, *7*, e42091. [CrossRef]
42. Yurkovetskiy, L.; Burrows, M.; Khan, A.A.; Graham, L.; Volchkov, P.; Becker, L.; Antonopoulos, D.; Umesaki, Y.; Chervonsky, A.V. Gender Bias in Autoimmunity Is Influenced by Microbiota. *Immunity* **2013**, *39*, 400–412. [CrossRef]
43. Markle, J.G.M.; Frank, D.N.; Mortin-Toth, S.; Robertson, C.E.; Feazel, L.M.; Rolle-Kampczyk, U.; Von Bergen, M.; McCoy, K.D.; Macpherson, A.J.; Danska, J.S. Sex Differences in the Gut Microbiome Drive Hormone-Dependent Regulation of Autoimmunity. *Science* **2013**, *339*, 1084–1088. [CrossRef]
44. Sartelli, M.; Di Bella, S.; McFarland, L.V.; Khanna, S.; Furuya-Kanamori, L.; Abuzeid, N.; Abu-Zidan, F.M.; Ansaloni, L.; Augustin, G.; Bala, M.; et al. 2019 Update of the WSES Guidelines for Management of Clostridioides (Clostridium) Difficile Infection in Surgical Patients. *World J. Emerg. Surg.* **2019**, *14*, 8. [CrossRef]
45. Herzog, T.; Deleites, C.; Belyaev, O.; Chromik, A.M.; Uhl, W. [Clostridium Difficile in Visceral Surgery]. *Chirurg.* **2015**, *86*, 781–786. [CrossRef]
46. Silva-Velazco, J.; Hull, T.L.; Craig Messick, J.M.C. Medical versus Surgical Patients with Clostridium Difficile Infection: Is There Any Difference? *Am Surg* **2016**, *82*, 1155–1159. [CrossRef]
47. Kimura, T.; Stanhope, S.; Sugitani, T. Excess Length of Hospital Stay, Mortality and Cost Attributable to Clostridioides (Clostridium) Difficile Infection and Recurrence: A Nationwide Analysis in Japan. *Epidemiol. Infect.* **2020**, *148*, e65. [CrossRef]
48. van Kleef, E.; Green, N.; Goldenberg, S.; Robotham, J.; Cookson, B.; Jit, M.; Edmunds, W.; Deeny, S. Excess Length of Stay and Mortality Due to Clostridium Difficile Infection: A Multi-State Modelling Approach. *J. Hosp. Infect.* **2014**, *88*, 213–217. [CrossRef]
49. Chalmers, J.D.; Akram, A.R.; Singanayagam, A.; Wilcox, M.H.; Hill, A.T. Risk Factors for Clostridium Difficile Infection in Hospitalized Patients with Community-Acquired Pneumonia. *J. Infect.* **2016**, *73*, 45–53. [CrossRef]
50. Ragusa, R.; Giorgianni, G.; Lupo, L.; Sciacca, A.; Rametta, S.; Verde, M.L.A.; Mulè, S.; Marranzano, M. Healthcare-Associated Clostridium Difficile Infection: Role of Correct Hand Hygiene in Cross-Infection Control. *J. Prev. Med. Hyg.* **2018**, *59*, E145.
51. Huang, Y.J.; Chen, J.S.; Luo, S.F.; Kuo, C.F. Comparison of Indexes to Measure Comorbidity Burden and Predict All-Cause Mortality in Rheumatoid Arthritis. *J. Clin. Med.* **2021**, *10*, 5460. [CrossRef]
52. Covino, M.; Gallo, A.; Pero, E.; Simeoni, B.; Macerola, N.; Murace, C.A.; Ibba, F.; Landi, F.; Franceschi, F.; Montalto, M. Early Prognostic Stratification of Clostridioides Difficile Infection in the Emergency Department: The Role of Age and Comorbidities. *J. Pers. Med.* **2022**, *12*, 1573. [CrossRef]
53. Charlson Comorbidity Index (CCI): An Independent Predictor of Outcomes in Clostridium Difficile Infection (CDI). Available online: https://journals.lww.com/ajg/fulltext/2018/10001/charlson_comorbidity_index__cci___an_independent.2742.aspx (accessed on 10 December 2023).
54. Study Details Risk of C Difficile with Clindamycin, Other Antibiotics. Available online: https://www.ajmc.com/view/study-details-risk-of-c-difficile-with-clindamycin-other-antibiotics (accessed on 18 January 2024).
55. Your Risk of C. Diff | CDC. Available online: https://www.cdc.gov/cdiff/risk.html (accessed on 18 January 2024).
56. Webb, B.J.; Subramanian, A.; Lopansri, B.; Goodman, B.; Jones, P.B.; Ferraro, J.; Stenehjem, E.; Brown, S.M. Antibiotic Exposure and Risk for Hospital-Associated Clostridioides Difficile Infection. *Antimicrob. Agents Chemother.* **2020**, *64*, e02169-19. [CrossRef]
57. Stevens, V.; Dumyati, G.; Fine, L.S.; Fisher, S.G.; Van Wijngaarden, E. Cumulative Antibiotic Exposures over Time and the Risk of Clostridium Difficile Infection. *Clin. Infect. Dis.* **2011**, *53*, 42–48. [CrossRef]
58. Hensgens, M.P.M.; Goorhuis, A.; Dekkers, O.M.; Kuijper, E.J. Time Interval of Increased Risk for Clostridium Difficile Infection after Exposure to Antibiotics. *J. Antimicrob. Chemother.* **2012**, *67*, 742–748. [CrossRef]

59. Del Mar Aldrete, S.; Magee, M.J.; Friedman-Moraco, R.J.; Chan, A.W.; Banks, G.G.; Burd, E.M.; Kraft, C.S. Characteristics and Antibiotic Use Associated With Short-Term Risk of Clostridium Difficile Infection Among Hospitalized Patients. *Am. J. Clin. Pathol.* **2015**, *143*, 895–900. [CrossRef]
60. Mishra, P.; Pandey, C.M.; Singh, U.; Gupta, A.; Sahu, C.; Keshri, A. Descriptive Statistics and Normality Tests for Statistical Data. *Ann. Card. Anaesth.* **2019**, *22*, 67. [CrossRef]
61. The Application of Statistical Analysis in the Biomedical Sciences | Basicmedical Key. Available online: https://basicmedicalkey.com/the-application-of-statistical-analysis-in-the-biomedical-sciences/ (accessed on 2 December 2023).
62. Miller, A.C.; Arakkal, A.T.; Sewell, D.K.; Segre, A.M.; Tholany, J.; Polgreen, P.M. Comparison of Different Antibiotics and the Risk for Community-Associated Clostridioides Difficile Infection: A Case–Control Study. *Open Forum Infect. Dis.* **2023**, *10*, 413. [CrossRef]
63. Slimings, C.; Riley, T.V. Antibiotics and Hospital-Acquired Clostridium Difficile Infection: Update of Systematic Review and Meta-Analysis. *J. Antimicrob. Chemother.* **2014**, *69*, 881–891. [CrossRef]
64. Schinas, G.; Polyzou, E.; Spernovasilis, N.; Gogos, C.; Dimopoulos, G.; Akinosoglou, K. Preventing Multidrug-Resistant Bacterial Transmission in the Intensive Care Unit with a Comprehensive Approach: A Policymaking Manual. *Antibiotics* **2023**, *12*, 1255. [CrossRef]
65. Karaoui, W.R.; Rustom, L.B.O.; Bou Daher, H.; Rimmani, H.H.; Rasheed, S.S.; Matar, G.M.; Mahfouz, R.; Araj, G.F.; Zahreddine, N.; Kanj, S.S.; et al. Incidence, Outcome, and Risk Factors for Recurrence of Nosocomial Clostridioides Difficile Infection in Adults: A Prospective Cohort Study. *J. Infect. Public Health* **2020**, *13*, 485–490. [CrossRef]
66. European Database of Suspected Adverse Drug Reaction Reports. Available online: https://www.adrreports.eu/en/ (accessed on 11 October 2023).
67. Medicines Agency, E. Introductory Cover Note, Last Updated with Chapter P.IV on Pharmacovigilance for the Paediatric Population Finalised Post-Public Consultation. In *Guidelines on Good Pharmacovigilance Practices (GVP)*; HMA: Brussels, Belgium, 2018.
68. Postigo, R.; Brosch, S.; Slattery, J.; van Haren, A.; Dogné, J.M.; Kurz, X.; Candore, G.; Domergue, F.; Arlett, P. EudraVigilance Medicines Safety Database: Publicly Accessible Data for Research and Public Health Protection. *Drug Saf.* **2018**, *41*, 665–675. [CrossRef]
69. Charlson Comorbidity Index (CCI). Available online: https://www.mdcalc.com/calc/3917/charlson-comorbidity-index-cci (accessed on 18 January 2024).
70. Charlson, M.E.; Pompei, P.; Ales, K.L.; MacKenzie, C.R. A New Method of Classifying Prognostic Comorbidity in Longitudinal Studies: Development and Validation. *J. Chronic Dis.* **1987**, *40*, 373–383. [CrossRef]

Disclaimer/Publisher's Note: The statements, opinions and data contained in all publications are solely those of the individual author(s) and contributor(s) and not of MDPI and/or the editor(s). MDPI and/or the editor(s) disclaim responsibility for any injury to people or property resulting from any ideas, methods, instructions or products referred to in the content.

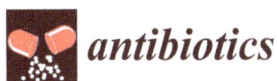

Article

Real-World Data in Pharmacovigilance Database Provides a New Perspective for Understanding the Risk of *Clostridium difficile* Infection Associated with Antibacterial Drug Exposure

Dongxuan Li [1,2,†], Yi Song [1,†], Zhanfeng Bai [1], Xin Xi [1], Feng Liu [3], Yang Zhang [3], Chunmeng Qin [1,2], Dan Du [1], Qian Du [1,4,*] and Songqing Liu [1,*]

1. Department of Pharmacy, The Third Affiliated Hospital of Chongqing Medical University, Chongqing 401120, China
2. College of Pharmacy, Chongqing Medical University, Chongqing 400016, China
3. Center for Medical Information and Statistics, The Third Affiliated Hospital of Chongqing Medical University, Chongqing 401120, China
4. Medical Data Science Academy, Chongqing Medical University, Chongqing 400016, China
* Correspondence: duqian@hospital.cqmu.edu.cn (Q.D.); liusq@hospital.cqmu.edu.cn (S.L.)
† These authors contributed equally to this work.

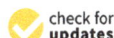

Citation: Li, D.; Song, Y.; Bai, Z.; Xi, X.; Liu, F.; Zhang, Y.; Qin, C.; Du, D.; Du, Q.; Liu, S. Real-World Data in Pharmacovigilance Database Provides a New Perspective for Understanding the Risk of *Clostridium difficile* Infection Associated with Antibacterial Drug Exposure. *Antibiotics* **2023**, *12*, 1109. https://doi.org/10.3390/antibiotics12071109

Academic Editors: Guido Granata and Mehran Monchi

Received: 24 May 2023
Revised: 20 June 2023
Accepted: 25 June 2023
Published: 27 June 2023

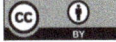

Copyright: © 2023 by the authors. Licensee MDPI, Basel, Switzerland. This article is an open access article distributed under the terms and conditions of the Creative Commons Attribution (CC BY) license (https://creativecommons.org/licenses/by/4.0/).

Abstract: Antibacterial drug exposure (ADE) is a well-known potential risk factor for *Clostridium difficile* infection (CDI), but it remains controversial which certain antibacterial drugs are associated with the highest risk of CDI occurrence. To summarize CDI risk associated with ADE, we reviewed the CDI reports related to ADE in the FDA Adverse Event Reporting System database and conducted disproportionality analysis to detect adverse reaction (ADR) signals of CDI for antibacterial drugs. A total of 8063 CDI reports associated with ADE were identified, which involved 73 antibacterial drugs. Metronidazole was the drug with the greatest number of reports, followed by vancomycin, ciprofloxacin, clindamycin and amoxicillin. In disproportionality analysis, metronidazole had the highest positive ADR signal strength, followed by vancomycin, cefpodoxime, ertapenem and clindamycin. Among the 73 antibacterial drugs, 58 showed at least one positive ADR signal, and ceftriaxone was the drug with the highest total number of positive signals. Our study provided a real-world overview of CDI risk for AED from a pharmacovigilance perspective and showed risk characteristics for different antibacterial drugs by integrating its positive–negative signal distribution. Meanwhile, our study showed that the CDI risk of metronidazole and vancomycin may be underestimated, and it deserves further attention and investigation.

Keywords: *Clostridium difficile* infection; antibacterial drug; FDA Adverse Event Reporting System; pharmacovigilance; disproportionality analysis; adverse reaction

1. Introduction

Clostridium difficile is an anaerobic, spore-forming Gram-positive bacillus that usually colonizes in the human gut [1]. It is an opportunistic pathogen that is able to abnormally proliferate, produce toxins and result in diarrhea, especially in patients with changes in the indigenous colonic microbiota following antibiotic use [2], and it is reported that the attributable mortality of *C. difficile* infection (CDI) should be at least 5.99% [3]. In recent decades, the increasing incidence, severity and mortality of CDI have made it a challenging clinical problem for medical personnel [4]. In response to this challenge, diagnosis and treatment guidelines have been developed in recent years to optimize the management of CDI [5–9]. In primary prevention for CDI, the careful selection of antibacterial drugs and, whenever possible, the avoidance of high-risk antibacterial drug exposure (ADE) is the mainstay because most cases of CDI are both iatrogenic and nosocomial [4]. Meanwhile, some studies have shown that strict antimicrobial stewardship is beneficial in reducing CDI rates [10–12], which also demonstrated the need to understand the CDI risk of different antibacterial agents to formulate management strategies. However, although it is well known that antibacterial therapy plays a central role in the pathogenesis of CDI [2,13], it remains controversial whether certain antibacterial drugs or classes of antibacterial drugs are potentially associated with an increased risk of CDI [14,15]. Therefore, there is a need to assess the potential risk of CDI caused by different antibacterial drugs with a uniform metric.

Currently, pharmacovigilance databases are widely used for real-world post-marketing studies and as a tool to summarize the real-time safety profile of medical products to provide information for clinical practice [16]. In pharmacovigilance practice, according to finding disproportionality between drug usage and adverse events (AEs) occurrence in the pharmacovigilance databases, these real-world AEs data can provide a reference for identifying the potential culprit drugs of specific AE, optimizing the drug selection for individual patients and exploring the interaction between drugs [17]. In terms of exploring the safety profile of antibiotics by using the pharmacovigilance database, Seo, H. and Kim, E. elaborated on the risk characteristics of electrolyte disorders associated with piperacillin/tazobactam and detected the significant signal of hypokalemia for piperacillin/tazobactam compared with other penicillins [18]; Patek, T.M. et al. investigated acute kidney injury reports related to antibiotics in the FDA Adverse Event Reporting System (FAERS) database and found 14 classes of antibiotics that were significantly associated with acute kidney injury [19]. CDI is a representative AE associated with ADE, so real-world AE information in pharmacovigilance databases can provide an unprecedented opportunity to understand the potential risk of CDI caused by different antibacterial drugs.

In this study, we summarized the report characteristics of antibacterial drug-associated CDI cases in the FAERS database and evaluated the statistical connection between ADE and CDI occurrence by using a well-established adverse reaction (ADR) signal detecting method, trying to distinguish the risk of CDI induced by different antibacterial drugs from the pharmacovigilance perspective, so as to provide a reference for better primary prevention for CDI and antimicrobial stewardship.

2. Results

2.1. Report Basic Information and Patient Characteristics

A total of 16,010,899 reports were recorded in the FAERS database from 1 January 2004 to 31 December 2022. Using the Preferred Terms (PTs) in Table 1 to retrieve target reports, a total of 30,937 reports considered CDI-related were returned and downloaded. As the culprit drug of CDI may be indecisive and can be attributed to multiple drugs, there were a total of 222,971 drugs contained in those CDI-related reports. After excluding drugs missing generic names, duplicated drugs and drugs that were not under J01 of the Anatomical Therapeutic Chemical (ATC) classification system, a total of 99 drug names were classified into "antibacterials for systemic use (J01)". The 99 drug names were used to match reports that CDI occurrence was related to antibacterial drug use, and finally, a total of 8063 (26.1%) reports were identified for further analysis. As some of the 99 drug names were synonymous (e.g., ampicillin and ampicillin sodium), we integrated drugs with the same ingredient manually, and finally, there were 73 drugs included in the final antibacterial drug list to detect ADR signals. The detailed processing flow is shown in Figure 1.

Information in the 8063 antibacterial drug use-related CDI reports was extracted and collected. The annual number of reports from 2004 to 2022 was presented in Figure 2A, among which 2019 was the year that FAERS received the greatest number of CDI reports associated with ADE. With regard to report sources, health professionals (73.8%) were the main submitters (Figure 2B), and the USA was the leading reporting country (Figure 2C). The demographic characteristics of patients were summarized, and the result showed that there were fewer male patients than female patients (Figure 2D) and the age of those patients was mainly located in the 71–80 age group (Figure 2E). In terms of patient outcome,

CDI usually resulted in hospitalization (67.3%), and even the death of 1282 (15.9%) patients were associated with CDI (Figure 2F).

Table 1. The narrow PT included in Standardized MedDRA Queries of pseudomembranous colitis.

PT	MedDRA Code
Antibiotic associated colitis	10052815
Clostridium bacteraemia	10058852
Clostridium colitis	10058305
Clostridium difficile colitis	10009657
Clostridium difficile infection	10054236
Clostridial infection	10061043
Clostridial sepsis	10078496
Clostridium test positive	10070027
Gastroenteritis clostridial	10017898
Pseudomembranous colitis	10037128

Abbreviations: PT, Preferred Term; MedDRA, Medical Dictionary for Drug Regulatory Activities.

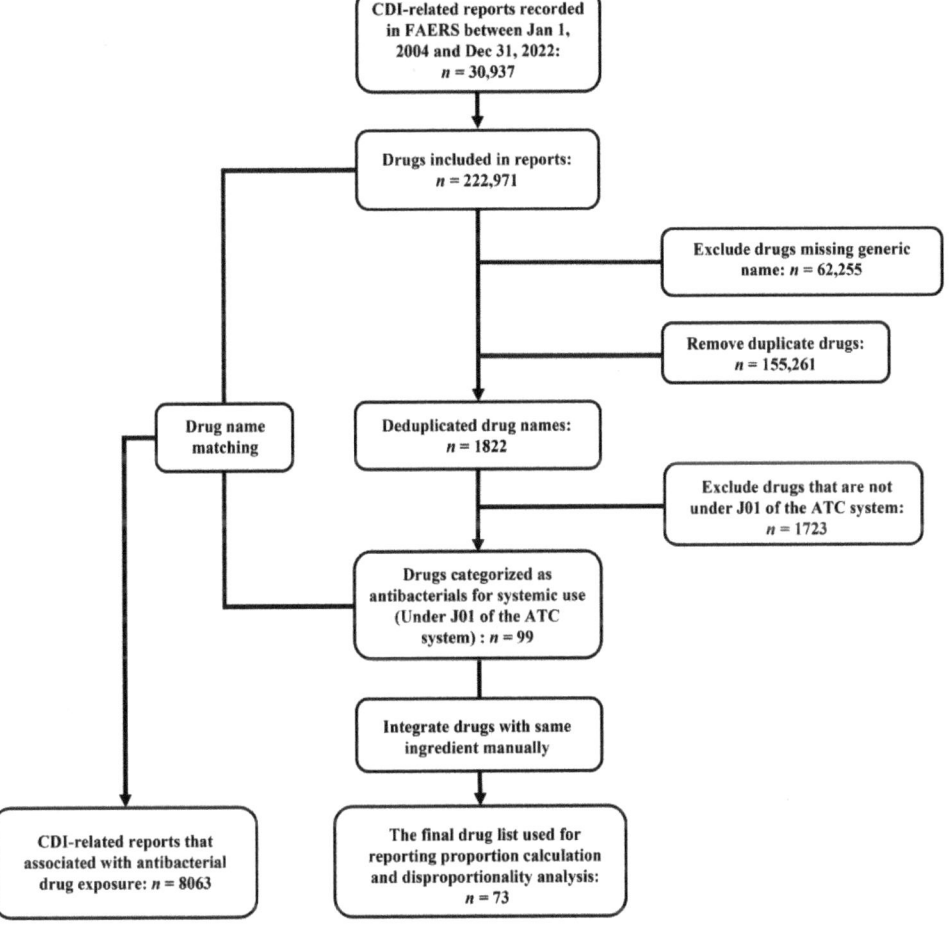

Figure 1. Flowchart of target reports identification. Abbreviations: ATC, Anatomical Therapeutic Chemical classification.

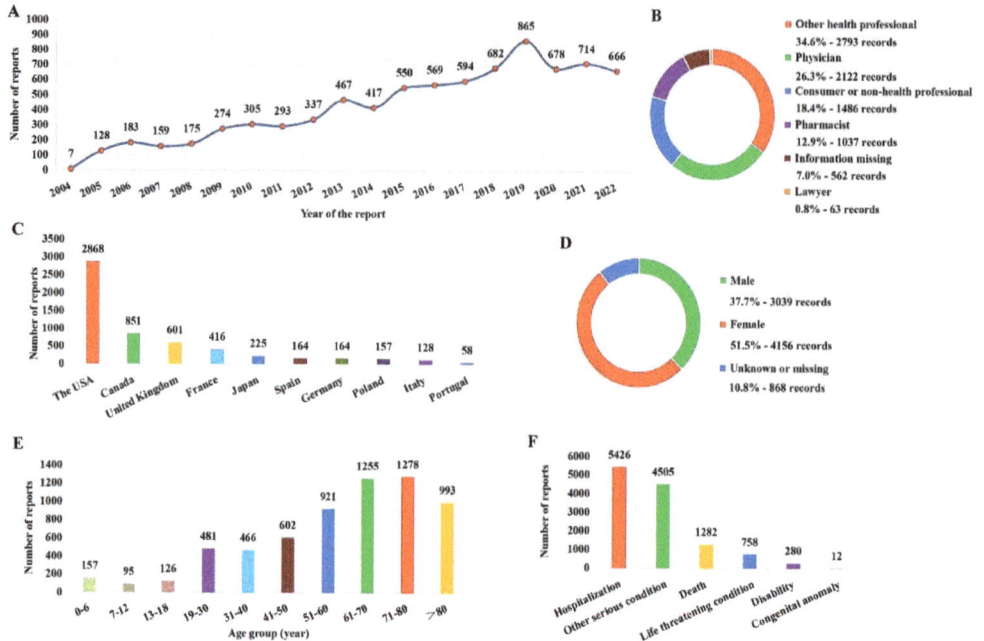

Figure 2. Report basic information and patient characteristics. (**A**) Distribution of the reporting year. (**B**) Distribution of reporter. (**C**) The top 10 countries with the most sources of reports. (**D**) Distribution of patient gender. (**E**) Distribution of patient age. (**F**) Distribution of patient outcome.

2.2. ADR Signal Detection Results

After integrating synonymous drugs, 73 antibacterial drugs were used to detect ADR signals at Standardized MedDRA Queries (SMQ) level and PT level. The signal detection results at the SMQ level are shown in Table 2, and it showed that metronidazole (a = 2004) was the most reported antibacterial drug followed by vancomycin (a = 1793), ciprofloxacin (a = 1176), clindamycin (a = 823) and amoxicillin (a = 566), while metronidazole (ROR = 22.10, 95% CI 21.10–23.14) had the highest positive signal strength followed by vancomycin (ROR = 21.30, 95% CI 20.29–22.36), cefpodoxime (ROR = 19.26, 95% CI 13.02–28.49), ertapenem (ROR = 16.69, 95% CI 14.30–19.49) and clindamycin (ROR = 16.29, 95% CI 15.18–17.47). In addition, the signal detection results for 10 different PT levels are shown in Tables S1–S10.

Table 2. Pharmacovigilance signal detection results at the SMQ level.

Medication	Drug of Interest with AE of Interest (a)	Other Drugs with AE of Interest (b)	Drug of Interest with Other AEs (c)	Other Drugs with Other AEs (d)	ROR (95% CI)
Tetracyclines (J01AA)					
Doxycycline	227	30,710	46,700	15,933,262	2.52 (2.21–2.87)
Tigecycline	78	30,859	4193	15,975,769	9.63 (7.70–12.05)
Minocycline	32	30,905	12,056	15,967,906	1.37 (0.97–1.94)
Combinations of tetracyclines	17	30,920	816	15,979,146	10.77 (6.66–17.41)
Tetracycline	2	30,935	371	15,979,591	2.78 (0.69–11.18)
Sarecycline	1	30,936	105	15,979,857	4.92 (0.69–35.25)
Amphenicols (J01BA)					
Chloramphenicol	1	30,936	26	15,979,936	19.87 (2.70–146.41)
Penicillins with extended spectrum (J01CA)					
Amoxicillin	566	30,371	57,359	15,922,603	5.17 (4.76–5.62)
Ampicillin	88	30,849	6189	15,973,773	7.36 (5.96–9.09)

Table 2. Cont.

Medication	Drug of Interest with AE of Interest (a)	Other Drugs with AE of Interest (b)	Drug of Interest with Other AEs (c)	Other Drugs with Other AEs (d)	ROR (95% CI)
Beta-lactamase sensitive penicillins (J01CE)					
Phenoxymethylpenicillin	10	30,927	1592	15,978,370	3.25 (1.74–6.04)
Benzylpenicillin	8	30,929	1613	15,978,349	2.56 (1.28–5.13)
Benzathine benzylpenicillin	1	30,936	559	15,979,403	0.92 (0.13–6.57)
Beta-lactamase resistant penicillins (J01CF)					
Oxacillin	10	30,927	893	15,979,069	5.79 (3.10–10.79)
Nafcillin	10	30,927	802	15,979,160	6.44 (3.45–12.02)
Dicloxacillin	1	30,936	116	15,979,846	4.45 (0.62–31.88)
Combinations of penicillins, incl. beta-lactamase inhibitors (J01CR)					
Piperacillin and beta-lactamase inhibitor	483	30,454	19,305	15,960,657	13.11 (11.97–14.36)
Amoxicillin and beta-lactamase inhibitor	326	30,611	21,834	15,958,128	7.78 (6.97–8.69)
Ampicillin and beta-lactamase inhibitor	51	30,886	2129	15,977,833	12.39 (9.39–16.36)
First-generation cephalosporins (J01DB)					
Cefazolin	162	30,775	8401	15,971,561	10.01 (8.56–11.7)
Cefalexin	150	30,787	15,184	15,964,778	5.12 (4.36–6.02)
Cefadroxil	12	30,925	1293	15,978,669	4.80 (2.72–8.47)
Second-generation cephalosporins (J01DC)					
Cefuroxime	311	30,626	11,920	15,968,042	13.60 (12.15–15.23)
Cefaclor	34	30,903	1157	15,978,805	15.19 (10.80–21.37)
Cefprozil	11	30,926	609	15,979,353	9.33 (5.14–16.94)
Cefoxitin	10	30,927	954	15,979,008	5.42 (2.90–10.10)
Cefotetan	2	30,935	101	15,979,861	10.23 (2.52–41.47)
Third-generation cephalosporins (J01DD)					
Ceftriaxone	548	30,389	25,953	15,954,009	11.09 (10.18–12.07)
Ceftazidime	126	30,811	5422	15,974,540	12.05 (10.09–14.38)
Cefdinir	89	30,848	5739	15,974,223	8.03 (6.51–9.90)
Cefotaxime	64	30,873	3257	15,976,705	10.17 (7.94–13.03)
Cefixime	50	30,887	1972	15,977,990	13.12 (9.90–17.37)
Cefpodoxime	26	30,911	698	15,979,264	19.26 (13.02–28.49)
Ceftazidime and beta-lactamase inhibitor	1	30,936	126	15,979,836	4.10 (0.57–29.33)
Fourth-generation cephalosporins (J01DE)					
Cefepime	288	30,649	10,696	15,969,266	14.03 (12.47–15.78)
Monobactams (J01DF)					
Aztreonam	42	30,895	6063	15,973,899	3.58 (2.64–4.85)
Carbapenems (J01DH)					
Meropenem	507	30,430	20,575	15,959,387	12.92 (11.83–14.12)
Ertapenem	166	30,771	5163	15,974,799	16.69 (14.30–19.49)
Imipenem and cilastatin	88	30,849	3343	15,976,619	13.63 (11.03–16.85)
Other cephalosporins and penems (J01DI)					
Ceftolozane and beta-lactamase inhibitor	7	30,930	749	15,979,213	4.83 (2.29–10.16)
Ceftaroline fosamil	5	30,932	501	15,979,461	5.16 (2.14–12.44)
Cefiderocol	1	30,936	112	15,979,850	4.61 (0.64–33.03)
Trimethoprim and derivatives (J01EA)					
Trimethoprim	165	30,772	8967	15,970,995	9.55 (8.18–11.14)
Intermediate-acting sulfonamides (J01EC)					
Sulfadiazine	4	30,933	1252	15,978,710	1.65 (0.62–4.40)
Combinations of sulfonamides and trimethoprim, incl. derivatives (J01EE)					
Sulfamethoxazole and trimethoprim	470	30,467	64,143	15,915,819	3.83 (3.49–4.19)
Macrolides (J01FA)					
Clarithromycin	300	30,637	26,676	15,953,286	5.86 (5.22–6.57)
Azithromycin	178	30,759	38,046	15,941,916	2.42 (2.09–2.81)
Erythromycin	118	30,819	14,595	15,965,367	4.19 (3.49–5.02)
Lincosamides (J01FF)					
Clindamycin	823	30,114	26,769	15,953,193	16.29 (15.18–17.47)
Lincomycin	7	30,930	230	15,979,732	15.72 (7.41–33.36)
Streptogramins (J01FG)					
Quinupristin/dalfopristin	2	30,935	102	15,979,860	10.13 (2.50–41.05)

Table 2. Cont.

Medication	Drug of Interest with AE of Interest (a)	Other Drugs with AE of Interest (b)	Drug of Interest with Other AEs (c)	Other Drugs with Other AEs (d)	ROR (95% CI)
Streptomycins (J01GA)					
Streptomycin	4	30,933	1002	15,978,960	2.06 (0.77–5.51)
Other aminoglycosides (J01GB)					
Gentamicin	210	30,727	12,309	15,967,653	8.87 (7.73–10.17)
Amikacin	142	30,795	11,578	15,968,384	6.36 (5.39–7.51)
Tobramycin	68	30,869	19,561	15,960,401	1.80 (1.42–2.28)
Fluoroquinolones (J01MA)					
Ciprofloxacin	1176	29,761	77,260	15,902,702	8.13 (7.67–8.63)
Levofloxacin	536	30,401	44,317	15,935,645	6.34 (5.82–6.91)
Moxifloxacin	75	30,862	11,887	15,968,075	3.26 (2.60–4.10)
Ofloxacin	39	30,898	5249	15,974,713	3.84 (2.80–5.26)
Gatifloxacin	33	30,904	1570	15,978,392	10.87 (7.70–15.34)
Delafloxacin	1	30,936	218	15,979,744	2.37 (0.33–16.9)
Glycopeptide antibacterials (J01XA)					
Vancomycin	1793	29,144	46,032	15,933,930	21.30 (20.29–22.36)
Dalbavancin	2	30,935	556	15,979,406	1.86 (0.46–7.45)
Telavancin	1	30,936	116	15,979,846	4.45 (0.62–31.88)
Oritavancin	1	30,936	791	15,979,171	0.65 (0.09–4.64)
Polymyxins (J01XB)					
Polymyxin B	14	30,923	975	15,978,987	7.42 (4.38–12.58)
Colistin	9	30,928	958	15,979,004	4.85 (2.52–9.36)
Imidazole derivatives (J01XD)					
Metronidazole	2004	28,933	49,926	15,930,036	22.10 (21.10–23.14)
Tinidazole	6	30,931	355	15,979,607	8.73 (3.90–19.57)
Nitrofuran derivatives (J01XE)					
Nitrofurantoin	15	30,922	2636	15,977,326	2.94 (1.77–4.88)
Other antibacterials (J01XX)					
Linezolid	168	30,769	20,272	15,959,690	4.30 (3.69–5.01)
Daptomycin	70	30,867	11,035	15,968,927	3.28 (2.59–4.15)
Fosfomycin	9	30,928	634	15,979,328	7.33 (3.80–14.16)
Tedizolid	3	30,934	499	15,979,463	3.11 (1.00–9.66)

Note: The classification of antibacterial agents is based on the Anatomical Therapeutic Chemical classification system, and the bold represents the drug category and its code. Abbreviations: AE, adverse event; CI, confidence interval; ROR, reporting odd ratio.

As metronidazole and vancomycin were usually used as therapeutic agents for CDI, we further reviewed the indications for metronidazole and vancomycin recorded in the "patient.drug.drugindication" field. In order to eliminate the influence of this factor on ADR signal detection results as much as possible, if the indication of metronidazole and vancomycin was related to the treatment of CDI, the report was excluded. The adjusted signal detection results for metronidazole and vancomycin at the SMQ level and PT level are shown in Tables 3 and 4, respectively.

2.3. Distribution of ADR Signals

There were 11 ADR signal detection results for each of the 73 antibacterial drugs, including one for the SMQ level and 10 for the PT level. In addition, signal detection results can be divided into three states, namely positive signals, negative signals and not reported for target drug-AE combinations. The distribution of signal detection results for 73 antibacterial drugs is presented in Figure 3. It showed that 58 antibacterial drugs had at least one positive ADR signal detection, while another 15 antibacterial drugs did not show any positive signals at the SMQ level or PT level, although there were CDI cases reported. Of these antibacterial drugs with positive signals, only ceftriaxone had 11 positive signals.

Table 3. Adjusted signal detection results for metronidazole at SMQ level and PT level.

Target PT	Drug of Interest with AE of Interest (a)	Other Drugs with AE of Interest (b)	Drug of Interest with Other AEs (c)	Other Drugs with Other AEs (d)	ROR (95% CI)
Antibiotic associated colitis	3	20	51,927	15,958,949	46.10 (13.70–155.14)
Clostridium bacteraemia	10	131	51,920	15,958,838	23.46 (12.33–44.64)
Clostridium colitis	49	750	51,881	15,958,219	20.10 (15.05–26.83)
Clostridium difficile colitis	535	7710	51,395	15,951,259	21.54 (19.72–23.52)
Clostridium difficile infection	725	15,071	51,205	15,943,898	14.98 (13.90–16.15)
Clostridial infection	140	2877	51,790	15,956,092	14.99 (12.65–17.77)
Clostridial sepsis	1	141	51,929	15,958,828	2.18 (0.30–15.58)
Clostridium test positive	104	1296	51,826	15,957,673	24.71 (20.23–30.18)
Gastroenteritis clostridial	4	277	51,926	15,958,692	4.44 (1.65–11.91)
Pseudomembranous colitis	140	1778	51,790	15,957,191	24.26 (20.42–28.82)
SMQ level	1863	29,074	50,067	15,929,895	20.39 (19.44–21.38)

Abbreviations: AE, adverse event; CI, confidence interval; PT, Preferred Term; ROR, reporting odd ratio.

Table 4. Adjusted signal detection results for vancomycin at SMQ level and PT level.

Target PT	Drug of Interest with AE of Interest (a)	Other Drugs with AE of Interest (b)	Drug of Interest with Other AEs (c)	Other Drugs with Other AEs (d)	ROR (95% CI)
Clostridium bacteraemia	10	131	47,815	15,962,943	25.48 (13.40–48.48)
Clostridium colitis	47	752	47,778	15,962,322	20.88 (15.55–28.04)
Clostridium difficile colitis	434	7811	47,391	15,955,263	18.71 (16.98–20.61)
Clostridium difficile infection	759	15,037	47,066	15,948,037	17.10 (15.89–18.41)
Clostridial infection	98	2919	47,727	15,960,155	11.23 (9.18–13.73)
Clostridial sepsis	8	134	47,817	15,962,940	19.93 (9.77–40.68)
Clostridium test positive	100	1300	47,725	15,961,774	25.73 (20.99–31.54)
Gastroenteritis clostridial	9	272	47,816	15,962,802	11.05 (5.69–21.46)
Pseudomembranous colitis	136	1782	47,689	15,961,292	25.54 (21.45–30.42)
SMQ level	1503	29,434	46,322	15,933,640	17.56 (16.66–18.51)

Note: There was no report of target drug-AE combination (a = 0) in antibiotic associated colitis (PT). Abbreviations: AE, adverse event; CI, confidence interval; PT, Preferred Term; ROR, reporting odd ratio.

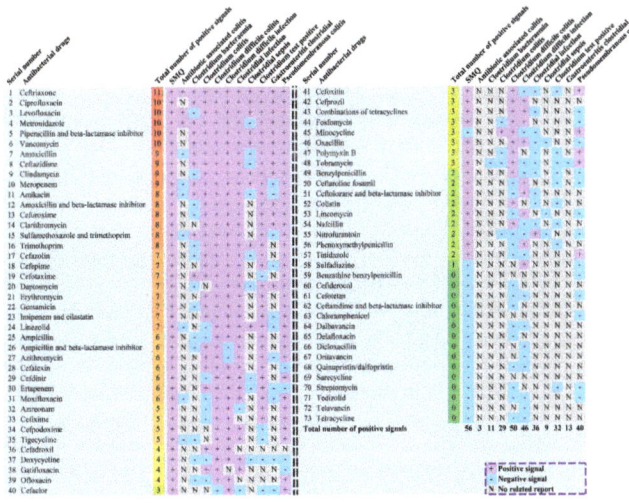

Figure 3. Pharmacovigilance signal distribution at the SMQ level and Preferred Term level. Note: the adjusted signal detection results for metronidazole and vancomycin at the SMQ level and PT level were used to show signal distribution. Abbreviations: SMQ, Standardized MedDRA Queries.

3. Discussion

Antibacterial drugs, one of the greatest achievements of human beings in the field of medicine, have played an extremely important role in improving human health level and ensuring life safety. However, with the extensive use of antibacterial drugs in clinical practices, various ADRs associated with antibacterial drugs have emerged, among which CDI is one of the most noteworthy potentially life-threatening ADRs [20]. Therefore, it is necessary to determine the risk of CDI induced by different antibacterial drugs. In this study, we reviewed CDI reports associated with ADE in the FAERS database between 2004 to 2022 and found that 73 antibacterial drugs were recorded as potential culprit drugs. At the same time, based on the aforementioned antibacterial drug list, we conducted a disproportionality analysis to evaluate the risk correlation between the occurrence of CDI and ADE. As far as we know, this is the first study using a pharmacovigilance database to evaluate the risk of CDI occurrence for ADE.

Although it is widely recognized that any antimicrobial therapy increases the risk of CDI and there is a difference among different antibiotics, it remains controversial which certain antibiotics or classes of antibiotics are related to the highest risk of CDI. A previous study showed that fluoroquinolones were the antibacterial agent most strongly associated with CDI, while all the third-generation of cephalosporins, macrolides, clindamycin and intravenous beta-lactam/beta-lactamase inhibitors were intermediate-risk antibacterial agent [13]. Another study showed that the risk of hospital-acquired CDI was greatest for cephalosporins and clindamycin, while the importance of fluoroquinolones should not be overemphasized [21]. A recent study suggested that the highest-risk antibacterial agents related to CDI occurrence included second-generation and later cephalosporins, carbapenems, fluoroquinolones and clindamycin, while doxycycline and daptomycin were related to a lower CDI risk [22]. However, due to the difference in the region, patient inclusion and exclusion criteria, study design, drugs involved in the evaluation and the definition of risk classification, it is difficult to unify the CDI risk of antibacterial agents. In this regard, by using a unified standard to detect the ADR signals for each antibacterial agent at the PT and SMQ level, our study added new evidence for understanding the risk of CDI induced by ADE from a pharmacovigilance perspective. In comparison to the studies mentioned above, the advantage of this study is that it makes full use of real-world data to get a complete antibiotics list leading to CDI occurrence, involving 73 antibiotics commonly used in clinical settings. Therefore, our study can provide a more comprehensive overview of the risk of antibacterial drugs, facilitating a comparison of risks between them and providing a reference for antimicrobial stewardship.

Consistent with previous studies [13,21,22], our ADR signal detection results showed a high risk of CDI in most fluoroquinolones, cephalosporins, carbapenems, macrolides, clindamycin and beta-lactam/beta-lactamase inhibitors, which proved the credibility of our results to some extent. However, it is noteworthy that, in ADR signal detection, metronidazole and vancomycin have a surprising number of reports and high signal strengths at the SMQ level and PT level, although they have been reported as possible causes of CDI in previous studies [23,24]. There are several possible explanations for this noteworthy result. First, metronidazole and vancomycin were used as therapeutic drugs for CDI [5–9], which may lead us to ignore their risk of inducing CDI, while our research detected this neglected risk relationship. Second, 26.2% of reporters in this study were non-health professionals, so they may confuse therapeutic and etiological drugs and misjudge culprit drugs, which may result in biased results. Third, due to FAERS being a database with a voluntary reporting nature, underreporting of other antibacterial agents may exist [25], which may highlight the CDI risks of metronidazole and vancomycin. In order to reduce the influence of misreporting due to the overlap of indications and AEs for metronidazole and vancomycin, we excluded the reports that the indication of metronidazole and vancomycin was related to the treatment of CDI, but the adjusted signal detection results for metronidazole and vancomycin still showed conspicuous high potential risk (Tables 3 and 4). In this regard, our results showed a warning that we should pay more attention to the CDI risk of metronidazole and vancomycin, which may have been previously neglected. Although the true relationship between CDI occurrence and vancomycin and metronidazole still needs a well-designed study to verify, we think there are two main potential values for these data. First, it provides evidence of the potential high risk of CDI induced by vancomycin and metronidazole, so it may help us identify previously neglected CDI cases induced by vancomycin and metronidazole. In this way, we can timely take measures, such as stopping taking medicine, changing medicine and etiological treatment, to protect patients from unnecessary sustained injury. Second, due to the potential high CDI risk signals of vancomycin and metronidazole, our results provided an opportunity to investigate further the CDI risks of vancomycin and metronidazole, which may affect future clinical practice in primary prevention of CDI and antimicrobial stewardship.

In addition to detecting ADR signals of 73 antibacterial drugs at the SMQ level and PT level and adjusting signal detection results for metronidazole and vancomycin, we also integrated the positive-negative distribution of their ADR signals, and the total number of positive signals was between 0 to 11 for each antimicrobial drug. If an antimicrobial drug has a relatively large total number of positive signals, it may mean that its risk of CDI is relatively high [26]. For example, in this study, ceftriaxone, one of the antimicrobial drugs belonging to the third generation of cephalosporins and one of the well-known high-CDI-risk antimicrobial agents, was the only drug showing 11 positive signals. In this regard, this indicator concisely summarized the CDI risk characteristics of antimicrobial drugs, facilitating to get a quick understanding of the risk of different antibacterial agents.

Although this study comprehensively summarized the CDI risk of antibacterial drugs by using a pharmacovigilance database, there were also some inevitable limitations in this study. First, due to the intrinsic limitations of the pharmacovigilance database, the fact that un-peer-reviewed data, underreporting, Weber effect and notoriety bias may lead to biased results [25,27,28]. Second, due to the total number of patients exposed to each antibacterial drug is unclear, the incidence of CDI for an antibacterial drug cannot be determined. Third, patient gender, age, concomitant therapeutic drugs, dose and duration of antibiotic use, and comorbidities may influence the occurrence of CDI, but it is almost impossible to shield the potential interference of those factors to our results due to the intrinsic limitations of the pharmacovigilance database. Fourth, the ADR signal result only represents the strength of the statistical association between the drug of interest and AE of interest, so a well-designed study is still needed to verify whether there is a true causality.

4. Materials and Methods

4.1. Data Source

The data in this study were obtained from the FAERS database, a large international pharmacovigilance database with voluntary reporting nature, which recorded ADRs information related to post-market, FDA-approved medications as well as natural substances, vaccines and medical devices [29]. It currently publicly opens more than 16 million drug post-marketing AEs records reported by manufacturers, consumers and healthcare professionals and updates quarterly. The recorded information in the database includes but is not limited to patient demographic information, report sources, medication information, AEs involved and patient outcomes [30]. Those data are highly structured and can be retrieved, collected and downloaded from the openFDA platform by constructing an appropriate retrieval statement through an application programming interface (API) [31]. In this study, we summarized and analyzed CDI reports related to ADE between 1 January 2004 and 31 December 2022 in FAERS.

4.2. Identification of CDI Reports Associated with Antibacterial Drug Use in FAERS

The FAERS reporting system uses the PTs in Medical Dictionary for Regulatory Activities (MedDRA) to standardize AEs occurring in patients [30]. SMQs are a series of PT sets that potentially indicate the same medical condition, which was developed to optimize data retrieval and signal detection in pharmacovigilance activity [32]. Within an SMQ, PTs can be further divided into narrow-scope PTs and broad-scope PTs according to the degree of association with the condition or area of interest [33]. Among them, the PTs with a narrow scope are closely related to the condition or area of interest, while such association is relatively weak for PTs with a broad scope.

Pseudomembranous colitis is an inflammatory condition of the colon characterized by the presence of yellow-white exudative plaques that coalesce to form pseudomembranes on the mucosa, and it is usually a marker of severe CDI [34]. Meanwhile, it is also one of the SMQs in MedDRA that includes many PTs potentially indicating CDI, so it can be used to identify CDI-related reports in FAERS. In order to improve the accuracy of case identification and signal detection, in this study, only narrow-scope PTs of pseudomembranous colitis (SMQ) in MedDRA 23.0 were selected to retrieve CDI-related reports in FAERS (Table 1). According to the ATC classification system, if one of the generic drug names recorded in the "patient.drug.openfda.generic_name" field can be classified into "antibacterials for systemic use (J01)" in a report, this report is considered CDI reports associated with ADE and included in the final analysis.

4.3. ADR Signal Detection Method

Disproportionality analysis is a kind of technology used to detect ADR signals at present. Based on the classical two-by-two contingency table (Table 5), researchers can compare the differences between the occurrence frequency and background frequency for target drugs and target AEs. The reporting odd ratio (ROR) is one of the well-established disproportionality analysis methods, which calculates the ratio of the odds of a selected drug versus all other drugs for a certain AEs compared to the odds of the same drugs for all other AEs recorded in FAERS to detect potential ADR signals [35]. In this study, we used the ROR and its corresponding 95% confidence intervals (CIs) to identify ADR signals, and the ROR and its 95% CI can be calculated by the following formula:

$$ROR = \frac{a/c}{b/d} = \frac{ad}{bc}, \quad (1)$$

$$95\% \ CI = e^{ln(ROR) \pm 1.96\sqrt{(\frac{1}{a}+\frac{1}{b}+\frac{1}{c}+\frac{1}{d})}}. \quad (2)$$

Table 5. Two-by-two contingency tables for disproportionality analysis.

	Drug of Interest	Other Drugs	Total
AE of interest	a	b	a + b
Other AEs	c	d	c + d
Total	a + c	b + d	a + b + c + d

Abbreviations: AE, adverse event.

When the lower-bound 95% CI of ROR was above 1.0 with at least three cases ($a \geq 3$ in Table 5), it was considered a positive signal, suggesting a potential risk of the target AE caused by the target drug; instead, if the lower-bound 95% CI of ROR and the number of cases cannot meet the above-mentioned threshold, it was regarded as a negative signal, suggesting the statistical connection between target AE occurrence and target drug use is weak [26,36]. To some extent, the ROR value represents a statistical correlation between the drug of interest and AE of interest, and the ROR value is larger, the stronger the statistical correlation. Using this indicator, we can highlight the AE that may be induced by a certain drug and conduct a further investigation so as to inform the possible risk; on the other hand, we can also use it to compare the risk of different drugs causing the same AE, so as to guide the selection of therapeutic drugs or discontinuation of a culprit drug [17].

4.4. Data Collection and Analysis

With reference to the API build guideline issued by the openFDA (https://open.fda.gov/apis/drug/event/how-to-use-the-endpoint/, accessed on 1 January 2023), we can retrieve and download the target reports for further analysis. The specific data collection and analysis steps of this study are as follows.

Firstly, by using the R package "httr" to call API, PTs in Table 1 were used to retrieve target reports in FAERS, and the returned dataset was downloaded in "json" format. Secondly, the R package "jsonlite" was used to read the downloaded dataset and extract the reports information, including Safety Report ID number, patient demographics, report time, report sources, medication use and outcomes. Thirdly, generic drug names recorded in the "patient.drug.openfda.generic_name" field were used to further identify reports associated with antibacterial drug use, and report characteristics were summarized. Fourthly, the ADR signals at the SMQ level and PT level were detected by calculating the *ROR* value and its 95% *CI* by using disproportionality analysis, and 11 signals were generated for each antibacterial drug. Finally, the positive-negative distribution of signals was summarized.

In this study, R version 4.1.0 (R Foundation for Statistical Computing, Vienna, Austria) was used for data processing and analysis.

5. Conclusions

The vastness, authenticity and accessibility of FAERS data have made it an important resource for evaluating drug safety cost-effectively. In this study, CDI reports associated with ADE in FAERS were summarized, and the CDI risk of different antibacterial agents was explored. As the first study to evaluate CDI risk related to antibacterial drug exposure using a pharmacovigilance database, our study provided a preliminary picture of CDI induced by antibacterial drugs in the real world that can help to better primary prevention for CDI and antimicrobial stewardship. Meanwhile, the potentially high CDI risk of metronidazole and vancomycin that may have been previously overlooked was detected, and it deserved further attention from regulators, health professionals and others involved in antimicrobial stewardship. Of particular note, however, our study as a pharmacovigilance study using the FAERS database only provided a statistical association between CDI occurrence and antibacterial drugs, so further well-designed study is still necessary to validate the causality.

Supplementary Materials: The following supporting information can be downloaded at: https://www.mdpi.com/article/10.3390/antibiotics12071109/s1, Table S1: Pharmacovigilance signal detection results for antibiotic associated colitis; Table S2: Pharmacovigilance signal detection results for clostridium bacteremia; Table S3: Pharmacovigilance signal detection results for clostridium colitis; Table S4: Pharmacovigilance signal detection results for clostridium difficile colitis; Table S5: Pharmacovigilance signal detection results for clostridium difficile infection; Table S6: Pharmacovigilance signal detection results for clostridial infection; Table S7: Pharmacovigilance signal detection results for clostridial sepsis; Table S8: Pharmacovigilance signal detection results for clostridium test positive; Table S9: Pharmacovigilance signal detection results for gastroenteritis clostridial; Table S10: Pharmacovigilance signal detection results for pseudomembranous colitis.

Author Contributions: Conceptualization, Q.D. and S.L.; methodology, D.L. and Y.S.; software, D.L. and Y.S.; data curation, D.L., Y.S., Z.B., X.X., F.L., Y.Z., C.Q. and D.D.; writing—original draft preparation, D.L. and Y.S.; writing—review and editing, D.L., Y.S., Z.B., X.X., F.L., Y.Z., C.Q., D.D., Q.D. and S.L.; funding acquisition, Q.D. All authors have read and agreed to the published version of the manuscript.

Funding: This research was funded by the Intelligent Medicine Research Project of Chongqing Medical University, grant number ZHYX202229.

Institutional Review Board Statement: Ethical review and approval were waived for this study due to the local legislation and institutional requirements, which were confirmed by the Institutional Review Board of The Third Affiliated Hospital of Chongqing Medical University.

Informed Consent Statement: A requirement for informed consent was waived because this study used an open database.

Data Availability Statement: Data are available on the FAERS database.

Acknowledgments: We acknowledge openFDA for providing their platforms and contributors for uploading their meaningful datasets.

Conflicts of Interest: The authors declare no conflict of interest.

References

1. Martin, J.S.; Monaghan, T.M.; Wilcox, M.H. Clostridium difficile infection: Epidemiology, diagnosis and understanding transmission. *Nat. Rev. Gastroenterol. Hepatol.* **2016**, *13*, 206–216. [CrossRef]
2. Owens, R.C., Jr.; Donskey, C.J.; Gaynes, R.P.; Loo, V.G.; Muto, C.A. Antimicrobial-associated risk factors for Clostridium difficile infection. *Clin. Infect. Dis.* **2008**, *46* (Suppl. 1), S19–S31. [CrossRef]
3. Karas, J.A.; Enoch, D.A.; Aliyu, S.H. A review of mortality due to Clostridium difficile infection. *J. Infect.* **2010**, *61*, 1–8. [CrossRef] [PubMed]
4. Kelly, C.P.; LaMont, J.T. Clostridium difficile—More difficult than ever. *N. Engl. J. Med.* **2008**, *359*, 1932–1940. [CrossRef] [PubMed]
5. Trubiano, J.A.; Cheng, A.C.; Korman, T.M.; Roder, C.; Campbell, A.; May, M.L.; Blyth, C.C.; Ferguson, J.K.; Blackmore, T.K.; Riley, T.V.; et al. Australasian Society of Infectious Diseases updated guidelines for the management of Clostridium difficile infection in adults and children in Australia and New Zealand. *Intern. Med. J.* **2016**, *46*, 479–493. [CrossRef] [PubMed]
6. McDonald, L.C.; Gerding, D.N.; Johnson, S.; Bakken, J.S.; Carroll, K.C.; Coffin, S.E.; Dubberke, E.R.; Garey, K.W.; Gould, C.V.; Kelly, C.; et al. Clinical Practice Guidelines for Clostridium difficile Infection in Adults and Children: 2017 Update by the Infectious Diseases Society of America (IDSA) and Society for Healthcare Epidemiology of America (SHEA). *Clin. Infect. Dis.* **2018**, *66*, e1–e48. [CrossRef] [PubMed]
7. Sartelli, M.; Di Bella, S.; McFarland, L.V.; Khanna, S.; Furuya-Kanamori, L.; Abuzeid, N.; Abu-Zidan, F.M.; Ansaloni, L.; Augustin, G.; Bala, M.; et al. 2019 update of the WSES guidelines for management of Clostridioides (Clostridium) difficile infection in surgical patients. *World J. Emerg. Surg.* **2019**, *14*, 8. [CrossRef]
8. Kelly, C.R.; Fischer, M.; Allegretti, J.R.; LaPlante, K.; Stewart, D.B.; Limketkai, B.N.; Stollman, N.H. ACG Clinical Guidelines: Prevention, Diagnosis, and Treatment of *Clostridioides difficile* Infections. *Am. J. Gastroenterol.* **2021**, *116*, 1124–1147. [CrossRef]
9. van Prehn, J.; Reigadas, E.; Vogelzang, E.H.; Bouza, E.; Hristea, A.; Guery, B.; Krutova, M.; Noren, T.; Allerberger, F.; Coia, J.E.; et al. European Society of Clinical Microbiology and Infectious Diseases: 2021 update on the treatment guidance document for *Clostridioides difficile* infection in adults. *Clin. Microbiol. Infect.* **2021**, *27* (Suppl. 2), S1–S21. [CrossRef]
10. Gaffin, N.; Spellberg, B. Sustained reductions in unnecessary antimicrobial administration and hospital *Clostridioides difficile* rates via stewardship in a nonacademic setting. *Infect. Control. Hosp. Epidemiol.* **2023**, *44*, 491–493. [CrossRef]
11. Hecker, M.T.; Son, A.H.; Alhmidi, H.; Wilson, B.M.; Wiest, P.M.; Donskey, C.J. Efficacy of a stewardship intervention focused on reducing unnecessary use of non-*Clostridioides difficile* antibiotics in patients with *Clostridioides difficile* infection. *Infect. Control. Hosp. Epidemiol.* **2020**, *41*, 216–218. [CrossRef] [PubMed]
12. Morgan, F.; Belal, M.; Lisa, B.; Ford, F.; LeMaitre, B.; Psevdos, G. Antimicrobial stewardship program achieved marked decrease in Clostridium difficile infections in a Veterans Hospital. *Am. J. Infect. Control.* **2020**, *48*, 1119–1121. [CrossRef]
13. Pepin, J.; Saheb, N.; Coulombe, M.A.; Alary, M.E.; Corriveau, M.P.; Authier, S.; Leblanc, M.; Rivard, G.; Bettez, M.; Primeau, V.; et al. Emergence of fluoroquinolones as the predominant risk factor for Clostridium difficile-associated diarrhea: A cohort study during an epidemic in Quebec. *Clin. Infect. Dis.* **2005**, *41*, 1254–1260. [CrossRef] [PubMed]
14. Weiss, K.; Bergeron, L.; Bernatchez, H.; Goyette, M.; Savoie, M.; Thirion, D. Clostridium difficile-associated diarrhoea rates and global antibiotic consumption in five Quebec institutions from 2001 to 2004. *Int. J. Antimicrob. Agents* **2007**, *30*, 309–314. [CrossRef] [PubMed]
15. Blondeau, J.M. What have we learned about antimicrobial use and the risks for Clostridium difficile-associated diarrhoea? *J. Antimicrob. Chemother.* **2009**, *63*, 238–242. [CrossRef] [PubMed]
16. Raschi, E.; La Placa, M.; Poluzzi, E.; De Ponti, F. The value of case reports and spontaneous reporting systems for pharmacovigilance and clinical practice. *Br. J. Dermatol.* **2021**, *184*, 581–583. [CrossRef]
17. Bohm, R.; von Hehn, L.; Herdegen, T.; Klein, H.J.; Bruhn, O.; Petri, H.; Hocker, J. OpenVigil FDA—Inspection of U.S. American Adverse Drug Events Pharmacovigilance Data and Novel Clinical Applications. *PLoS ONE* **2016**, *11*, e0157753. [CrossRef]
18. Seo, H.; Kim, E. Electrolyte Disorders Associated with Piperacillin/Tazobactam: A Pharmacovigilance Study Using the FAERS Database. *Antibiotics* **2023**, *12*, 240. [CrossRef]
19. Patek, T.M.; Teng, C.; Kennedy, K.E.; Alvarez, C.A.; Frei, C.R. Comparing Acute Kidney Injury Reports Among Antibiotics: A Pharmacovigilance Study of the FDA Adverse Event Reporting System (FAERS). *Drug Saf.* **2020**, *43*, 17–22. [CrossRef]
20. Calderwood, S.B.; Moellering, R.C., Jr. Common adverse effects of antibacterial agents on major organ systems. *Surg. Clin. N. Am.* **1980**, *60*, 65–81. [CrossRef]
21. Slimings, C.; Riley, T.V. Antibiotics and hospital-acquired Clostridium difficile infection: Update of systematic review and meta-analysis. *J. Antimicrob. Chemother.* **2014**, *69*, 881–891. [CrossRef]

22. Webb, B.J.; Subramanian, A.; Lopansri, B.; Goodman, B.; Jones, P.B.; Ferraro, J.; Stenehjem, E.; Brown, S.M. Antibiotic Exposure and Risk for Hospital-Associated *Clostridioides difficile* Infection. *Antimicrob. Agents Chemother.* **2020**, *64*, e02169-19. [CrossRef] [PubMed]
23. Schechner, V.; Fallach, N.; Braun, T.; Temkin, E.; Carmeli, Y. Antibiotic exposure and the risk of hospital-acquired diarrhoea and *Clostridioides difficile* infection: A cohort study. *J. Antimicrob. Chemother.* **2021**, *76*, 2182–2185. [CrossRef] [PubMed]
24. Forster, A.J.; Daneman, N.; van Walraven, C. Influence of antibiotics and case exposure on hospital-acquired Clostridium difficile infection independent of illness severity. *J. Hosp. Infect.* **2017**, *95*, 400–409. [CrossRef] [PubMed]
25. Alatawi, Y.M.; Hansen, R.A. Empirical estimation of under-reporting in the U.S. Food and Drug Administration Adverse Event Reporting System (FAERS). *Expert. Opin. Drug Saf.* **2017**, *16*, 761–767. [CrossRef]
26. Li, D.; Gou, J.; Zhu, J.; Zhang, T.; Liu, F.; Zhang, D.; Dai, L.; Li, W.; Liu, Q.; Qin, C.; et al. Severe cutaneous adverse reactions to drugs: A real-world pharmacovigilance study using the FDA Adverse Event Reporting System database. *Front. Pharmacol.* **2023**, *14*, 1117391. [CrossRef]
27. Hoffman, K.B.; Dimbil, M.; Erdman, C.B.; Tatonetti, N.P.; Overstreet, B.M. The Weber effect and the United States Food and Drug Administration's Adverse Event Reporting System (FAERS): Analysis of sixty-two drugs approved from 2006 to 2010. *Drug Saf.* **2014**, *37*, 283–294. [CrossRef]
28. Neha, R.; Subeesh, V.; Beulah, E.; Gouri, N.; Maheswari, E. Existence of Notoriety Bias in FDA Adverse Event Reporting System Database and Its Impact on Signal Strength. *Hosp. Pharm.* **2021**, *56*, 152–158. [CrossRef]
29. Wichelmann, T.A.; Abdulmujeeb, S.; Ehrenpreis, E.D. Bevacizumab and gastrointestinal perforations: A review from the FDA Adverse Event Reporting System (FAERS) database. *Aliment. Pharmacol. Ther.* **2021**, *54*, 1290–1297. [CrossRef]
30. Altebainawi, A.F.; Alfaraj, L.A.; Alharbi, A.A.; Alkhuraisi, F.F.; Alshammari, T.M. Association between proton pump inhibitors and rhabdomyolysis risk: A post-marketing surveillance using FDA adverse event reporting system (FAERS) database. *Ther. Adv. Drug Saf.* **2023**, *14*, 20420986231154075. [CrossRef]
31. Kass-Hout, T.A.; Xu, Z.; Mohebbi, M.; Nelsen, H.; Baker, A.; Levine, J.; Johanson, E.; Bright, R.A. OpenFDA: An innovative platform providing access to a wealth of FDA's publicly available data. *J. Am. Med. Inform. Assoc.* **2016**, *23*, 596–600. [CrossRef] [PubMed]
32. Ma, P.; Pan, X.; Liu, R.; Qu, Y.; Xie, L.; Xie, J.; Cao, L.; Chen, Y. Ocular adverse events associated with anti-VEGF therapy: A pharmacovigilance study of the FDA adverse event reporting system (FAERS). *Front. Pharmacol.* **2022**, *13*, 1017889. [CrossRef] [PubMed]
33. Mozzicato, P. Standardised MedDRA queries: Their role in signal detection. *Drug. Saf.* **2007**, *30*, 617–619. [CrossRef] [PubMed]
34. Farooq, P.D.; Urrunaga, N.H.; Tang, D.M.; von Rosenvinge, E.C. Pseudomembranous colitis. *Dis. Mon.* **2015**, *61*, 181–206. [CrossRef] [PubMed]
35. Sakaeda, T.; Tamon, A.; Kadoyama, K.; Okuno, Y. Data mining of the public version of the FDA Adverse Event Reporting System. *Int. J. Med. Sci.* **2013**, *10*, 796–803. [CrossRef]
36. Lin, X.; Lin, W.; Yang, J.; Weng, L. Differences in Hypersensitivity Reactions to Iodinated Contrast Media: Analysis of the FDA Adverse Event Reporting System Database (FAERS). *J. Allergy Clin. Immunol. Pract.* **2023**, *11*, 1494–1502.e6. [CrossRef]

Disclaimer/Publisher's Note: The statements, opinions and data contained in all publications are solely those of the individual author(s) and contributor(s) and not of MDPI and/or the editor(s). MDPI and/or the editor(s) disclaim responsibility for any injury to people or property resulting from any ideas, methods, instructions or products referred to in the content.

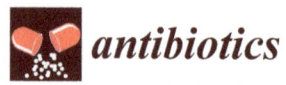

Article

Clinical Determinants Predicting *Clostridioides difficile* Infection among Patients with Chronic Kidney Disease

Łukasz Lis [1,2], Andrzej Konieczny [3,*], Michał Sroka [1], Anna Ciszewska [4], Kornelia Krakowska [3], Tomasz Gołębiowski [3] and Zbigniew Hruby [1,5]

1. Research and Development Center, Department of Nephrology, Provincial Specialist Hospital, Kamienskiego 73a, 51-124 Wroclaw, Poland; lislukasz@ymail.com (Ł.L.); michal.sroka@wssk.wroc.pl (M.S.); zhruby@wssk.wroc.pl (Z.H.)
2. Department of Internal Medicine, University Hospital, Witosa 23, 45-401 Opole, Poland
3. Department of Nephrology and Transplantation Medicine, Wroclaw Medical University, Borowska 213, 50-556 Wroclaw, Poland; korneliakrakowska006@gmail.com (K.K.); tomasz.golebiowski@umw.edu.pl (T.G.)
4. Department of Intensive Care and Anesthesiology, Provincial Specialist Hospital, Kamienskiego 73a, 51-124 Wroclaw, Poland; aniaa.ciszewska@gmail.com
5. Department of Clinical Nursing, Wroclaw Medical University, Bartla 5, 51-618 Wroclaw, Poland
* Correspondence: andrzej.konieczny@umw.edu.pl; Tel.: +48-717332536

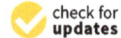

Abstract: The majority of recently published studies indicate a greater incidence rate and mortality due to Clostridioides difficile infection (CDI) in patients with chronic kidney disease (CKD). The aim of this study was to assess the clinical determinants predicting CDI among hospitalized patients with CKD and refine methods of prevention. We evaluated the medical records of 279 patients treated at a nephrological department with symptoms suggesting CDI, of whom 93 tested positive for CDI. The survey showed that age, poor kidney function, high Padua prediction score (PPS) and patients' classification of care at admission, treatment with antibiotics, and time of its duration were significantly higher or more frequent among patients who suffered CDI. Whereas BMI, Norton scale (ANSS) and serum albumin concentration were significantly lowered among CDI patients. In a multivariate analysis we proved the stage of CKD and length of antibiotics use increased the risk of CDI, whereas higher serum albumin concentration and ANSS have a protective impact.

Keywords: *Clostridioides difficile*; chronic kidney disease; malnutrition; pseudomembranous enterocolitis

Citation: Lis, Ł.; Konieczny, A.; Sroka, M.; Ciszewska, A.; Krakowska, K.; Gołębiowski, T.; Hruby, Z. Clinical Determinants Predicting *Clostridioides difficile* Infection among Patients with Chronic Kidney Disease. *Antibiotics* **2022**, *11*, 785. https://doi.org/10.3390/antibiotics11060785

Academic Editor: Guido Granata

Received: 10 May 2022
Accepted: 8 June 2022
Published: 8 June 2022

Publisher's Note: MDPI stays neutral with regard to jurisdictional claims in published maps and institutional affiliations.

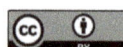

Copyright: © 2022 by the authors. Licensee MDPI, Basel, Switzerland. This article is an open access article distributed under the terms and conditions of the Creative Commons Attribution (CC BY) license (https://creativecommons.org/licenses/by/4.0/).

1. Introduction

Clostridioides difficile infection (CDI) is caused by a Gram-positive, anaerobic, spore-forming bacillus, the most prevalent cause of a nosocomial diarrhea worldwide [1]. It is transferred by a fecal–oral route and can have either a mild course or progress to a life-threatening colitis, with diarrhea, abdominal pain, dehydration, fever, and subsequent circulatory shock [2].

Antibiotic treatment, older age, and hospitalization belong to the most significant risk factors for CDI [3,4]. The other well-defined clinical conditions, predisposing to CDI, include an inflammatory bowel disease, malignant tumors, transplantations, and chronic kidney disease (CKD) [3,5].

The influence of proton pump inhibitors (PPI) on the incidence of CDI remains controversial. Several studies have found a significant association between PPI treatment and CDI [6,7]; however, there are also a number of papers where such correlation was not proven [8,9].

Although the estimated burden of *Clostridioides difficile* (CD) health care-associated infections decreased in the United States by an adjusted 24% from 2011 to 2017 [10], it has been still recognized as a leading cause of infection among hospitalized patients and a considerable threat to public health globally [11].

Some of the most vulnerable patients are those suffering from CKD and in particular with end-stage renal disease (ESRD), despite the implementation of CDI prevention strategies [12]. The majority of recently published studies indicate a greater incidence rate and mortality due to CDI in CKD, especially among those with ESRD, in comparison to the general population [13–15]. It also results in a significant increase in the treatment costs and prolonged hospitalization time [16].

The main aim of this paper was to assess clinical determinants for predicting CDI among hospitalized patients with CKD and refine methods of prevention to combat the epidemic of nosocomial infections with CD etiology.

2. Materials and Methods

This was a single center, retrospective study, including data of 15,389 patients hospitalized in a department of nephrology, between 1 January 2016 and 31 December 2020, who developed symptoms indicating CDI. A flowchart presenting initial qualification, the screening of patients, and assignment to CDI positive and CDI negative groups is presented in Figure 1.

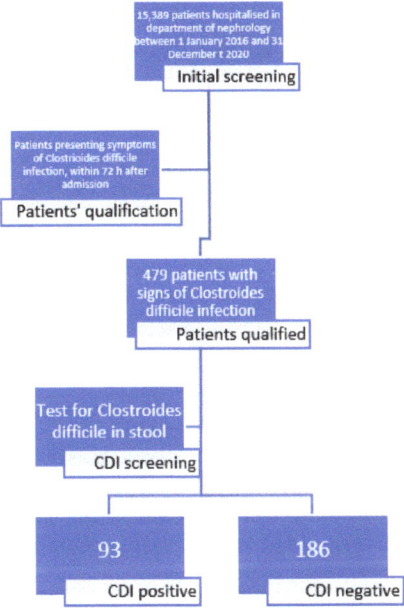

Figure 1. Patients' screening and recruitment.

Qualifying symptoms were diarrhea (>3 stools per day) and abdominal pain and/or fever [2]. Although we based on definition of CDI provided by the Infectious Diseases Society of America (IDSA) and Society for Healthcare Epidemiology of America (SHEA), we included only patients who developed the symptoms within at least 72 h after admission.

In all patients a rapid enzyme cassette immunoassay was performed, detecting the antigens of toxins A and B of CD in stool (TOX A/B QUIK CHEK®; Techlab, Blackburg, VA, USA).

The exclusion criteria were missing clinical data, length of stay (LOS) shorter than 3 days, or admission from another hospital.

The following data were assessed: patients' age; gender; body mass index (BMI); presence of concomitant diseases; length of stay (LOS); stay in an emergency department (ER) directly before admission; presence of acute kidney injury (AKI), defined according to the KDIGO [17]; and pharmacotherapy with the emphasis on antibiotics, proton pump inhibitors (PPI), statins, probiotics, and immunosuppression.

At admission each patient was assessed using the Norton scale (ANSS) and the classification of patient care, evaluated by the ward nurse, and the Padua prediction score (PPS), assessed by the physician.

ANSS assesses the risk of pressure sores during hospitalization. It consists of five variables: physical and mental condition, activity, mobility, and incontinence. Each domain is graded from 1 to 4 points and final admission ANSS ranges between 5 and 20 points and an ANSS ≤ 14 is considered as being low [16].

The classification of patient care is a clinical tool used for managing and planning the allocation of nursing staff in accordance with the nursing care needs. It is subdivided into four classifications, namely: 1—self-care patient, 2—partial care patient, 3—complete care patient, 4—critical care patient.

The PPS identifies admitted patients at a high risk for venous thromboembolism (VTE) and who would benefit from thromboprophylaxis. In the PPS, the risk profile for VTE is calculated using 11 common risk factors [18]. Each risk factor is weighted according to a point scale. A high risk of VTE is defined as a cumulative score ≥ 4 and a low risk as < 4 [18].

Laboratory tests were performed in the hospital laboratory using standard methods, including the concentration of serum creatinine (sCr), serum urea, and albumin (ALB). The shortened Modification of Diet in Renal Disease (MDRD) equation was used to calculate the estimated glomerular filtration rate (eGFR) [18].

Statistical analysis was performed utilizing the STATISTICA ver. 12 software (StatSoft Inc., Tulsa, OK, USA). Numerical data were expressed as mean and standard deviations (SD). Normal distribution was verified with the Kolmogorov–Smirnov test, which enabled the assessment of the differences between the two groups with Student's t test, the homogeneity of variations being checked with Fisher's test. In case of non-linear distribution, statistical importance of the differences was evaluated with the use of the U Mann–Whitney test. For quantitative data, χ^2 analysis was performed. The influence of the parameters of CDI occurrence was tested with the implementation of logistic regression. The statistical significance cut-off level was set at $p = 0.05$.

3. Results

3.1. Patients' Baseline Characteristic

A total number of 279 patients, aged 68 years, 124 (44%) women and 155 (66%) men, were enrolled in the study, of whom 93 (33%) had proven CDI and 186 were without CDI. All patients presented symptoms suggesting CDI, e.g., diarrhea and abdominal pain, whereas 45 in group of CDI positive patients and 76 of CDI negative patients had fever additionally.

3.2. Differences between CDI and Control Group

Patients who suffered from CDI were significantly older and displayed poor kidney function. They were more frequently treated with PPIs and antibiotics, for a significantly prolonged time. Moreover, they presented with higher PPS and patients' care classifications at admission and were more frequently hospitalized in the ER before admission. Patients with CDI had higher mortality and required longer LOS. CDI-patients presented lower albumin concentration and ANSS.

It was not revealed whether treatment with statins, immunosuppression, probiotics, or the presence of diabetes, neoplasm significantly affects the risk of CDI. Comparison of differences in clinical data are presented in Table 1.

Table 1. Comparison of clinical parameters between CDI-patients and non-CDI.

Parameter	CDI (N = 93)	Non-CDI (N = 186)	p * Chi^2-Test
Age [years]	72.1 ± 13.8	65.6 ± 16.1	0.001
BMI	23.6 ± 5.6	26.7 ± 4.6	<0.0001
LOS [days]	30.7 ± 18.5	8.9 ± 6.3	<0.0001
sCr at admission [mg/dL]	3.8 ± 3.9	2.3 ± 1.7	0.0002
Urea concentration at admission [mg/dL]	144.6 ± 102.6	84.2 ± 56.1	<0.0001
CKD stage	4.3 ± 1.1	3.6 ± 1.4	<0.0001
HD treatment	36 (39%)	46 (25%)	0.016 *
ALB at admission [g/dL]	2.8 ± 0.6	3.7 ± 0.5	<0.0001
Use of antibiotics	89 (96%)	54 (29%)	<0.0001 *
Number of antibiotics used	2 ± 1	0.4 ± 0.7	<0.0001
Length of antibiotics treatment [days]	15.7 ± 8.7	2.6 ± 4.4	<0.0001
PPS	4.6 ± 1.9	1.6 ± 1.5	<0.0001
ANSS	12.5 ± 3.3	17.5 ± 2.2	<0.0001
Patients' care class 1/2/3/4	2.7 ± 0.5	1.8 ± 0.6	<0.0001
Presence of neoplasm	11 (12%)	18 (10%)	0.6 *
DM	29 (31%)	52 (28%)	0.58 *
PPI treatment	65 (70%)	92 (49%)	0.002 *
Use of probiotics	42 (45%)	14 (8%)	<0.0001 *
Use of statins	24 (25%)	63 (34%)	0.17 *
Immunosuppression use	17 (18%)	47 (25%)	0.19 *
Death	18 (19%)	9 (5%)	0.0001 *
ER stay	89 (96%)	71 (38%)	<0.0001 *
AKI at admission	35 (38%)	19 (10%)	<0.0001 *

Abbreviations: LOS—length of stay; CKD—chronic kidney disease; sCr—serum creatinine concentration; ALB—serum albumin concentration; CDI—Clostridioides difficile infection; HD—hemodialysis; PPI—proton pump inhibitor; DM—diabetes mellitus; ER—emergency department; AKI—acute kidney injury; ANSS—the Norton scale; PPS—the Padua prediction score; *—for non parametric variables Chi^2 was applied.

3.3. Univariate Logistic Regression Predicting CDI

Using univariate logistic regression models (as shown in Table 2), we have found that age, CKD stage, both serum creatinine and urea concentrations, number of antibiotics used in therapy, time of treatment, assessment in PPS, and higher patients' care class significantly increased the risk of CDI. Whereas serum albumin concentration at admission, ANSS, and BMI lowered the risk of CDI.

Table 2. Univariate logistic regression in predicting CDI.

Variable	Estimate	Odds Ratio	95% Confidence Interval		p-Value
Age	0.03	1.03	1.01	1.05	0.001
CKD Stage	0.45	1.57	1.26	1.96	0.001
sCr at admission [mg/dL]	0.24	1.27	1.09	1.47	0.002
Urea at admission [mg/dL]	0.01	1.01	1.006	1.02	0.001
ALB at admission [g/dL]	−2.27	0.1	0.06	0.18	0.001
Number of antibiotics	1.91	6.8	4.4	10.4	0.001
Length of antibiotics use [days]	0.33	1.38	1.28	1.49	0.001
PPS	0.82	2.26	1.89	2.71	0.001
ANSS	−0.57	0.56	0.5	0.64	0.001
Patients' care class	2.4	11.04	6.25	19.5	0.001
BMI	−0.14	0.87	0.82	0.94	0.001

Abbreviations: CKD—chronic kidney disease; sCr—serum creatinine concentration; ALB—serum albumin concentration; ANSS—the Norton scale; PPS—the Padua prediction score; BMI—body mass index.

In a multivariate model, CKD stage and the length of antibiotics treatment had a significant impact on CDI, whereas albumin concentration and Norton score lowered the risk, as presented in Table 3.

Table 3. Multivariate logistic regression in predicting CDI.

Variable	Estimate	Odds Ratio	95% Confidence Interval		p-Value
CKD Stage	0.53	1.7	1.01	2.7	0.02
ALB at admission [g/dL]	−1.4	0.25	0.1	0.58	0.001
Length of antibiotics use [days]	0.26	1.3	1.19	1.42	0.001
ANSS	−0.39	0.68	0.57	0.82	0.001

Abbreviations: CKD—chronic kidney disease; ALB—serum albumin concentration; ANSS—the Norton scale.

4. Discussion

Our study showed that age, declined kidney function (expressed by both serum creatinine and urea concentration and subsequently by CKD stage), higher PPS, patients' care classification at admission, treatment with antibiotics and length of its duration were significantly higher or more frequent among patients who suffered from CDI. Whereas BMI, ANSS, and serum albumin concentration were significantly lower among CDI patients.

In a multivariate analysis both the stage of CKD and length of antibiotics use increased the risk of CDI, whereas higher serum albumin concentration and ANSS lowered the CDI risk. These factors are the best clinical determinants for predicting the presence of CDI among patients with CKD. No effect was found for other factors, including treatment with statins, immunosuppression, probiotics, or presence of diabetes and neoplasm.

Age is the most frequently reported risk factor for CDI [12,13]. It is associated with an increased number of comorbidities, malnutrition, and reduced psychomotor skills. These may result in a lower ANSS ($\leq$14 is considered as being low) and higher PPS (high risk of VTE is defined as a cumulative score $\geq$ 4) or care classification (III—complete care patient and IV critical care patient), which were proven to be significant factors for CDI, to our knowledge probably first time in the literature.

These findings might be applied to screen the most vulnerable patients and to shorten their hospitalization, ER stay, or time of laboratory tests and to increase vigilance of medical personnel for aseptic behavior. The ANSS, PPS, and care classification is easy to learn, easy to use, and, most importantly, it is already being used successfully throughout the world to assess the risk of pressure ulcers, venous thromboembolism, or patient nursing care needs.

It is worth underlining that ER stays before admission were an independent risk factor for CDI patients with CKD in our survey. Moreover, in one of recent study it has been suggested that ER may be one of the main reservoirs of CDI [19].

Lower BMI and albumin concentration were definitive clinical determinants for predicting CDI. This fact has been confirmed in other papers and is associated with malnutrition and secondary immunodeficiency due to deproteinization [15,20]. Bearing in mind that lower albumin concentration was one of the best determinants for predicting CDI in our study, improvements in diagnosing and treating hospital malnutrition are needed, the effects of which could benefit both patients and healthcare providers.

It has been reported that the use of antibiotics and, in particular, the length of antibiotic treatment significantly increased the risk of CDI. Antibiotics policy seems to be the most important factors, influencing a significant reduction in CDI frequency. The importance of the problem is crucial because it is estimated that approximately 50% of antibiotics used in hospitals are considered unnecessary [21].

Most studies have confirmed that PPIs increase the risk of CDI. The risk is estimated to be 1.7–2.3 times higher [6,7]. Given the widespread abuse of the above-mentioned drugs, caution in their use seems to be indispensable.

Patients with advanced stage of CKD (especially those in the ESRD phase) and with the presence of AKI at admission were also at risk of CDI, according to our results. Several studies have found a significant association between advanced CKD, AKI, and CDI [22–24], but, on the other hand, there are papers where such correlation was not proven [25,26]. In our previous study, it was not documented that reduced eGFR augmented the risk of the CDI [15]. This may be attributable to the fact that the control group in this study consisted of

CD-negative patients with diarrhea and the investigated group of patients was dominated by those with class 5 CKD: 137 of 207 (65.7%) with 77 (37.2%) of them chronically dialyzed. On the other hand, in our study, the control group consisted of 186 patients with signs of infection but without CDI, who were admitted to the same department and hospitalized at the same time as patients with CDI. The investigated group was not dominated by patients with CKD class 5: 128 of 279 (45.8%) with 82 (29.4%) of them undergoing dialysis.

It was also found that patients with CDI had higher mortality and required longer LOS and most of recent publications have confirmed that correlation. Pant et al. showed that if the average duration of hospitalization is longer than 9 days, then its costs rise additionally on 68 thousand dollars, and mortality is twice as high [16,22].

Clinicians should be aware of these clinical determinants predicting CDI in CKD patients, because some of them are modifiable and amenable to effective interventions. Special attention should be devoted to the rapid diagnosis of CDI and rational antibiotics policy, aimed at reducing the use of unwarranted antibiotic therapy, avoiding drugs increasing the risk of CDI, and shorten the time of treatment duration. Furthermore, aseptic behavior, the proper nutrition of malnourished patients; systematic education and control of medical personnel; and cautious use PPIs, limiting them to situations where they are necessary, especially in patients with low albumin concentration, ANSS, and advanced CKD, could significantly reduce CDI-associated morbidity and mortality among adults, particularly those with CKD.

Our study has some limitations. Firstly, all patients who were enrolled in the study were of Caucasian origin. Secondly, analysis was based on patients' data over a 5-year period. The survey relies only on the single center experience. To provide a robust clinical tool, allowing the identification of individuals at high risk of CDI among CKD patients, a long-term multicenter study, including larger cohort, is required.

5. Conclusions

The best clinical determinants predicting the presence or absence of CDI among patients with CKD are stage of CKD and the length of antibiotics use, increasing the risk of CDI, whereas higher serum albumin concentration and ANSS have a principal protective impact.

Author Contributions: Conceptualization, Ł.L. and A.K.; methodology, formal analysis, Ł.L., A.K., M.S. and T.G.; investigation, Ł.L., A.C. and M.S.; resources, Ł.L., A.C. and M.S.; data curation, Ł.L., A.C., M.S. and A.K.; writing—original draft preparation, Ł.L., A.K., K.K. and T.G.; writing—review and editing, Ł.L., A.K., M.S., K.K., T.G. and Z.H.; supervision, A.K., T.G. and Z.H.; funding acquisition, A.K. All authors have read and agreed to the published version of the manuscript.

Funding: This research received no external funding.

Institutional Review Board Statement: The study was conducted according to the guidelines of the Declaration of Helsinki and approved by the Institutional Review Board of Regional Specialistic Specialist Hospital in Wroclaw (KB 32/2020).

Informed Consent Statement: Informed consent was obtained from all subjects involved in the study.

Data Availability Statement: Data are contained within the article.

Conflicts of Interest: The authors declare no conflict of interest.

References

1. Czepiel, J.; Dróżdż, M.; Pituch, H.; Kuijper, E.J.; Perucki, W.; Mielimonka, A.; Goldman, S.; Wultańska, D.; Garlicki, A.; Biesiada, G. *Clostridium difficile* infection: Review. *Eur. J. Clin. Microbiol.* **2019**, *38*, 1211–1221. [CrossRef] [PubMed]
2. McDonald, L.C.; Gerding, D.N.; Johnson, S.; Bakken, J.S.; Carroll, K.C.; Coffin, S.E.; Dubberke, E.R.; Garey, K.W.; Gould, C.V.; Kelly, C.; et al. Clinical Practice Guidelines for *Clostridium difficile* Infection in Adults and Children: 2017 Update by the Infectious Diseases Society of America (IDSA) and Society for Healthcare Epidemiology of America (SHEA). *Clin. Infect. Dis.* **2018**, *66*, e1–e48. [CrossRef] [PubMed]
3. Leffler, D.A.; Lamont, J.T. *Clostridium difficile* Infection. *N. Engl. J. Med.* **2015**, *373*, 287–288. [CrossRef] [PubMed]

guidelines do not offer guidance on the use of metronidazole (MNZ), which was previously advocated as first-line therapy for CDI. Nonetheless, MNZ has long been employed in CDI treatment due to its cost-effectiveness compared to VCM and its reduced likelihood of promoting VCM-resistant organisms. Japanese and Australian CDI guidelines recommend MNZ as the first-line therapy for non-severe CDI [8,9].

A retrospective nationwide cohort study demonstrated no improvement in treatment failure or probable recurrence between the pre- and post-guideline cohorts in the US, wherein MNZ usage was reduced [10]. Unfortunately, real-world comparative studies assessing the clinical efficacy of MNZ and FDX, along with their associated recurrence rates, remain limited. Thus, further research is necessary to determine the optimal treatment strategy for CDI.

This study aimed to comprehensively evaluate the clinical efficacy of FDX and oral MNZ in the treatment of CDI and the associated recurrence rates. By directly comparing these two treatment modalities, we aimed to elucidate the potential advantages and disadvantages of each regimen, which might aid clinicians in making informed decisions regarding CDI management.

2. Results

During the study period, 264 patients were assessed for eligibility (Figure 1). Of these, 166 were excluded based on the exclusion criteria. Thus, 105 patients were included in this study. Of these, 75 and 30 were assigned to the oral MNZ and FDX groups, respectively. The demographic and baseline characteristics of the study population are shown in Table 1. In both groups, the median age was 76 years, and most patients were male. The two groups were well matched in terms of baseline characteristics such as age, sex, and comorbidities. Patient conditions at the time of CDI diagnosis, such as body temperature, bowel movements, and bloody stool, were similar in both groups. Intergroup differences in hospitalization within the past 1 year, use of enteral feeding, a history of abdominal surgery, and the types of antimicrobials used were not significant. The FDX group had a significantly higher proportion of patients using potassium-competitive acid blockers (FDX, 36.7% vs. MNZ, 8.0%, $p < 0.01$), whereas the MNZ group had a significantly higher proportion of patients using probiotics before CDI diagnosis (MNZ, 18.7% vs. FDX, 3.3%, $p = 0.04$). The proportions of non-severe cases based on the IDSA/SHEA criteria were 70.7% and 60.0% in the MNZ and FDX groups, respectively ($p = 0.29$). The rates of intensive care unit admission at the time of CDI diagnosis were similar between the two groups.

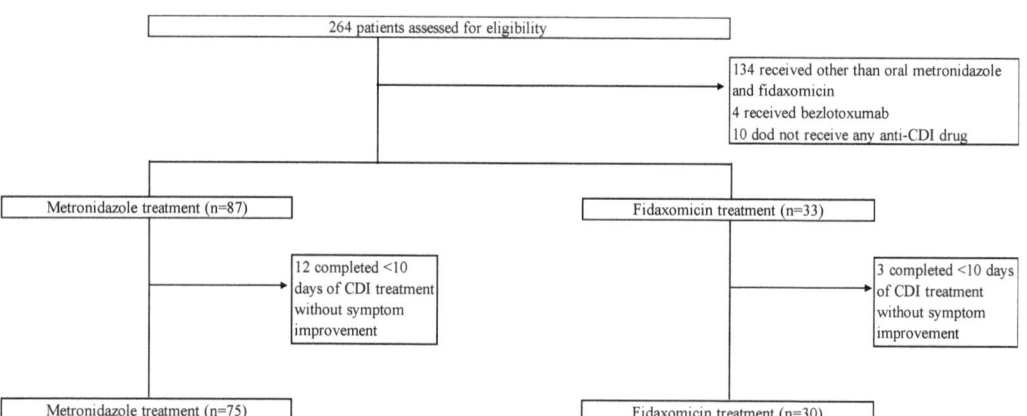

Figure 1. Study flow chart.

Table 1. Baseline characteristics of patients having CDI with and without recurrence.

Variables	Total (n = 105)	Metronidazole Group (n = 75)	Fidaxomicin Group (n = 30)	p-Value
Age (years), median (IQR)	76 (68–83)	76 (70–85)	76 (57–81)	0.17
Female sex, no. (%)	49 (46.7)	36 (48.0)	13 (43.3)	0.83
Body mass index, median (IQR)	18.4 (16.4–21.3)	18.3 (16.4–20.5)	18.5 (16.8–22.0)	0.26
Temperature at the time of CDI diagnosis, median (IQR)	37.6 (37.1–38.2)	37.7 (37.1–38.2)	37.6 (37.1–38.2)	0.82
Bowel movements at the time of CDI diagnosis, median (IQR)	4 (3–7)	4 (3–7)	4 (3–6)	0.93
Bloody stool at the time of CDI diagnosis, median (IQR)	12 (11.4)	10 (13.3)	2 (6.7)	0.33
Comorbidities, no. (%)				
Diabetes mellitus	36 (34.3)	24 (32.0)	12 (40.0)	0.50
Chronic kidney disease	28 (25.7)	16 (21.3)	12 (40.0)	0.09
Heart failure/ischemic heart disease	25 (23.8)	17 (22.7)	8 (26.7)	0.80
Chronic liver disease	2 (1.9)	1 (1.3)	1 (3.3)	0.50
Chronic obstructive pulmonary disease	7 (6.7)	5 (6.7)	2 (6.7)	1.00
Cerebrovascular disease	25 (23.8)	21 (28.0)	4 (13.3)	0.13
Inflammatory bowel disease	4 (3.8)	3 (4.0)	1 (3.3)	1.00
Solid malignancy	26 (24.8)	17 (22.7)	9 (30.0)	0.46
Hematologic malignancy	6 (5.7)	5 (6.7)	1 (3.3)	0.67
Enteral feeding, no. (%)	24 (22.9)	20 (26.7)	4 (13.3)	0.20
Past hospitalization within 1 year, no. (%)	61 (58.1)	40 (53.3)	21 (70.0)	0.13
History of abdominal surgery, no. (%)	23 (21.9)	13 (17.3)	10 (33.3)	0.12
ICU admission at the time of CDI diagnosis, no. (%)	10 (9.5)	8 (19.7)	2 (6.7)	0.72
Non-severe CDI, no. (%)				
IDSA/SHEA criteria	71 (67.6)	53 (70.7)	18 (60.0)	0.35
Laboratory data, median (IQR)				
White blood cell count (/μL)	9100 (5500–12,700)	8000 (5000–11,600)	10,550 (5800–14,500)	0.05
Albumin (mg/dL)	2.4 (2.1–2.9)	2.4 (2.2–2.8)	2.5 (1.6–3.1)	0.98
Creatinine (mg/dL)	0.74 (0.5–1.46)	0.7 (0.48–1)	0.8 (0.54–1.61)	0.30
C-reactive protein (mg/dL)	4.1 (1.3–7.0)	4.01 (1.18–7.05)	4.44 (1.27–6.78)	0.44
Antibiotics, no. (%)				
Penicillin	3 (2.9)	2 (2.7)	1 (3.3)	1.00
Cephalosporin	52 (49.5)	33 (44.0)	19 (63.0)	0.09
Carbapenem	24 (22.9)	17 (22.7)	7 (23.3)	1.00
Fluoroquinolone	13 (12.4)	8 (10.7)	5 (16.7)	0.51
Clindamycin	1 (0.9)	1 (1.3)	0 (0.0)	1.00
β-Lactam/β-Lactamase inhibitor	60 (57.1)	44 (58.7)	16 (53.3)	0.67
Antiviral agents	6 (5.7)	6 (8.0)	0 (0.0)	0.18
Antifungal agents	5 (4.8)	5 (6.7)	0 (0.0)	0.32
Concomitant medication use, no. (%)				
PPIs	49 (46.7)	35 (46.7)	14 (46.7)	1.00
H2RAs	5 (4.8)	5 (6.7)	0 (0.0)	0.32
P-CABs	17 (16.2)	6 (8.0)	11 (36.7)	0.001
Immunosuppression therapy	20 (19.0)	13 (17.3)	7 (23.3)	0.58
Anticancer chemotherapy	7 (6.7)	5 (6.7)	2 (6.7)	1.00
Probiotics used before CDI diagnosis, no. (%)	40 (38.1)	27 (36.0)	13 (43.3)	0.51

CDI: *Clostridioides difficile* infection; IQR: interquartile range; ICU: intensive care unit; PPI: proton pump inhibitor; H2RA: histamine 2 blocker; P-CAB: potassium-competitive acid blocker.

In the univariate analysis, there was no difference in the primary outcome, i.e., the global cure rate between the MNZ and FDX groups (53.3% vs. 70.0%, $p = 0.12$). Furthermore, the groups did not differ in terms of clinical cure (78.7% (MNZ) vs. 86.7% (FDX), $p = 0.35$), recurrence rate (25.3% (MNZ) vs. 16.7% (FDX), $p = 0.34$), and cause of death within 30 days (1.4% (MNZ) vs. 3.4% (FDX), $p = 0.50$) (Table 2). However, there were significantly more first-line drug changes during CDI treatment in the MNZ group than in the FDX group (18.7% vs. 0.0%, $p = 0.01$). In the MNZ group, 12 patients were switched to VCM or FDX after the initial treatment failed, and 2 were switched to intravenous MNZ. Two patients in the MNZ group were switched to vancomycin due to adverse events. These events included nausea and a decrease in blood count. No adverse events were observed in the FDX group.

Table 2. Outcomes of metronidazole and fidaxomicin treatments for CDI.

Variables	Metronidazole Group (n = 75)	Fidaxomicin Group (n = 30)	p-Value
Global cure, no. (%)	40 (53.3)	21 (70.0)	0.13
Clinical cure, no. (%)	59 (78.7)	26 (86.7)	0.42
Recurrence, no. (%)	19 (25.3)	5 (16.7)	0.44
Change in the initial CDI treatment, no. (%)	14 (18.7)	0 (0.0)	0.01
Adverse effect, no. (%)	2 (2.7)	0 (0.0)	1.00
All-cause mortality within 30 days, no. (%)	1 (1.4)	1 (3.4)	0.49

CDI: *Clostridioides difficile* infection.

The global and non-global cure rates for all patients are compared in Table 3. Although the non-global cure group had a significantly higher proportion of patients with hematological malignancies (p = 0.003), there were no significant differences in other factors between the groups. In multivariate analysis of the global cure rate in the total population, FDX treatment, severe CDI, proton pump inhibitor (PPI) use, and age were not associated with a global cure (Table 4).

Table 3. Comparison of global cure and non-global cure in patients with CDI.

Variables	Global Cure Group (n = 61)	Non-Global Cure Group (n = 44)	p-Value
Age (years), median (IQR)	77 (70–84)	76 (66–86)	0.93
Male sex, no. (%)	36 (59.0)	20 (45.5)	0.23
Body mass index, median (IQR)	18.3 (16.2–20.4)	18.6 (16.1–21.2)	0.76
Temperature at the time of CDI diagnosis, median (IQR)	37.4 (36.3–38.5)	37.9 (37.2–38.6)	0.09
Bowel movements at the time of CDI diagnosis, median (IQR)	4 (2.5–5.5)	5 (2.5–7.5)	0.08
Bloody stool at the time of CDI diagnosis, no. (%)	8 (13.1)	4 (9.1)	0.76
Comorbidities, no. (%)			
Diabetes mellitus	19 (31.1)	17 (38.6)	0.53
Chronic kidney disease	16 (26.2)	12 (27.3)	1.00
Heart failure/ischemic heart disease	15 (24.6)	10 (22.7)	1.00
Chronic liver disease	2 (3.3)	0 (0.0)	0.50
Chronic obstructive pulmonary disease	3 (4.9)	4 (9.1)	0.45
Cerebrovascular disease	14 (23.0)	11 (25.0)	0.82
Inflammatory bowel disease	3 (4.9)	1 (2.3)	0.64
Solid malignancy	14 (23.0)	12 (27.3)	0.65
Hematologic malignancy	0 (0.0)	6 (13.6)	0.004
Enteral feeding, no. (%)	10 (16.4)	51 (83.6)	0.10
Past hospitalization within 1 year, no. (%)	35 (57.4)	26 (59.1)	1.00
History of abdominal surgery, no. (%)	14 (23.0)	9 (20.5)	0.82
ICU admission at the time of CDI diagnosis, no. (%)	5 (50.0)	56 (91.8)	0.74
Severe CDI, no. (%)	18 (29.5)	16 (36.4)	0.53
Antibiotics, no. (%)			
Penicillin	1 (1.7)	2 (4.5)	0.57
Cephalosporin	31 (59.6)	30 (56.6)	0.84
Carbapenem	10 (41.7)	51 (63.0)	0.10
Fluoroquinolone	7 (11.5)	6 (13.6)	0.77
Clindamycin	0 (0.0)	1 (2.3)	0.42
β-Lactam/β-Lactamase inhibitor	36 (59.0)	24 (54.5)	0.69
Antiviral agents	4 (6.6)	2 (4.5)	1.00
Antifungal agents	2 (3.3)	3 (6.8)	0.65
Concomitant medication use, no. (%)			
PPIs	30 (49.2)	19 (43.2)	0.56
H2RAs	3 (4.9)	2 (4.5)	1.00
P-CAB	12 (19.7)	5 (11.4)	0.29
Immunosuppression therapy	10 (16.4)	10 (22.7)	0.46
Anticancer chemotherapy	3 (4.9)	4 (9.1)	0.45
Probiotics, no. (%)	21 (34.4)	19 (43.2)	0.42
FDX treatment, no. (%)	21 (34.4)	9 (20.5)	0.13

CDI: *Clostridioides difficile* infection; IQR: interquartile range; ICU: intensive care unit; PPI: proton pump inhibitor; H2RA: histamine 2 blocker; P-CAB: potassium-competitive acid blocker.

Table 4. Multivariable analysis of factors associated with the global cure of *Clostridioides difficile* infection.

Variable	Odds Ratio	95% CI	p-Value
Fidaxomicin treatment	1.49	0.94–2.37	0.09
Age	1.01	0.98–1.04	0.66
Severe *Clostridioides difficile* infection	0.68	0.29–1.58	0.37
Use of proton pump inhibitor	1.24	0.56–2.77	0.6

3. Discussion

This retrospective study showed no significant difference between the FDX and oral MNZ treatments in terms of global cure rates in the univariate analysis, although the global cure rate tended to be higher in the FDX treatment group than in the MNZ treatment group. The multivariate analysis did not reveal a significant increase in the global cure rate associated with FDX treatment. Notably, approximately 19% of patients in the MNZ group were switched to other agents during the treatment period because of treatment failure. These findings provide a basis for understanding the comparative efficacy of FDX and oral MNZ in CDI treatment.

The clinical cure and recurrence rates were better in the FDX group than in the MNZ group; however, these differences were not significant. The multivariate analysis revealed that FDX treatment compared to oral MNZ treatment did not significantly affect the global cure rate. Since WBC, which is included in the IDSA/SHEA severity criteria, was significantly higher in the FDX group than in the MNZ group, it is important to consider the possibility that many patients may have been severely ill despite not meeting the severity criteria. Potassium-competitive acid blocker (P-CAB) users were also statistically more prevalent in the FDX group than the MNZ group; P-CABs have been reported to cause more changes in intestinal flora than PPIs [11], which might have influenced the treatment response. Literature searches conducted using PubMed, Google Scholar, and Web of Science did not reveal any direct studies comparing FDX and oral MNZ. However, some studies have compared FDX and VCM, as well as MNZ and VCM, for the treatment of CDI. Several studies have evaluated the clinical efficacy of FDX versus MNZ for CDI treatment through indirect comparisons and meta-network analyses [12–14]. A meta-network analysis showed a significant difference in favor of FDX compared with MNZ for sustained cure (clinical cure without recurrence) (odds ratio (OR): 2.39; 95% CI: 1.65–3.47), clinical cure (OR: 1.77; 95% CI: 1.11–2.83), and recurrence (OR: 0.44; 95% CI: 0.27–0.72) [12]. However, another meta-analysis and indirect treatment comparison revealed that FDX led to improved sustained cure rates (clinical cure without recurrence during follow-up; OR: 2.55; 95% CI: 1.44–4.51) and recurrence rates (OR: 0.42; 95% CI: 0.18–0.96) in patients with CDI compared to MNZ. Nevertheless, the intergroup difference in clinical cure was not significant [14]. Additionally, a meta-analysis of real-world data demonstrated no significant differences in recurrence rates between the two groups (OR: 0.71; 95% CI: 0.05–9.47) [13]. While considering differences in study methods and heterogeneity among the articles, it is noteworthy that FDX did not show markedly different results, and there was variability in the findings. Although MNZ treatment has been associated with poorer outcomes compared to VCM treatment, a large cohort study [15] reported that the clinical outcomes achieved with MNZ were comparable to those with VCM if the patients had non-severe CDI and were younger than 65 years, suggesting that oral MNZ may be as effective as other CDI treatment drugs depending on the patient's background. Therefore, the initial treatment drug for CDI may not necessarily be FDX; however, it may be selected later based on indications, patient background, and economic considerations.

Our findings suggest the need for caution in the therapeutic management of CDI by using oral MNZ. Although there was no significant difference in the global cure rate between the oral MNZ and FDX groups in this study, it should be considered that the initial treatment failed in approximately 18% of the patients in the MNZ group, resulting in a change in the treatment drug. Previous retrospective cohort studies showed that the rate of switching from MNZ to VCM was 15.9–32% [16,17]. There are several possible reasons for the failure of the initial treatment with oral MNZ. First, the systemic bioavailability of oral MNZ is very high (>90%) [18], with most of it readily absorbed in the gastrointestinal tract, and the drug does not reach particularly high concentrations in the intestinal lumen itself. In contrast, FDX is poorly absorbed from the intestinal tract, and one study reported mean fecal concentrations more than 5000 times the minimum inhibitory concentration of 0.25 µg/mL against *C. difficile* [19]. Notably, the effect of FDX persists on *C. difficile* spores, preventing subsequent growth and toxin production in vitro [20], whereas MNZ does not. Second, the percentage of *C. difficile* strains with reduced susceptibility to MNZ has gradually increased globally [21]. According to a pan-European longitudinal surveillance study, between 2011 and 2012, 18% of *C. difficile* clinical isolates were resistant to MNZ (based on the European Committee on Antimicrobial Susceptibility Testing breakpoint) [22]. However, it is worth noting that *C. difficile* strains resistant to MNZ have never been isolated in Japan [23–25], and there have been limited reports of *C. difficile* strains resistant to FDX [26]. Therefore, the effect of MNZ-resistant bacteria on treatment failure in our study was likely small. In cases where the response to initial treatment with oral MNZ is poor, immediate consideration should be given to making necessary changes.

This study has some limitations. First, because this was a single-center retrospective study, the number of patients analyzed was small. Second, it has inherent limitations such as potential selection bias and confounding factors that could not be accounted for. Third, we were unable to assess the differences in the therapeutic efficacy against strains because ribotyping analysis was not performed in this study, although there have been a few reports on ribotype 027 strain isolates in Japan [27]. Despite these limitations, there have been no reports comparing the therapeutic outcomes of FDX and oral MNZ treatments for CDI. Therefore, this study will help clinicians make informed decisions regarding the management of CDI.

In conclusion, both FDX and oral MNZ demonstrated comparable therapeutic efficacy as initial therapy for CDI. MNZ could potentially serve as a suitable treatment option for initial CDI. However, it necessitates more careful observation since some patients may experience treatment failure and require a change in medication. Further investigations with larger patient cohorts are warranted to thoroughly compare the efficacy of both treatment approaches.

4. Materials and Methods

4.1. Study Design

This study used a retrospective cohort design and involved the use of the medical records of patients diagnosed with CDI between January 2015 and March 2023 at Aichi Medical University Hospital, a 900-bed tertiary-care hospital located in Aichi, Japan. Ethical approval was granted by the institutional review board of Aichi Medical University (2023-042). Patients ≥ 2 years old with symptomatic primary CDI who were treated with either FDX or oral MNZ were included. Patients were excluded if they died during CDI treatment or did not show improvement in CDI symptoms and were treated in <10 days or received bezlotoxumab.

The following data were collected from the patient's electronic medical records: age; sex; body mass index; body temperature and bowel movements at the time of CDI diagnosis; bloody stool; nutrition mode (whether enteral tube feeding was used or not); underlying disease; past hospitalization within 1 year; history of abdominal surgery; intensive care unit admission at the time of CDI diagnosis; laboratory data (white blood cell (WBC) counts and levels of albumin, creatinine (Cr), and C-reactive protein); type of antibiotics administered within 2 months of CDI diagnosis; use of acid suppressants (histamine 2 blockers, PPIs, and potassium-competitive acid blockers), immunosuppressants, anticancer drugs, and prescribed probiotics; severity of CDI; change in anti-CDI medication from the initial treatment; clinical cure; recurrence; and all-cause mortality within 30 days after CDI diagnosis.

4.2. Outcomes

The primary outcome was the difference in the global cure rates of CDI between FDX and MNZ. The secondary outcome was the identification of factors associated with the global cure of patients with CDI as determined using multivariate logistic regression. A systematic review [28] and network meta-analysis [12] showed that advanced age, the use of PPIs, severe CDI, and anti-CDI treatment were associated with poor CDI prognosis. Therefore, these factors were included as explanatory variables. In addition, the rate of medication change due to initial treatment failure and incidence rates of clinical cure, recurrence, adverse effects, and all-cause mortality within 30 days were recorded.

4.3. Variable Definition

CDI was defined as follows: (1) the presence of ≥ 3 diarrheal bowel movements (type 5–7 stool on the Bristol Stool Scale) in the 24 h preceding stool collection, or diarrhea plus patient-reported abdominal pain or cramping, and (2) a positive result for *C. difficile* toxins in a rapid immunoenzyme test for glutamate dehydrogenase (GDH) and a toxin assay (C. DIFF QUIK CHEK COMPLETE; TechLab, Blacksburg, VA, USA or GE Test Immunochromato-CD GDH/TOX; Nissui Pharmaceutical Co., Ltd., Tokyo, Japan) or polymerase chain reaction of the toxin B gene using the Cepheid GeneXpert *C. difficile* Assay (Beckman Coulter Inc., Tokyo, Japan). The C. DIFF QUIK CHEK COMPLETE kit (TechLab) was used between January 2015 and March 2022, whereas the GE test immunochromatography-CD GDH/TOX was used from March 2023. Severe CDI was defined as a WBC count of >15,000 cells/mL or serum Cr level of ≥ 1.5 mg/dL based on the guidelines released by the IDSA and SHEA [5]. Global cure was defined as clinical cure, no recurrence, and no change in medication owing to a poor response to the initial treatment during the treatment period. We defined the global cure rate as the percentage of patients who completed treatment with MNZ and FDX and met the criteria for global cure. Clinical cure was defined as an improvement in stool characteristics within 2 days of the end of CDI treatment. Recurrent CDI was defined as the re-administration of the initial treatment for diarrhea and a confirmatory positive test up to 8 weeks after the treatment of the initial CDI episode.

4.4. Statistical Analysis

Discrete variables such as age are expressed as medians and interquartile ranges (IQRs). Mann–Whitney U and Fisher's exact tests were used for continuous and two categorical variables, respectively. The significance level was set at 0.05, and a p-value < 0.05 was considered statistically significant. Stata version 14.2 (STATA Inc., College Station, TX, USA) was used for statistical analyses.

Author Contributions: N.M.: data curation, formal analysis, and writing—original draft. J.H.: data curation and writing—review and editing. W.O.: formal analysis and methodology and writing—review and editing. N.A.: writing—review and editing. Y.S.: writing—review and editing. H.M.: writing—review and editing, and supervision. All authors have read and agreed to the published version of the manuscript.

Funding: This research received no external funding.

Institutional Review Board Statement: Ethical approval was granted by the institutional review board of Aichi Medical University (2023-042).

Informed Consent Statement: The need for patient consent was waived owing to this study's retrospective nature. An online opt-out option was clearly described and made available to all patients.

Data Availability Statement: The data presented in this study are available on request from the corresponding author.

Conflicts of Interest: N.M., J.H., W.O., N.A., and Y.S. have no conflicts of interest. H.M. received research funding from Asahi Kasei Pharma Corporation, FUJIFILM Toyama Chemical Co., Ltd., Shionogi & Co., Ltd., Daiichi Sankyo Co., Ltd., and Sumitomo Dainippon Pharma Co., Ltd.

References

1. Liu, C.; Monaghan, T.; Yadegar, A.; Louie, T.; Kao, D. Insights into the Evolving Epidemiology of *Clostridioides difficile* Infection and Treatment: A Global Perspective. *Antibiotics* **2023**, *12*, 1141. [CrossRef] [PubMed]
2. Lessa, F.C.; Mu, Y.; Bamberg, W.M.; Beldavs, Z.G.; Dumyati, G.K.; Dunn, J.R.; Farley, M.M.; Holzbauer, S.M.; Meek, J.I.; Phipps, E.C.; et al. Burden of *Clostridium difficile* Infection in the United States. *N. Engl. J. Med.* **2015**, *372*, 825–834. [CrossRef]
3. Guh, A.Y.; Mu, Y.; Winston, L.G.; Johnston, H.; Olson, D.; Farley, M.M.; Wilson, L.E.; Holzbauer, S.M.; Phipps, E.C.; Dumyati, G.K.; et al. Trends in U.S. Burden of *Clostridioides difficile* Infection and Outcomes. *N. Engl. J. Med.* **2020**, *382*, 1320–1330. [CrossRef] [PubMed]
4. Zhang, D.; Prabhu, V.S.; Marcella, S.W. Attributable Healthcare Resource Utilization and Costs for Patients with Primary and Recurrent *Clostridium difficile* Infection in the United States. *Clin. Infect. Dis.* **2018**, *66*, 1326–1332. [CrossRef]
5. Johnson, S.; Lavergne, V.; Skinner, A.M.; Gonzales-Luna, A.J.; Garey, K.W.; Kelly, C.P.; Wilcox, M.H. Clinical Practice Guideline by the Infectious Diseases Society of America (IDSA) and Society for Healthcare Epidemiology of America (SHEA): 2021 Focused Update Guidelines on Management of *Clostridioides difficile* Infection in Adults. *Clin. Infect. Dis.* **2021**, *73*, 755–757. [CrossRef] [PubMed]
6. Louie, T.J.; Miller, M.A.; Mullane, K.M.; Weiss, K.; Lentnek, A.; Golan, Y.; Gorbach, S.; Sears, P.; Shue, Y.-K. Fidaxomicin versus Vancomycin for *Clostridium difficile* Infection. *N. Engl. J. Med.* **2011**, *364*, 422–431. [CrossRef]
7. Cornely, O.A.; Crook, D.W.; Esposito, R.; Poirier, A.; Somero, M.S.; Weiss, K.; Sears, P.; Gorbach, S.; for the OPT-80-004 Clinical Study Group. Fidaxomicin versus Vancomycin for Infection with *Clostridium difficile* in Europe, Canada, and the USA: A Double-Blind, Non-Inferiority, Randomised Controlled Trial. *Lancet Infect. Dis.* **2012**, *12*, 281–289. [CrossRef]
8. Kunishima, H.; Ohge, H.; Suzuki, H.; Nakamura, A.; Matsumoto, K.; Mikamo, H.; Mori, N.; Morinaga, Y.; Yanagihara, K.; Yamagishi, Y.; et al. Japanese Clinical Practice Guidelines for Management of Clostridioides (Clostridium) Difficile Infection. *J. Infect. Chemother.* **2022**, *28*, 1045–1083. [CrossRef]
9. Trubiano, J.A.; Cheng, A.C.; Korman, T.M.; Roder, C.; Campbell, A.; May, M.L.A.; Blyth, C.C.; Ferguson, J.K.; Blackmore, T.K.; Riley, T.V.; et al. Australasian Society of Infectious Diseases Updated Guidelines for the Management of *Clostridium difficile* Infection in Adults and Children in Australia and New Zealand. *Intern. Med. J.* **2016**, *46*, 479–493. [CrossRef]
10. Gentry, C.A.; Campbell, D.L.; Williams, R.J., II. Outcomes Associated with Recent Guideline Recommendations Removing Metronidazole for Treatment of Non-Severe *Clostridioides difficile* Infection: A Retrospective, Observational, Nationwide Cohort Study. *Int. J. Antimicrob. Agents* **2021**, *66*, 106282. [CrossRef]
11. Otsuka, T.; Sugimoto, M.; Inoue, R.; Ohno, M.; Ban, H.; Nishida, A.; Inatomi, O.; Takahashi, S.; Naito, Y.; Andoh, A. Influence of Potassium-Competitive Acid Blocker on the Gut Microbiome of Helicobacter Pylori-Negative Healthy Individuals. *Gut* **2017**, *66*, 1723–1725. [CrossRef] [PubMed]
12. Okumura, H.; Fukushima, A.; Taieb, V.; Shoji, S.; English, M. Fidaxomicin Compared with Vancomycin and Metronidazole for the Treatment of Clostridioides (Clostridium) Difficile Infection: A Network Meta-Analysis. *J. Infect. Chemother.* **2020**, *26*, 43–50. [CrossRef] [PubMed]
13. Dai, J.; Gong, J.; Guo, R. Real-World Comparison of Fidaxomicin versus Vancomycin or Metronidazole in the Treatment of *Clostridium difficile* Infection: A Systematic Review and Meta-Analysis. *Eur. J. Clin. Pharmacol.* **2022**, *78*, 1727–1737. [CrossRef]
14. Cornely, O.A.; Nathwani, D.; Ivanescu, C.; Odufowora-Sita, O.; Retsa, P.; Odeyemi, I.A.O. Clinical Efficacy of Fidaxomicin Compared with Vancomycin and Metronidazole in *Clostridium difficile* Infections: A Meta-Analysis and Indirect Treatment Comparison. *J. Antimicrob. Chemother.* **2014**, *69*, 2892–2900. [CrossRef]
15. Appaneal, H.J.; Caffrey, A.R.; LaPlante, K.L. What Is the Role for Metronidazole in the Treatment of *Clostridium difficile* Infection? Results From a National Cohort Study of Veterans With Initial Mild Disease. *Clin. Infect. Dis.* **2019**, *69*, 1288–1295. [CrossRef]
16. Jacobson, S.M.; Slain, D. Evaluation of a Bedside Scoring System for Predicting Clinical Cure and Recurrence of *Clostridium difficile* Infections. *Am. J. Health. Syst. Pharm.* **2015**, *72*, 1871–1875. [CrossRef] [PubMed]
17. Sugimoto, H.; Yoshihara, A.; Yamamoto, T.; Sugimoto, K. A Preliminary Study of Bowel Rest Strategy in the Management of *Clostridioides difficile* Infection. *Sci. Rep.* **2020**, *10*, 22061. [CrossRef] [PubMed]
18. Lamp, K.C.; Freeman, C.D.; Klutman, N.E.; Lacy, M.K. Pharmacokinetics and Pharmacodynamics of the Nitroimidazole Antimicrobials. *Clin. Pharmacokinet.* **1999**, *36*, 353–373. [CrossRef]
19. Sears, P.; Crook, D.W.; Louie, T.J.; Miller, M.A.; Weiss, K. Fidaxomicin Attains High Fecal Concentrations with Minimal Plasma Concentrations Following Oral Administration in Patients with *Clostridium difficile* Infection. *Clin. Infect. Dis.* **2012**, *55* (Suppl. S2), S116–S120. [CrossRef]
20. Chilton, C.H.; Crowther, G.S.; Ashwin, H.; Longshaw, C.M.; Wilcox, M.H. Association of Fidaxomicin with *C. difficile* Spores: Effects of Persistence on Subsequent Spore Recovery, Outgrowth and Toxin Production. *PLoS ONE* **2016**, *11*, e0161200. [CrossRef]
21. Spigaglia, P. Recent Advances in the Understanding of Antibiotic Resistance in *Clostridium difficile* Infection. *Ther. Adv. Infect. Dis.* **2016**, *3*, 23–42. [CrossRef]
22. Freeman, J.; Vernon, J.; Morris, K.; Nicholson, S.; Todhunter, S.; Longshaw, C.; Wilcox, M.H.; Pan-European Longitudinal Surveillance of Antibiotic Resistance among Prevalent *Clostridium difficile* Ribotypes' Study Group. Pan-European Longitudinal Surveillance of Antibiotic Resistance among Prevalent *Clostridium difficile* Ribotypes. *Clin. Microbiol. Infect.* **2015**, *21*, 248.e9–248.e16. [CrossRef]

23. Aoki, K.; Takeda, S.; Miki, T.; Ishii, Y.; Tateda, K. Antimicrobial Susceptibility and Molecular Characterisation Using Whole-Genome Sequencing of *Clostridioides difficile* Collected in 82 Hospitals in Japan between 2014 and 2016. *Antimicrob. Agents Chemother.* **2019**, *63*, 10–1128. [CrossRef] [PubMed]
24. Kunishima, H.; Chiba, J.; Saito, M.; Honda, Y.; Kaku, M. Antimicrobial Susceptibilities of *Clostridium difficile* Isolated in Japan. *J. Infect. Chemother.* **2013**, *19*, 360–362. [CrossRef]
25. Kato, H.; Senoh, M.; Honda, H.; Fukuda, T.; Tagashira, Y.; Horiuchi, H.; Chiba, H.; Suzuki, D.; Hosokawa, N.; Kitazono, H.; et al. Clostridioides (Clostridium) Difficile Infection Burden in Japan: A Multicenter Prospective Study. *Anaerobe* **2019**, *60*, 102011. [CrossRef]
26. Freeman, J.; Vernon, J.; Pilling, S.; Morris, K.; Nicolson, S.; Shearman, S.; Clark, E.; Palacios-Fabrega, J.A.; Wilcox, M.; Pan-European Longitudinal Surveillance of Antibiotic Resistance among Prevalent *Clostridium difficile* Ribotypes' Study Group. Five-Year Pan-European, Longitudinal Surveillances of *Clostridium difficile* Ribotype Prevalence and Antimicrobial Resistance: The Extended ClosER Study. *Eur. J. Clin. Microbiol. Infect. Dis.* **2020**, *39*, 169–177. [CrossRef] [PubMed]
27. Senoh, M.; Kato, H. Molecular Epidemiology of Endemic *Clostridioides difficile* Infection in Japan. *Anaerobe* **2022**, *74*, 102510. [CrossRef] [PubMed]
28. van Rossen, T.M.; Ooijevaar, R.E.; Vandenbroucke-Grauls, C.M.J.E.; Dekkers, O.M.; Kuijper, E.J.; Keller, J.J.; van Prehn, J. Prognostic Factors for Severe and Recurrent *Clostridioides difficile* Infection: A Systematic Review. *Clin. Microbiol. Infect.* **2022**, *28*, 321–331. [CrossRef] [PubMed]

Disclaimer/Publisher's Note: The statements, opinions and data contained in all publications are solely those of the individual author(s) and contributor(s) and not of MDPI and/or the editor(s). MDPI and/or the editor(s) disclaim responsibility for any injury to people or property resulting from any ideas, methods, instructions or products referred to in the content.

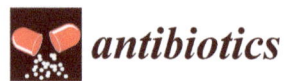

Review

Clostridioides Difficile Enteritis: Case Report and Literature Review

Artsiom Klimko [1,†], Cristian George Tieranu [2,3,*,†], Ana-Maria Curte [4], Carmen Monica Preda [2,5], Ioana Tieranu [6], Andrei Ovidiu Olteanu [2,3] and Elena Mirela Ionescu [2,3]

1. Division of Physiology and Neuroscience, "Carol Davila" University of Medicine and Pharmacy, 050747 Bucharest, Romania; artsiom.klimko@stud.umfcd.ro
2. Department of Gastroenterology, "Carol Davila" University of Medicine and Pharmacy, 020021 Bucharest, Romania; carmenmonica.preda@gmail.com (C.M.P.); dr.olteanuandrei@gmail.com (A.O.O.); mirela.ionescu@umfcd.ro (E.M.I.)
3. Department of Gastroenterology, "Elias" Emergency University Hospital, 011461 Bucharest, Romania
4. Department of Pathology, "Elias" Emergency University Hospital, 011461 Bucharest, Romania; anma.pop@gmail.com
5. Department of Gastroenterology, Fundeni Clinical Institute, 022328 Bucharest, Romania
6. Department of Pediatrics, "Carol Davila" University of Medicine and Pharmacy, 020021 Bucharest, Romania; Ioana.tieranu1@drd.umfcd.ro
* Correspondence: cristian.tieranu@umfcd.ro; Tel.: +40-765-490-005
† These authors contributed equally to this work.

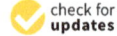

Citation: Klimko, A.; Tieranu, C.G.; Curte, A.-M.; Preda, C.M.; Tieranu, I.; Olteanu, A.O.; Ionescu, E.M. Clostridioides Difficile Enteritis: Case Report and Literature Review. *Antibiotics* 2022, 11, 206. https://doi.org/10.3390/antibiotics11020206

Academic Editor: Guido Granata

Received: 2 January 2022
Accepted: 2 February 2022
Published: 6 February 2022

Publisher's Note: MDPI stays neutral with regard to jurisdictional claims in published maps and institutional affiliations.

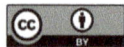

Copyright: © 2022 by the authors. Licensee MDPI, Basel, Switzerland. This article is an open access article distributed under the terms and conditions of the Creative Commons Attribution (CC BY) license (https://creativecommons.org/licenses/by/4.0/).

Abstract: Background: *Clostridioides Difficile* is a well-known pathogen causing diarrhea of various degrees of severity through associated infectious colitis. However, there have been reports of infectious enteritis mainly in patients with ileostomy, causing dehydration through high-output volume; Case presentation: We report the case of a 46-year-old male patient, malnourished, who presented with high-output ileostomy following a recent hospitalization where he had suffered an ileo-colic resection with ileal and transverse colon double ostomy, for stricturing Crohn's disease. *Clostridioides Difficile* toxin A was identified in the ileal output confirming the diagnosis of acute enteritis. Treatment with oral Vancomycin was initiated with rapid reduction of the ileostomy output volume; Conclusion: We report a case of *Clostridioides Difficile* enteral infection as a cause for high-output ileostomy, successfully treated with oral Vancomycin. We also review the existing literature data regarding this specific localized infection.

Keywords: Clostridioides difficile; enteritis; ileostomy; dehydration

1. Introduction

Clostridioides Difficile (CD) is a challenging global healthcare issue—CD is the leading cause of healthcare-associated infection, with a variable clinical course that ranges from mild disease to severe colitis and toxic megacolon with a 5.9% mortality rate [1]. Conventionally, CD is limited to the large bowel which has been attributed to molecular and physiologic differences between the small and large bowel [2]. However, there is increasing evidence indicating CD may also affect the small bowel, termed CD enteritis (CDE), which is associated with a protracted clinical course and mortality rates approaching 30% [3]. We present a case of CDE and conduct a literature review and pooled analysis of all documented CDE cases to provide contemporary information pertaining to patient characteristics, management consideration, and mortality rates.

2. Case Presentation

A 46-year-old male patient was admitted to the Gastroenterology Department of the "Elias" Emergency University Hospital in Bucharest for high-output ileostomy (approximately 1500 mL/24 h), oliguria, and diffuse colicky abdominal pain. His symptoms gradually worsened over the preceding two weeks and were accompanied by a 6 kg weight loss. He had long-standing history of neglected stricturing ileal Crohn's disease and he had undergone laparotomy for intestinal obstruction secondary to ileal strictures several weeks prior to current hospital admission. The patient was immunocompetent, with negative molecular tests for human immunodeficiency virus. Additionally, he had HLA-B27-associated ankylosing spondylitis treated sporadically with non-steroidal anti-inflammatory drugs. His family history was negative for inflammatory bowel disease (IBD) and colorectal cancer. He denied the use of illicit substances, alcohol consumption or smoking prior to the hospital admission. Upon hospitalization, he was underweight, with a body mass index of 17 kg/m^2.

Clinical examination upon admission revealed normal hemodynamic and respiratory parameters, normal temperature, with diffuse pain upon palpation without acute peritoneal signs.

Laboratory data showed mild leukocytosis (14.000/mmc) with neutrophilia, elevated C-reactive protein at 15-fold increase above the upper limit of normal (75 mg/dL, normal value < 5 mg/dL), hyperkalemia (6.3 mmol/L), hyponatremia (132 mmol/L), elevated serum urea (97 mg/dL) and creatinine levels (1.7 mg/dL). Ileal output obtained from the ostomy bag was used for further bacterial and parasitic testing. Ova and parasite analysis was performed via microscopy, as this is routine in our practice, and test was negative. Bacterial cultures were negative but enzyme immunoassays for toxins A and glutamate dehydrogenase (GDH) for the detection of CD infection (CDI) came back positive. The patient was started, immediately after diagnosis, on day 1 of hospitalization, on oral 125 mg of vancomycin dosed every 6 h and intravenous crystalloid rehydration therapy with 1000 mL Sodium Chloride 0.9% solution, supplemented with intravenous analgesics—Metamizole 1000 mg/2 mL twice daily.

Response to treatment was evaluated based on the dynamics of ileal output volume and clinical parameters such as urinary output volume and pain. Ileostomy volume was measured using a graded plastic recipient every 12 h, and daily total volumes were noted.

Ileal endoscopic evaluation was performed by introducing the gastroscope through the ileostomy orifice and advanced approximately 30 cm upwards, revealing diffuse erythema with several superficial, linear ulcerations and fibrin deposits (Figure 1a,b).

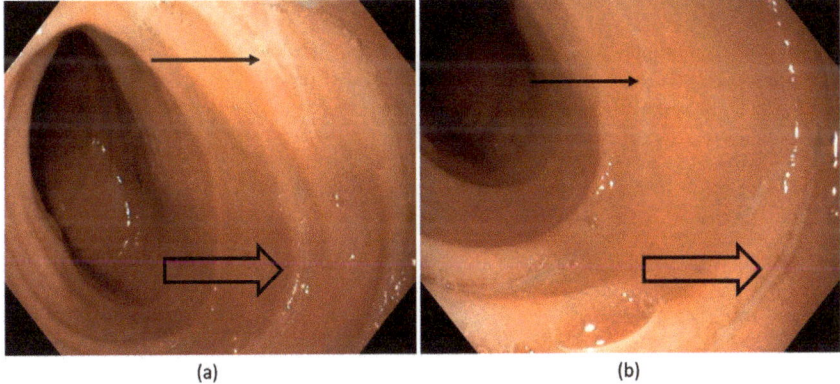

Figure 1. Small bowel endoscopy (**a**,**b**) showing diffuse ileal erythema with transverse superficial linear ulcerations (thick arrows) and fibrin deposits (small arrows).

Given the previous diagnosis of Crohn's disease, multiple biopsies were obtained for further evaluation and differential diagnosis, to exclude an underlying active Crohn's disease as a cause for high ostomy volumes.

The histological examination concluded over an acute, non-specific, moderate severity erosive enteritis based on the absence of architectural disruptions, frequent mucosal erosions, mucus depletion, fibrin deposits and intraepithelial neutrofilic infiltrate (Figure 2).

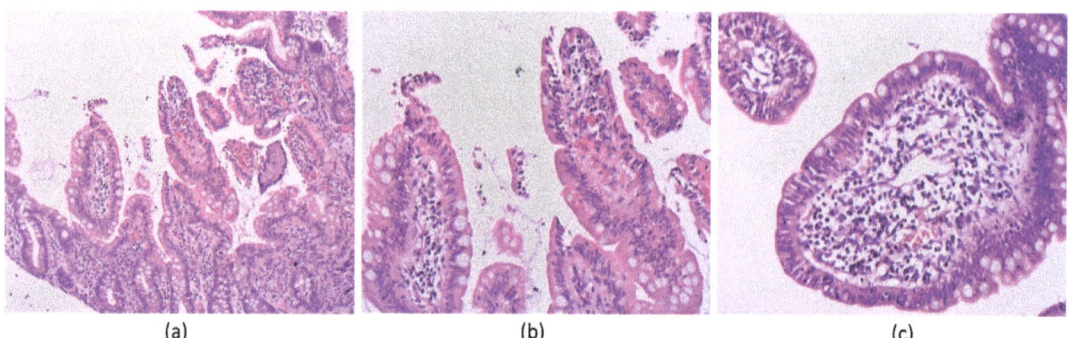

Figure 2. H&E stain, 10×. (**a**) Intestinal mucosa showing erosions, focal edema and moderate acute inflammatory infiltrate in lamina propria; (**b**), H&E stain, 20×. Intestinal mucosa showing superficial erosions, and focal edema and moderate acute inflammatory infiltrate within lamina propria; (**c**) H&E stain, 20×. Intestinal mucosa showing intraepithelial polymorphonuclear infiltrate, mucin depletion of the intestinal epithelium, edema and moderate acute inflammatory infiltrate within.

Consequently, we continued to investigate the patient with computed tomography (CT) in order to exclude intraabdominal abscess or upstream bowel lesions of active Crohn's disease, as causes for high output stoma, which showed a symmetric, diffuse thickening of the small-bowel wall, without obvious stenosis, without dilated enteric segments and no intraabdominal collections. The small-bowel vascularization on CT scan was negative for arterial or venous thromboses and the presence of the Comb sign was supportive of a local inflammatory process.

By the fourth day of treatment, the patient was rapidly recovering—the ileostomy volumes were decreasing and abdominal pain was absent. Rehydration therapy and analgesics were stopped on day 6 of treatment. In hospital evolution of altered laboratory parameters and ileal output volume are presented in Figure 3. The patient was happy to be discharged after 14 days of treatment with low-volume output (<500 mL/24 h) and normalized serum ion concentrations and renal function tests.

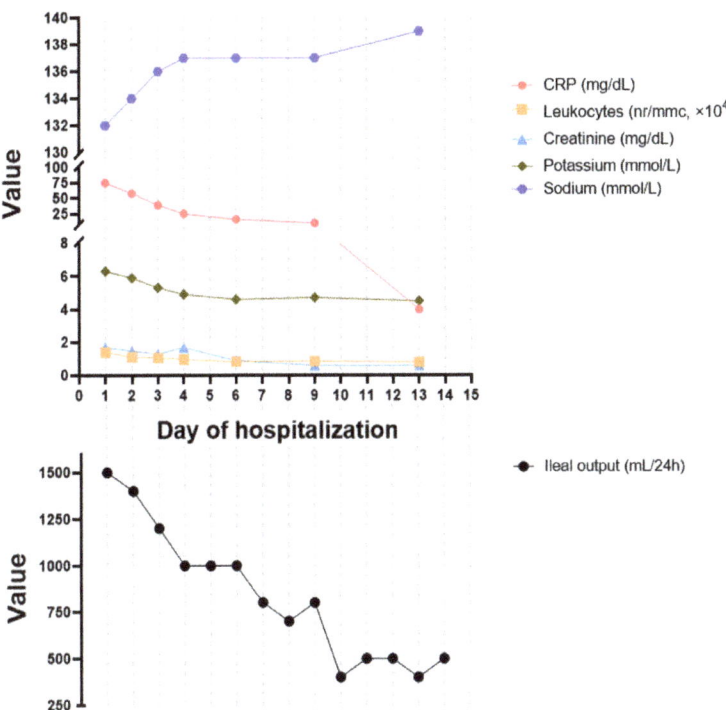

Figure 3. Evolution of relevant laboratory parameters and ileal output during hospitalization.

3. Discussion

We presented a case of CDE in a patient with previously diagnosed stricturing Crohn's disease. The particular feature of our case resides on the coexistence of IBD with CDE, especially in the postoperative setting, when high-output volume of stomas is difficult to interpret, thus making differential diagnosis of utmost importance. Moreover, there is a conventional paradigm correlating CD with colitis, this contributing to delays in diagnosis and adapted management, that can negatively impact the outcome.

In our case report, the difficulty of differential diagnosis relies on the lack of previous data regarding the small-bowel extension of Crohn's disease, upstream active disease being able to reproduce the same clinical scenario as CDE.

To further explore patient characteristics, management considerations, and outcome trajectories in patients with CDE, we conducted a literature review using the PubMed database. Key terms included "Clostridium difficile", "Clostridioides difficile", "small bowel", "enteritis", "enteral", and "pouchitis" were identified either as medical subject heading (MeSH) terms or within the title and/or abstract. All cases published in the last 20 years were included in our review for pooled analysis. Veterinary studies were excluded, as were basic science studies and articles focusing on pediatric patients (age <18 years). Per our selection strategy, 77 reported cases were identified in 49 publications and our results are presented in Table 1 [3–50].

Table 1. Pooled analysis of reviewed cases, detailing differing patient characteristics in survivors and non-survivors of CDE.

	Survived CDE (n = 54)	Did Not Survive CDE (n = 23)	p-Value
Sex			
Male	26 (48.1%)	14 (60.9%)	0.331
Female	28 (51.9%)	9 (39.1%)	
Age (Years)			
Mean (SD)	49.0 (18.6)	70.2 (10.5)	<0.001
Median [Min, Max]	49.0 [18.0, 83.0]	69.0 [53.0, 91.0]	
Inflammatory bowel disease			
Crohn's Disease	8 (14.8%)	1 (4.3%)	0.049
Ulcerative colitis	23 (42.6%)	5 (21.7%)	
None	23 (42.6%)	17 (73.9%)	
Gastrointestinal cancer (previously or concurrent)			
No	50 (92.6%)	14 (60.9%)	0.00157
Yes	4 (7.4%)	9 (39.1%)	
Recent hospitalization			
Surgical admission	42 (77.8%)	19 (82.6%)	0.903
Non-surgical admission	7 (13.0%)	3 (13.0%)	
No recent hospitalization	5 (9.3%)	1 (4.3%)	
History of surgery			
IPAA	25 (46.3%)	2 (8.7%)	0.0171
Total colectomy	7 (13.0%)	4 (17.4%)	
Hemicolectomy	6 (11.1%)	5 (21.7%)	
Non-GI	1 (1.9%)	2 (8.7%)	
Other	11 (20.4%)	7 (30.4%)	
None	4 (7.4%)	3 (13.0%)	
Concurrent CD colitis			
Yes	9 (16.7%)	4 (17.4%)	1
No	45 (83.3%)	19 (82.6%)	
Was CDE caused by surgery for which the patient was admitted?			
Yes	29 (53.7%)	14 (60.9%)	0.835
No, other surgery	16 (29.6%)	6 (26.1%)	
No, non-surgical	9 (16.7%)	3 (13.0%)	
Predisposing antibiotic use			
Yes	39 (72.2%)	16 (69.6%)	0.913
No	3 (5.6%)	2 (8.7%)	
Unknown	12 (22.2%)	5 (21.7%)	
Immunosuppressed			
Yes	15 (27.8%)	8 (34.8%)	0.894
No	29 (53.7%)	11 (47.8%)	
Unknown	10 (18.5%)	4 (17.4%)	
Treatment administered			
Metronidazole with vancomycin	24 (44.4%)	13 (56.5%)	0.626
Metronidazole	13 (24.1%)	4 (17.4%)	
Vancomycin	11 (20.4%)	2 (8.7%)	
Other	3 (5.6%)	2 (8.7%)	
Unknown	3 (5.6%)	2 (8.7%)	

Table 1. Cont.

	Survived CDE (n = 54)	Did Not Survive CDE (n = 23)	p-Value
Surgical treatment of CDE			
Yes	14 (25.9%)	9 (39.1%)	0.283
No	40 (74.1%)	14 (60.9%)	
ICU transfer			
Yes	17 (31.5%)	22 (95.7%)	<0.001
No	37 (68.5%)	1 (4.3%)	
Time to outcome (Resolution of infection or death)			
<2 weeks	27 (50.0%)	9 (39.1%)	0.766
>2 weeks	24 (44.4%)	13 (56.5%)	
Unknown	3 (5.6%)	1 (4.3%)	
Readmission			
Yes	4 (7.4%)	0 (0%)	-
No	50 (92.6%)	0 (0%)	
Not applicable	0 (0%)	23 (100%)	

CD: *Clostridioides Difficile*; CDE: *Clostridioides Difficile* enteritis; SD: standard deviation; IPAA: ileal pouch–anal anastomosis; GI: gastrointestinal; ICU: intensive care unit.

Within the identified cases, the following parameters were examined: age, sex, inflammatory bowel disease (IBD) status, gastrointestinal (GI) cancer history, recent hospitalization, previous surgery, predisposing antibiotic use, immunosuppression, treatment administered (conservative and/or surgical), intensive care unit (ICU) transfer, time to outcome (defined as either infection resolution of patient death), and readmission. In all patients, the diagnosis of CDE was confirmed via positive CD toxin assays and supplemented with either: (i) CT scans revealing inflammatory changes (e.g., bowel wall thickening, intramural air, etc.) localized to the small bowel or (ii) direct visualization of small bowel pseudomembranes. In some cases, the diagnosis was made postmortem on autopsy results, where there was histologic evidence of CDI localized to the small bowel. In a subset of patients who underwent restorative proctocolectomy with ileal pouch-anal anastomosis for IBD, CDE was treated as a diagnosis of exclusion as most patient did not have a colon. Out of 77 cases evaluated, 54 survived and 23 patients had a lethal outcome—the mortality rate of CDE in this pooled analysis is 29.8%.

For the survivors' cohort, the mean age of the patients was 49.0 years (standard deviation 18.6), and of the 54 patients, 26 were male and 28 were female. For the non-survivor cohort, the mean age of the patients was 70.2 years (standard deviation 10.5), and of the 23 patients, 14 were male and nine were female. There was a slight predilection within the survivors' cohort to have a diagnosis of IBD (57.4%)—23 (42.6%) and eight (14.8%) patients had a history of ulcerative colitis and Crohn's disease, respectively. Virtually all patients (92.2%) suffered from hospital acquired CDE, where infection arose in a backdrop of hospitalization. Statistically significant differences between the two patient groups included age, IBD diagnosis, history of prior surgery, and ICU transfer.

Given the accentuated coexistence of IBD in CDE patients, positive CDE toxin assays should aid in contrasting CDE against a flare of IBD, especially in patients with previous GI-altering surgery. Although the endoscopy results in our patients helped cement the diagnosis, indeterminate features (e.g., superficial ulcerations, fibrin deposits) could raise suspicion for prestomial Crohn's disease, with upstream disease also potentially explaining high-ouput from the ileostomy site. As such, predisposing history of recent hospitalization and antibiotics use, coupled with positive diagnostic tests for CD, may be advantageous for prompt diagnosis.

Surgery frequently initiated CDE (79.2%), where infection arose either immediately after proctocolectomy with ileostomy or after ileostomy takedown. In a minority of cases, patients had already undergone GI surgery and CDE arose independently of that initial hospitalization. GI procedures, which were implicated, include hernia repair, GU cancer-motivated resection, ileostomy closer, laparotomy for adhesiolysis, selective vagotomy, cholecystectomy, and anastomosis. Non-GI procedures, which precipitated CDE, include hemodialysis, nephrectomy, prostatectomy, aortic embolectomy, and pelvic evisceration. Non-surgical indications for admission, which instigated CDE, included pneumonia, urinary tract infections, closed non-displaced fractures, and soft tissue infections.

Antimicrobial agent use is a canonical catalyst for CDI through dysbiosis of colonic microbiota, which enables either seeding or spore germination in newly exposed or carrier patients, respectively. A detailed analysis of the antibiotics implicated in predisposing to CDE is summarized in Table 2.

Table 2. Classes of antibiotics predisposing to CDE.

Antibiotic	Case Load
Cephalosporins	21 (27.3%)
Fluoroquinolones	10 (13.0%)
Penicillins	9 (11.7%)
Carbapenems	2 (2.6%)
Metronidazole	2 (2.6%)
Trimethoprim / Sulfamethoxazole	2 (2.6%)
Doxycycline	1 (1.3%)
Vancomycin	1 (1.3%)
Rifampin	1 (1.3%)
Clindamycin	1 (1.3%)
Unknown	22 (28.6%)
None	5 (6.5%)

In our review, only five patients (6.5%) developed CDE spontaneously without prior documented antibiotic exposure or recent hospitalization. The three most common cephalosporins included cefuroxime ($n = 6$), cefazolin ($n = 6$), and cefoxitin ($n = 6$) –in this review, second generation drugs of this class carried the highest risk of triggering CDE. The most common fluoroquinolones included ciprofloxacin ($n = 6$) and levofloxacin ($n = 4$). The most common ampicillins implicated included amoxicillin ($n = 4$), ampicillin ($n = 2$), and penicillin ($n = 2$). Multiple meta-analyses quantified antibiotic exposure and risk of CD infection—clindamycin is firmly cemented as the most frequently implicated antibiotic, followed by fluoroquinolones, cephalosporins, and penicillins [51,52]. For CDE, this pattern is somewhat upended, with cephalosporins being most commonly inculpated while clindamycin is significantly underrepresented. Cephalosporins are commonly given as part of preoperative prophylaxis; it is likely the high surgical admission rates of patients we reviewed reflect predisposing antibiotic use

In the majority of patients in this review, CDE arose in context of surgically altered GI anatomy—48 patients underwent colectomy with ileostomy. CD may colonize the large bowel—intestinal resection, which disrupts the ileocecal valve, may therefore facilitate bacterial translocation to the small bowel, leading to CDE [8]. However, CDE can affect patients with an anatomically normal GI tract and an intact ileocecal valve, as was reported in the case series by Lavallee and colleagues. [26]. Why certain patients suffer from a particularly deleterious progression of CD with severe features, such as ischemic colitis or enteritis is unclear [53]. Lack of immortalized appropriate cell lines (human small bowel intestinal epithelium) complicates elucidation of pathophysiologic mechanisms underlying CDE. Concomitant involvement of the small and large bowel in CDE has also been reported in 13 cases. Kurtz et al. documented a patient who underwent proctocolectomy, in addition to progressive small bowel resections due to recalcitrant Crohn's disease—despite less than four feet of small bowel remaining, the patient still developed CDE [33].

It is challenging to accurately depict the exact treatment regimen—for most cases, the cornerstone of therapy was parenteral metronidazole with enteral vancomycin. However, it was administered with considerable variation. In some cases, antibiotic therapy was sequential, beginning with metronidazole and after several days transitioning to exclusively vancomycin. If the patients could not tolerate combinatorial therapy, they were administered intravenous fluids with metronidazole until they were able to tolerate oral metronidazole with vancomycin. For patients with stomas, vancomycin could also be administered as enemas per the distal limb of the conduit. In instances where CDE resulted in diffuse mucosal bleeding, vancomycin-soaked tamponade use was also reported. Adjunctive treatments included total parenteral nutrition, loperamide, fiber, oral fluid restriction, and in severe cases, other antibiotics were added—most commonly carbapenems.

As patients improved, there was a general trend to switch them to enteral vancomycin and continue therapy for up to four weeks in an outpatient setting. In approximately one third of patients, infection trajectory necessitated therapeutic subtotal resection of the colon and terminal ileum, in addition to antibiotics. "Unknown" treatments, as denoted in Table 1, most often referred to broad-spectrum antibiotics, which were not specified by the authors. "Other" treatments included streptomycin (n = 1), supportive treatment (n = 2) or combinatorial therapy (e.g., tobramycin, teicoplanin, or gentamicin combined with metronidazole), which were chosen to either circumvent patient antibiotic allergies or cover for a co-infection, such as pneumonia or a lower urinary tract infection. In a pediatric cohort of 18 patients (average age 4.8 years), majority of cases (72.2%) did not require dedicated treatment and were managed via antibiotic discontinuation and observation—a stark contrast to adult patients in our study, where only two patients were managed with antibiotics [50].

Grouping patients by strictly by presence or absence of prior abdominal surgery was found to be misleading, as it disrupted the temporal relationship of events that led up to the CDE infection. Majority of CDE cases arose in patients who underwent prior GI surgery, usually for IBD. However, in a minority of cases, there was history of GI surgery and therefore, altered bowel anatomy—however, hospitalization that incited CDE was unrelated to the original GI procedure. For example, a patient underwent complication-free IPAA for recalcitrant UC and six months later underwent elective hernia repair, which ultimately precipitated CDE. In order to highlight this important distinction, we additionally created the "Was CDE caused by surgery for which the patient was admitted" column. Indications for ICU transfer included hemodynamic decompensation, bowel perforation, sepsis, and multiorgan dysfunction. Virtually all patients who survived CDE were discharged in good health. One patient survived CDE, but had a complicated course and could not be weaned of ventilatory support—she was discharged to a chronic care facility. Cause of death was generally attributed to either protracted hospitalization, such as respiratory failure due to ventilator-associated pneumonia, or directly to sepsis and multiorgan failure induced by CDE.

Mortality rates for CDE demonstrate considerable variability. For case report-based pooled reviews, mortality attributed to CDE has been stabilizing at approximately 30% (Table 3).

Table 3. Review of historically conducted literature reviews of *Clostridioides Difficile* enteritis and the evolution of the associated mortality rate, as case number increased.

Author and Year	Cases Reviewed	Case Year Range	CDE Mortality Rate
Freiler et al., 2001 [12]	10	1980–2001	60%
Lundeen et al., 2007 [18]	20	1980–2007	45%
Holmer et al., 2011 [36]	56	1980–2011	32.1%
Beal et al., 2015 [3]	63	1980–2015	30.1%
Present study	77	2001–2021	29.8%

In our review, mortality rates can be further decreased to 23.1%, if cases older than 20 years old are excluded. Ulrich et al. identified 44 cases in 855 postcolectomy patients—regarding outcome measures, only one patient expired due to CDE, leading to a mortality rate of 2% [48]. Furthermore, Park et al. retrospectively identified 18 pediatric cases of CDE—in their cohort, there were no reported deaths [50]. It can be conjectured that the mortality rate of CDE is likely lower than reported, in part due to case report bias and underreported incidence of CDE.

4. Conclusions

CDE becomes more frequently diagnosed possibly due to an increase in colectomy rates for different indications. There is a need for an elevated degree of suspicion to differentiate from other cause of intraabdominal sepsis like acute mesenteric ischemia, intestinal obstruction, or postsurgical complications. Its high fatality rate, even though lower than previously described, makes rapid diagnosis of utmost importance to initiate adequate treatment for better outcome.

Author Contributions: A.K., C.G.T. conceptualization, methodology, validation, writing–original draft preparation; A.O.O., C.M.P., I.T. conceptualization, methodology, formal analysis, writing–review and editing, A.-M.C., E.M.I. methodology, validation, formal analysis, data curation and supervision. All authors have read and agreed to the published version of the manuscript.

Funding: This research received no external funding.

Institutional Review Board Statement: Ethical review and approval were waived for this study because the manuscript consists of only a case presentation which does not fulfill the criteria for research studies involving humans.

Informed Consent Statement: Informed consent was obtained from the patient for research use of any pictures from imaging/endoscopy/histology examinations.

Data Availability Statement: The raw data is available at the corresponding author upon reasonable request.

Conflicts of Interest: The authors declare no conflict of interest.

References

1. Balsells, E.; Shi, T.; Leese, C.; Lyell, I.; Burrows, J.; Wiuff, C.; Campbell, H.; Kyaw, M.H.; Nair, H. Global burden of *Clostridium difficile* infections: A systematic review and meta-analysis. *J. Glob. Health* **2019**, *9*, 010407. [CrossRef]
2. Seril, D.N.; Shen, B. *Clostridium difficile* infection in the postcolectomy patient. *Inflamm. Bowel Dis.* **2014**, *20*, 2450–2469. [CrossRef]
3. Beal, E.W.; Bass, R.; Harzman, A.E. Two Patients with Fulminant *Clostridium difficile* Enteritis Who Had Not Undergone Total Colectomy: A Case Series and Review of the Literature. *Case Rep. Surg.* **2015**, *2015*, 957257. [CrossRef]
4. LaMont, J.T.; Trnka, Y.M. Therapeutic implications of *Clostridium difficile* toxin during relapse of chronic inflammatory bowel disease. *Lancet* **1980**, *315*, 381–383. [CrossRef]
5. Shortland, J.R.; Spencer, R.C.; Williams, J.L. Pseudomembranous colitis associated with changes in an ileal conduit. *J. Clin. Pathol.* **1983**, *36*, 1184–1187. [CrossRef] [PubMed]
6. Miller, D.L.; Sedlack, J.D.; Holt, R.W. Perforation complicating rifampin-associated pseudomembranous enteritis. *Arch. Surg.* **1989**, *124*, 1082. [CrossRef]
7. Kuntz, D.P.; Shortsleeve, M.J.; Kantrowitz, P.A.; Gauvin, G.P. *Clostridium difficile* enteritis. A cause of intramural gas. *Dig. Dis. Sci.* **1993**, *38*, 1942–1944. [CrossRef] [PubMed]
8. Tsutaoka, B.; Hansen, J.; Johnson, D.; Holodniy, M. Antibiotic-associated pseudomembranous enteritis due to *Clostridium difficile*. *Clin. Infect. Dis.* **1994**, *18*, 982–984. [CrossRef]
9. Yee, H.F., Jr.; Brown, R.S., Jr.; Ostroff, J.W. Fatal *Clostridium difficile* enteritis after total abdominal colectomy. *J. Clin. Gastroenterol.* **1996**, *22*, 45–47. [CrossRef] [PubMed]
10. Kralovich, K.A.; Sacksner, J.; Karmy-Jones, R.A.; Eggenberger, J.C. Pseudomembranous colitis with associated fulminant ileitis in the defunctionalized limb of a jejunal-ileal bypass. Report of a case. *Dis. Colon Rectum* **1997**, *40*, 622–624. [CrossRef]
11. Vesoulis, Z.; Williams, G.; Matthews, B. Pseudomembranous enteritis after proctocolectomy: Report of a case. *Dis. Colon Rectum* **2000**, *43*, 551–554. [CrossRef] [PubMed]
12. Freiler, J.F.; Durning, S.J.; Ender, P.T. *Clostridium difficile* small bowel enteritis occurring after total colectomy. *Clin. Infect. Dis.* **2001**, *33*, 1429–1431. [CrossRef] [PubMed]
13. Jacobs, A.; Barnard, K.; Fishel, R.; Gradon, J.D. Extracolonic manifestations of *Clostridium difficile* infections. Presentation of 2 cases and review of the literature. *Medicine* **2001**, *80*, 88–101. [CrossRef] [PubMed]
14. Tjandra, J.J.; Street, A.; Thomas, R.J.; Gibson, R.; Eng, P.; Cade, J. Fatal *Clostridium difficile* infection of the small bowel after complex colorectal surgery. *ANZ J. Surg.* **2001**, *71*, 500–503. [CrossRef]

15. Mann, S.D.; Pitt, J.; Springall, R.G.; Thillainayagam, A.V. *Clostridium difficile* infection—An unusual cause of refractory pouchitis: Report of a case. *Dis. Colon Rectum* **2003**, *46*, 267–270. [CrossRef]
16. Hayetian, F.D.; Read, T.E.; Brozovich, M.; Garvin, R.P.; Caushaj, P.F. Ileal perforation secondary to *Clostridium difficile* enteritis: Report of 2 cases. *Arch. Surg.* **2006**, *141*, 97–99. [CrossRef]
17. Kim, K.A.; Wry, P.; Hughes, E., Jr.; Butcher, J.; Barbot, D. *Clostridium difficile* small-bowel enteritis after total proctocolectomy: A rare but fatal, easily missed diagnosis. Report of a case. *Dis. Colon Rectum* **2007**, *50*, 920–923. [CrossRef]
18. Lundeen, S.J.; Otterson, M.F.; Binion, D.G.; Carman, E.T.; Peppard, W.J. *Clostridium difficile* enteritis: An early postoperative complication in inflammatory bowel disease patients after colectomy. *J. Gastrointest. Surg.* **2007**, *11*, 138–142. [CrossRef]
19. Boland, E.; Thompson, J.S. Fulminant *Clostridium difficile* enteritis after proctocolectomy and ileal pouch-anal anastamosis. *Gastroenterol. Res. Pract.* **2008**, *2008*, 985658. [CrossRef]
20. El Muhtaseb, M.S.; Apollos, J.K.; Dreyer, J.S. *Clostridium difficile* enteritis: A cause for high ileostomy output. *ANZ J. Surg.* **2008**, *78*, 416. [CrossRef]
21. Follmar, K.E.; Condron, S.A.; Turner, I.I.; Nathan, J.D.; Ludwig, K.A. Treatment of metronidazole-refractory *Clostridium difficile* enteritis with vancomycin. *Surg. Infect.* **2008**, *9*, 195–200. [CrossRef]
22. Wood, M.J.; Hyman, N.; Hebert, J.C.; Blaszyk, H. Catastrophic *Clostridium difficile* enteritis in a pelvic pouch patient: Report of a case. *J. Gastrointest. Surg.* **2008**, *12*, 350–352. [CrossRef]
23. Yafi, F.A.; Selvasekar, C.R.; Cima, R.R. *Clostridium difficile* enteritis following total colectomy. *Tech. Coloproctol.* **2008**, *12*, 73–74.
24. Causey, M.W.; Spencer, M.P.; Steele, S.R. *Clostridium difficile* enteritis after colectomy. *Am. Surg.* **2009**, *75*, 1203–1206. [CrossRef] [PubMed]
25. Fleming, F.; Khursigara, N.; O'Connell, N.; Darby, S.; Waldron, D. Fulminant small bowel enteritis: A rare complication of *Clostridium difficile*-associated disease. *Inflamm. Bowel Dis.* **2009**, *15*, 801–802. [CrossRef] [PubMed]
26. Lavallée, C.; Laufer, B.; Pépin, J.; Mitchell, A.; Dubé, S.; Labbé, A.C. Fatal *Clostridium difficile* enteritis caused by the BI/NAP1/027 strain: A case series of ileal *C. difficile* infections. *Clin. Microbiol. Infect.* **2009**, *15*, 1093–1099. [CrossRef] [PubMed]
27. Peacock, O.; Speake, W.; Shaw, A.; Goddard, A. *Clostridium difficile* enteritis in a patient after total proctocolectomy. *BMJ Case Rep.* **2009**, *2009*, bcr1020081165. [CrossRef]
28. Shen, B.; Remzi, F.H.; Fazio, V.W. Fulminant *Clostridium difficile*-associated pouchitis with a fatal outcome. *Nat. Rev. Gastroenterol. Hepatol.* **2009**, *6*, 492–495. [CrossRef]
29. Wee, B.; Poels, J.A.; McCafferty, I.J.; Taniere, P.; Olliff, J. A description of CT features of *Clostridium difficile* infection of the small bowel in four patients and a review of literature. *Br. J. Radiol.* **2009**, *82*, 890–895. [CrossRef]
30. Williams, R.N.; Hemingway, D.; Miller, A.S. Enteral *Clostridium difficile*, an emerging cause for high-output ileostomy. *J. Clin. Pathol.* **2009**, *62*, 951–953. [CrossRef]
31. Gagandeep, D.; Ira, S. *Clostridium difficile* enteritis 9 years after total proctocolectomy: A rare case report. *Am. J. Gastroenterol.* **2010**, *105*, 962–963. [CrossRef] [PubMed]
32. Khan, M.S.; Levy, D.; Mann, S. *Clostridium difficile* infection in the absence of a colon. *BMJ Case Rep.* **2010**, *2010*, bcr0220102728. [CrossRef]
33. Kurtz, L.E.; Yang, S.S.; Bank, S. *Clostridium difficile*-associated small bowel enteritis after total proctocolectomy in a Crohn's disease patient. *J. Clin. Gastroenterol.* **2010**, *44*, 76–77. [CrossRef] [PubMed]
34. Malkan, A.D.; Pimiento, J.M.; Maloney, S.P.; Palesty, J.A.; Scholand, S.J. Unusual manifestations of *Clostridium difficile* infection. *Surg. Infect.* **2010**, *11*, 333–337. [CrossRef] [PubMed]
35. Hariri, S.; Gouin, P.; Tuech, J.J.; Veber, B.; Dureuil, B. *Clostridium difficile* infection causing multiple organ failure and small-bowel enteritis. *Clin. Res. Hepatol. Gastroenterol.* **2011**, *35*, 142–144. [CrossRef] [PubMed]
36. Holmer, C.; Zurbuchen, U.; Siegmund, B.; Reichelt, U.; Buhr, H.J.; Ritz, J.P. *Clostridium difficile* infection of the small bowel—Two case reports with a literature survey. *Int. J. Colorectal Dis.* **2011**, *26*, 245–251. [CrossRef]
37. Ramos Martínez, A.; Romero Pizarro, Y.; Martínez Arrieta, F.; Balandín Moreno, B.; Múñez Rubio, E.; Cuiñas León, K.; Sánchez Romero, I.; Cantos López de Ibargüen, B.; Asensio Vegas, A. *Clostridium difficile* enteritis. *Gastroenterol. Hepatol.* **2011**, *34*, 539–545. [CrossRef]
38. Thomas, K.; Taylor, J.; Everitt, L.; Nelson, R. *Clostridium difficile* does not only affect the colon: A case series. *Colorectal Dis.* **2011**, *13*, e156–e157. [CrossRef]
39. Wiggelinkhuizen, M.; Gerrits, M.A. *Clostridium difficile*-induced necrotizing enteritis. *Ned. Tijdschr. Geneeskd.* **2011**, *155*, A2414.
40. Dineen, S.P.; Bailey, S.H.; Pham, T.H.; Huerta, S. *Clostridium difficile* enteritis: A report of two cases and systematic literature review. *World J. Gastrointest. Surg.* **2013**, *5*, 37–42. [CrossRef]
41. Thai, H.; Guerron, A.D.; Bencsath, K.P.; Liu, X.; Loor, M. Fulminant *Clostridium difficile* enteritis causing abdominal compartment syndrome. *Surg. Infect.* **2014**, *15*, 821–825. [CrossRef]
42. Khan, S.A.; Towheed, A.; Tul Llah, S.; Bin Abdulhak, A.; Tilson-Mallett, N.R.; Salkind, A. Atypical Presentation of *C. Difficile* Infection: Report of a Case with Literature Review. *Cureus* **2016**, *8*, e563. [CrossRef]
43. Tarasiuk-Rusek, A.; Shah, K.J. *Clostridium difficile* ileitis in a patient, after total colectomy. *BMJ Case Rep.* **2016**, *2016*, bcr2015214319. [CrossRef] [PubMed]
44. Siddiqui, J.; Campion, T.; Wei, R.; Kuzmich, S. *Clostridium difficile* enteritis: Diffuse small bowel radiological changes in a patient with abdominal sepsis. *BMJ Case Rep.* **2018**, *2018*, bcr2017222209. [CrossRef]

45. Abid, H.; Bischof, E. An Unusual Presentation of Severe Sepsis Due to *Clostridium difficile* Enteritis. *Cureus* **2019**, *11*, e4162. [CrossRef] [PubMed]
46. Aujla, A.K.; Averbukh, L.D.; Potashinsky, A.; Rossi, L. A Rare Case of *Clostridium difficile* Enteritis: A Common Bug in an Uncommon Place. *Cureus* **2019**, *11*, e4519. [CrossRef] [PubMed]
47. Nasser, H.; Munie, S.; Shakaroun, D.; Ivanics, T.; Nalamati, S.; Killu, K. *Clostridium difficile* Enteritis after Total Abdominal Colectomy for Ulcerative Colitis. *Case Rep. Crit. Care* **2019**, *2019*, 2987682. [CrossRef]
48. Ulrich, R.J.; Bott, J.; Imlay, H.; Lopez, K.; Cinti, S.; Rao, K. *Clostridioides difficile* Enteritis in Patients Following Total Colectomy—A Rare but Genuine Clinical Entity. *Open Forum Infect. Dis.* **2019**, *6*, ofz409. [CrossRef]
49. Velez, D.R.; Ahmeti, M. *Clostridioides difficile* Enteritis Induced Anastomotic Rupture: A Case Report and Literature Review. *Case Rep. Surg.* **2020**, *2020*, 9794823. [CrossRef]
50. Park, S.W.; Lee, Y.J.; Ryoo, E. Difference in Vitamin D Levels between Children with *Clostridioides difficile* Enteritis and Those with Other Acute Infectious Enteritis. *Pediatr. Gastroenterol. Hepatol. Nutr.* **2021**, *24*, 81–89. [CrossRef]
51. Deshpande, A.; Pasupuleti, V.; Thota, P.; Pant, C.; Rolston, D.D.; Sferra, T.J.; Hernandez, A.V.; Donskey, C.J. Community-associated *Clostridium difficile* infection and antibiotics: A meta-analysis. *J. Antimicrob. Chemother.* **2013**, *68*, 1951–1961. [CrossRef] [PubMed]
52. Brown, K.A.; Khanafer, N.; Daneman, N.; Fisman, D.N. Meta-analysis of antibiotics and the risk of community-associated *Clostridium difficile* infection. *Antimicrob. Agents Chemother.* **2013**, *57*, 2326–2332. [CrossRef] [PubMed]
53. Ionescu, E.M.; Curte, A.M.; Olteanu, A.O.; Preda, C.M.; Tieranu, I.; Klimko, A.; Tieranu, C.G. Rare Clinical Association between *Clostridioides difficile* Infection and Ischemic Colitis: Case Report and Literature Review. *Medicina* **2021**, *57*, 705. [CrossRef] [PubMed]

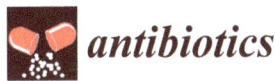

Article

Impact of Subinhibitory Concentrations of Metronidazole on Morphology, Motility, Biofilm Formation and Colonization of *Clostridioides difficile*

Tri-Hanh-Dung Doan [1], Marie-Françoise Bernet-Camard [2], Sandra Hoÿs [2], Claire Janoir [2] and Séverine Péchiné [2,*]

1. UniCancer Group, 94270 Le Kremlin-Bicêtre, France; th-dungdoan@unicancer.fr
2. Université Paris-Saclay, INRAE, AgroParisTech, Micalis Institute, 78350 Jouy-en-Josas, France; marie-francoise.bernet-camard@universite-paris-saclay.fr (M.-F.B.-C.); sandra.hoys@universite-paris-saclay.fr (S.H.); claire.janoir-jouveshomme@universite-paris-saclay.fr (C.J.)
* Correspondence: severine.pechine@universite-paris-saclay.fr; Tel.: +0033-146-835-883

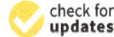

Citation: Doan, T.-H.-D.; Bernet-Camard, M.-F.; Hoÿs, S.; Janoir, C.; Péchiné, S. Impact of Subinhibitory Concentrations of Metronidazole on Morphology, Motility, Biofilm Formation and Colonization of *Clostridioides difficile*. *Antibiotics* **2022**, *11*, 624. https://doi.org/10.3390/antibiotics11050624

Academic Editor: Guido Granata

Received: 25 March 2022
Accepted: 27 April 2022
Published: 5 May 2022

Publisher's Note: MDPI stays neutral with regard to jurisdictional claims in published maps and institutional affiliations.

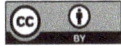

Copyright: © 2022 by the authors. Licensee MDPI, Basel, Switzerland. This article is an open access article distributed under the terms and conditions of the Creative Commons Attribution (CC BY) license (https://creativecommons.org/licenses/by/4.0/).

Abstract: *Clostridioides difficile* infection (CDI) is the primary cause of health-care-associated infectious diarrhea. Treatment requires mostly specific antibiotics such as metronidazole (MTZ), vancomycin or fidaxomicin. However, approximately 20% of treated patients experience recurrences. Treatment with MTZ is complicated by reduced susceptibility to this molecule, which could result in high failure and recurrence rates. However, the mechanism remains unclear. In this study, we investigated the impact of subinhibitory concentrations of MTZ on morphology, motility, biofilm formation, bacterial adherence to the intestinal Caco-2/TC7 differentiated monolayers, and colonization in monoxenic and conventional mouse models of two *C. difficile* strains (VPI 10463 and CD17-146), showing different susceptibility profiles to MTZ. Our results revealed that in addition to the inhibition of motility and the downregulation of flagellar genes for both strains, sub-inhibitory concentrations of MTZ induced various in vitro phenotypes for the strain CD17-146 exhibiting a reduced susceptibility to this antibiotic: elongated morphology, enhanced biofilm production and increased adherence to Caco-2/TC7 cells. Weak doses of MTZ induced higher level of colonization in the conventional mouse model and a trend to thicker 3-D structures entrapping bacteria in monoxenic mouse model. Thus, sub-inhibitory concentrations of MTZ can have a wide range of physiological effects on bacteria, which may contribute to their persistence after treatment.

Keywords: *Clostridioides difficile*; metronidazole; biofilm; motility; morphology; adherence; colonization

1. Introduction

Clostridioides difficile (CD) is a Gram-positive, spore forming and obligate anaerobic bacilli, responsible for various intestinal symptoms from mild diarrhea to severe pseudomembranous colitis and is the primary cause of antibiotic-associated diarrhea in developed countries [1].

For decades, vancomycin and MTZ were widely used as first-line therapy. However, the emergence and spread of *C. difficile* clinical isolates resistant to MTZ led to a recent update guideline to recommend MTZ only as an alternative to vancomycin or fidaxomicin for an initial non-severe *Clostridioides difficile* infection (CDI) treatment due to its high failure and high recurrence rates (20–25%) [2,3]. One possible factor that may explain MTZ treatment failure is pharmacokinetics of the antibiotic. Indeed, when MTZ is administered orally, at least 80 percent of the drug is absorbed in one hour. Fecal elimination and colonic (*C. difficile* infection site) concentrations are low [4]. In symptomatic patients, stool concentrations of MTZ were detected with a mean concentration of 9.3 µg/g in watery stool and 1.2 µg/g in formed stool. In asymptomatic patients, MTZ were undetectable [5]. The poor fecal concentrations of MTZ might result in insufficient antibiotic concentrations to inhibit vegetative bacteria, promoting the development of adaptation and resistance mechanisms of *C. difficile*.

Indeed, some studies indicate that MTZ resistance in *C. difficile* is heterogeneous, which means that growth in the presence of MTZ may select slow growing subclones with higher MTZ minimum inhibitory concentrations (MIC) from a population with low MIC [6]. The slowly growing or non-growing state of bacterial persisters is due to a general arrest in metabolic activity which is thought to give them the ability to survive exposure to antibiotics [7]. Moura et al. also found that following the exposure to subinhibitory concentrations of this antibiotic, *C. difficile* strains PCR ribotype 001 and 010 showed increased MIC [8]. MTZ heteroresistant *C. difficile* can obviously be a matter of concern, resulting in therapeutic failures.

In addition, the production of *C. difficile* biofilm is proved to be induced by the exposure to MTZ at subinhibitory concentrations [9]. In vitro, biofilm formation has been reported to be an important factor contributing to antimicrobial resistance of *C. difficile* by forming a multilayered structure encased in a matrix containing proteins, DNA, and polysaccharides [10]. In particular, cells of toxigenic *C. difficile* strains NAP1/027 R20291 grown in biofilm showed a 100-fold increase in the resistance to antibiotic compared to planktonic cells [10]. Higher biofilm formation could participate to better colonization and persistence in vivo and so far, persistent recurring *C. difficile* infections have been a major challenge in the treatment of CDI [11]. Indeed, recurrent bacterial infections occur with the ability to produce resilient biofilms by various pathogens [12].

Exposure to sub-MIC levels of antibiotics has been found to cause substantial increase in bacterial adherence to eukaryotic host cells and induced biofilm formation for several pathogenic species. Subinhibitory concentrations of ciprofloxacin were shown to increase bacterial adherence to host tissue by upregulating the expression of fibronectin-binding proteins in *S. aureus*. This increased expression involves two pathways: upregulation of the stress-response sigma factor SigB and induction of the SOS response (RecA and LexA) [13]. Moreover, in *P. aeruginosa*, aminoglycoside antibiotics have been shown to induce biofilm formation. This response requires a functional *arr* gene, which encodes an inner membrane phosphodiesterase, whose substrate is cyclic di-guanosine monophosphate (c-di-GMP), a second messenger that inhibits bacterial motility and promotes cell surface adherence and biofilm formation [14].

Thus, we thought of great interest to examine impacts of low doses of MTZ on the ability of *C. difficile* strains to form a biofilm and to colonize mice.

In this study, we compare characteristics (morphology, motility, in vitro bacterial adherence, and biofilm production) of two strains of *C. difficile*, the CD17-146 with reduced susceptibility to MTZ and the VPI 10463 sensitive to MTZ, in absence and presence of MTZ at subinhibitory concentrations. Besides, we also determine in vivo the effect of low doses of MTZ on the colonization process of these strains in a conventional mouse model. Finally, distributions of each strain over the cecal tissue in a mono-associated mouse model were visualized by confocal laser scanning microscopy.

2. Results

2.1. Impact of MTZ on the Morphology of C. difficile

The VPI 10463 *C. difficile* strain, isolated from an abdominal wound, is Tcd A and Tcd B positive, and belongs to PCR-ribotype 087. The CD17-146 isolate is a non-toxigenic strain from PCR ribotype 596, displaying reduced susceptibility to MTZ. The MIC values for MTZ determined as described in Material and Method section, were 1 µg/mL for CD17-146 and 0.5 µg/mL for VPI 10463. Morphological analyses were performed on the untreated cultures (without MTZ) as well as cultures exposed to MTZ at concentration of MIC/4 and MIC/2. Morphological analyses were performed on the untreated cultures (without MTZ) as well as cultures exposed to MTZ at concentration of MIC/4 and MIC/2. Optical microscopic observation on Gram staining showed that CD17-146 strain was grown into filaments with subinhibitory concentrations of MTZ. On the contrary, this morphology change was not observed in VPI 10463 cultures treated with MTZ whatever the subinhibitory concentration used (Figure 1).

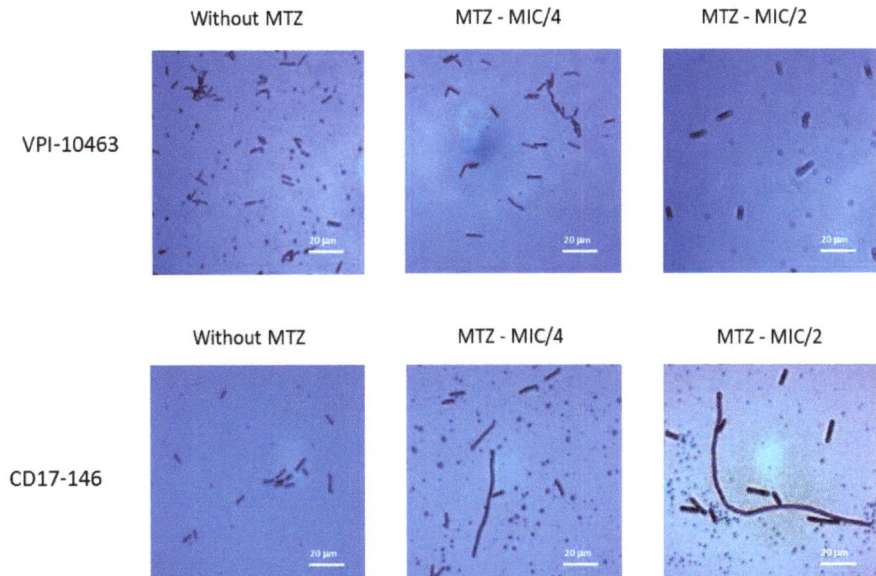

Figure 1. Morphology of bacterial cells at subinhibitory concentrations of MTZ. VPI 10463 and CD17-146 were grown in BHI-SG broth without MTZ or with MTZ at MIC/4 and MIC/2 until OD600 nm of cultures reached 0.4. Gram-stain images of CD17-146 at 100× magnification demonstrated an elongation of bacterial cells.

2.2. C. difficile Biofilm Production in Absence and Presence of MTZ

Biofilm formation has been reported to be induced by subinhibitory concentrations of MTZ in three *C. difficile* isolates belonging to PCR-ribotype 010 [9]. To study whether MTZ stimulates biofilm formation of VPI 10463 and CD17-146 strains in vitro, bacteria were grown in BHISG with a range of concentrations of MTZ (0 to 2 µg/mL) and biofilm formation was measured after 48 h by crystal violet staining and viable cell and spore enumeration.

In the absence of MTZ, a significant higher biofilm production was observed in VPI 10463 strain compared to CD17-146 strain. We found a declining trend of biomass and vegetative forms in VPI 10463 strain at MTZ subinhibitory concentrations (Figure 2A,C). However, differences observed were not statically significant. Interestingly, there were no spores in biofilm of VPI 10463 at MIC/4 and MIC/2. (A570 values were 4.44 ± 1.69 and 1.35 ± 0.22 in VPI 10463 and CD17-146, respectively). Differently, when MTZ was added, a significant 4-fold increase of biomass (A570 value 4.08 ± 0.87) was observed in the CD17-146 strain at MIC/2 (0.5 µg/mL) (Figure 2A), indicating a strong induction of biofilm formation in this strain by MTZ. In accordance with results of the quantitative biofilm assay by crystal violet, the viable cells and spores of this strain went up dramatically at MIC/2 with an increase of two log (Figure 2B).

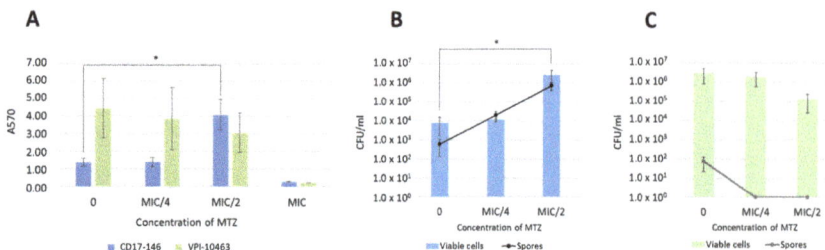

Figure 2. Biofilm quantification of VPI 10463 and CD17-146 at subinhibitory concentrations of MTZ. Bacteria were cultivated in BHI-SG broth without or with MTZ at MIC/4 and MIC/2 at 37 °C under anaerobic conditions to form biofilms. After 48 h, the biofilm mass was quantified by crystal violet staining. A 4-fold increase of biomass was observed in the CD17-146 strain at MIC/2 (**A**). Panels (**B**) and (**C**) depicts enumeration of vegetative forms and spores included in biofilms formed the two strains CD17-146 and VPI 10463, respectively. Data are means of at least three independent experiments, each performed in triplicate. The error bars represent standard deviation. Significantly different ($p < 0.05$) ratios are indicated by asterisks (Man-Whitney test).

These results highlight different behaviors of two strains in presence of MTZ.

2.3. Impact of MTZ on the Motility of C. difficile and Transcriptions of Flagellar Genes

As the motility and bacterial flagella are known to modulate attachment and biofilm production, we used a semi-soft agar assay to monitor the effect of MTZ on motility of *C. difficile*. We observed a significant decrease in the mobility of both *C. difficile* strains through soft agar and the effect is concentration dependent. The motility of *C. difficile* decreased with increasing concentrations of MTZ. This suggested that MTZ might impede transcription of flagellar genes (Figure 3). For this study, the flagellated 630 flagellated and the unflagellated 630Δ*fliC* (deletion mutant for *fliC* gene resulting in lack of the flagellar filament production) strains were used as positive and negative controls for motility assay, respectively.

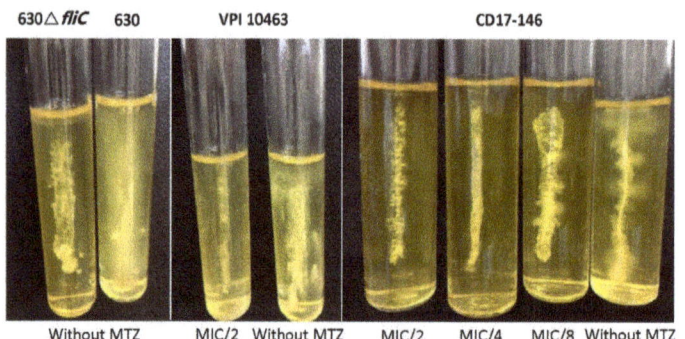

Figure 3. Motility of VPI 10463 (VPI) and CD17-146 (146) at subinhibitory concentrations of MTZ. Bacterial strains were inoculated in BHI medium containing 0.3% agar without or with MTZ at the concentrations 0.125, 0.25 or 0.5 µg/mL and grown anaerobically at 37 °C for 48 h. MTZ reduced the motility of both *C. difficile* strains through soft agar and this effect is concentration dependent.

To test this, *C. difficile* strains were cultured in the presence or absence of MTZ, and the levels of flagellar gene transcripts were measured by qRT-PCR. In both strains, subinhibitory concentrations of MTZ reduced the levels of fliC, flgB and fliA mRNAs, compared to the cultures without MTZ (Figure 4). The levels of transcription at MIC/4 were quite similar to the levels at MIC/2 for the two strains. For CD17-146 strain, the expression of *fliC* and *fliA* decreased around 2-fold, while *flgB* went down 3-fold at MIC/4 and 4-fold at MIC/2.

For VPI 10463 the expression of these genes decreased more drastically: 10-fold, 3-fold and 5-fold for *fliA*, *flgB* and *fliC*, respectively. Furthermore, *gluD* (reference gene) transcript levels were equivalent in both strains grown with or without MTZ. Therefore, subinhibitory concentrations of MTZ had a global negative effect on transcription of flagellar genes.

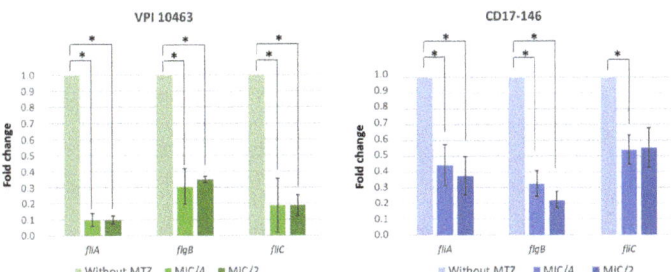

Figure 4. Expression of flagellar genes of VPI 10463 (VPI, green) and CD17-146 (146, blue) at subinhibitory concentrations of MTZ. Bacteria were grown in BHI-SG broth without or with MTZ at MIC/4 and MIC/2 at 37 °C under anaerobic conditions until OD600 nm reached 0.7. Using qRT-PCR, transcripts levels of *fliA*, *flgB* and *fliC* were measured. MTZ repressed the expression of flagellar genes in the two strains. Data are representative of three independent experiments, each performed in triplicate. The error bars represent standard errors of mean (SEM). Significantly different ($p < 0.05$) ratios are indicated by asterisks (Man-Whitney test).

2.4. Effect of Subinhibitory Concentrations of MTZ on C. difficile Adherence

Since the first step of infection is the colonization process which may include adherence to epithelial cells, we studied the impact of exposure to MTZ on *C. difficile* adherence to an intestinal cell Caco-2/TC7, a simple and human in vitro model.

Counts of cell adherent bacteria showed that exposure to MTZ at MIC/2 increased significantly the adherence of CD17-146 to Caco-2/TC7 cells. On the contrary, there were no significant changes in the number of adherent bacteria observed in VPI 1043 whatever the sub-inhibitory concentrations of MTZ. Despite having the similar level of adherence without MTZ, the two strains responded differently to MTZ pressure (Figure 5).

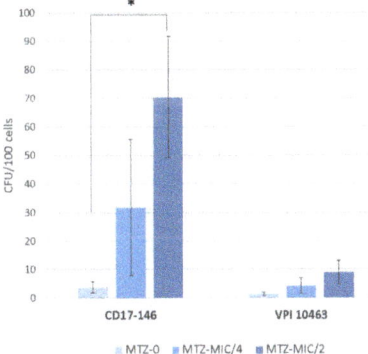

Figure 5. Impact of MTZ on adherence of VPI 10463 and CD17-146 strains to Caco-2TC7 cells. Overnight cultures of each *C. difficile* strain in BHISG broth, with or without subinhibitory concentrations of antibiotics, were pelleted and washed once with PBS, then incubated with Caco-2/TC7 cells in DMEM for 1 h 30 at 37 °C under anaerobic conditions. The adhesion ability was expressed as the number of adherent bacteria per 100 Caco-2/TC7 cells. The adherence to Caco-2/TC7 cells of CD17-146 exposure to MTZ at MIC/2 increased significantly. Data are representative of at least three independent experiments, each performed in triplicate. The error bars represent standard error of the mean (SEM). Significantly differences ($p < 0.05$) are indicated by asterisks (Man-Whitney test).

2.5. Subinhibitory Concentrations of MTZ Stimulate Cecum Colonization by CD17-146 in the Conventional Mouse Model

After having observed different impacts of MTZ on in vitro biofilm formation and on the adherence to a human intestinal cell model for the two *C. difficile* strains, we decided to study their colonization fitness in conventional mice receiving different regimen of MTZ. The experiment design is described in Figure 6.

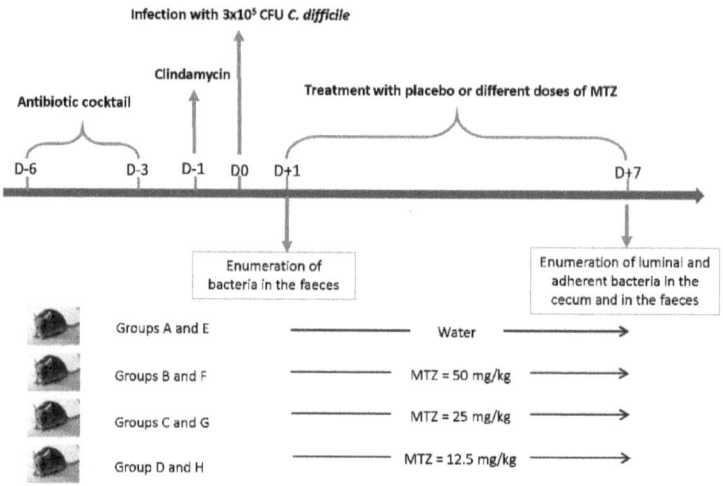

Figure 6. Experimental design of the conventional mouse model to study the impact of different doses of MTZ on the cecum colonization by VPI 10463 and CD17-146. The antibiotic cocktail contained kanamycin (40 mg/kg), gentamycin (3.5 mg/kg), colistin (8.5mg/kg), MTZ (21.5 mg/kg) and vancomycin (4.5 mg/kg). The clindamycin was administrated intraperitoneally (10 mg/kg). The mice were divided into 8 groups, 6 mice per group: four groups (A–D) infected with VPI-10463 and four groups (E–H) infected with CD17-146.

The bacterial burden was quantified by seeding fecal (on days 1 and 7 post-infection) and cecal (on day 7 post-infection) samples on selective plates.

After infection, both strains proliferated and reached a bacterial burden of approximately 3×10^7 bacteria per gram of feces after 24 h. As expected, mice infected by VPI 10463 showed signs of clinical illness with weight loss and severe diarrhea, especially from 48 h to 72 h post-challenge. Approximately 80% of mice died in group A non treated with MTZ and only two mice survived after 7 days. In group C treated with a half and D treated with a quarter of usual dose, mortality rates were about 30–40%. In contrast, there were no deaths in the group B treated with usual dose. On the other hand, mice infected with CD17-146 did not have any signs of illness, consistent with the non-toxigenic status of this strain.

The levels of intestinal colonization reached by each strain at day 7 are shown in Figure 7. Overall, without MTZ, VPI 10463 strain significantly colonized better than CD17-146 ($p = 0.025$) but their rates of colonization were similar in presence of MTZ. Indeed, the treatment of MTZ did not impact the colonization of VPI 10463 strain: number of spores and vegetative cells in cecum and feces were similar between the non-treated group and groups treated with MTZ, even with the group treated with the highest dose of MTZ (50 mg/kg).

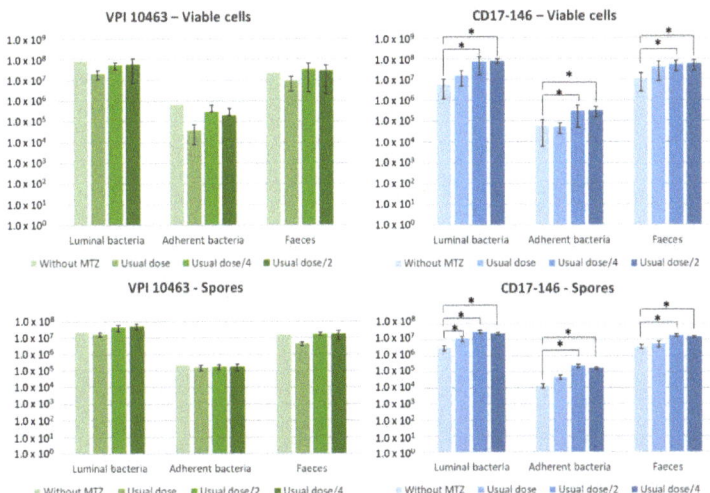

Figure 7. Impact of MTZ on cecum colonization of *C. difficile* in conventional mice, 7 days post-infection. Conventional mice were infected by either VPI 10463 (green) or CD17-146 (blue) with equivalent number of vegetative cells. Colonization process and bacterial burden were monitored by seeding fecal, cecal contents (luminal bacteria) and homogenized mucosal tissues (adherent bacteria) on selective plates at day 7 post-infection. Low doses (usual dose/4 and usual dose/2) of MTZ stimulated the colonization of CD17-146. Data generated from two independent experiments. The error bars represent standard error of the mean (SEM). Significant differences ($p < 0.05$) compared to group without treatment are indicated by asterisks (Man-Whitney test).

For the groups infected by CD17-146, we observed a 10-fold significant increase of bacterial burden in cecum (for both luminal and adherent bacteria) and in feces after treatment of MTZ with doses of 12.5 (group H) and 25 (group G) mg/kg. In contrast, there were no significant differences between the bacterial burden in mice treated with usual dose and non-treated. Our results suggest that subinhibitory concentrations of MTZ stimulated the mouse intestinal colonization by CD17-146 *C. difficile* strain.

2.6. Visualisation of Bacterial Distribution in the Cecum by CLSM

Our results in conventional mouse model showed that doses lower than the usual one of MTZ had the same impacts on the colonization of CD17-146 for usual dose/4 and usual dose/2. To study the spatial organization of the two strains in the cecum, we then chose the usual dose/4 (12.5 mg/kg) for visualization of bacterial distribution by confocal laser microscopy in a monoxenic mice model. One mouse in the group A infected by VPI 10463 and treated with water died 3 days post-infection. In the other groups, all three mice survived after 7 days.

The distribution of *C. difficile* in the cecum was heterogeneous. Irrespective of strain, we observed areas without and with bacteria associated with tissues. The cecal mucosa-associated bacteria were entrapped in a 3-D structure and displayed mainly isolated bacteria. (Figure S1).

We estimated the thickness of the bacterial layer present in tissues at different regions of the cecum. For VPI 10463 strain, without MTZ the thickness varies from 32.5 μm to 81.6 μm (average: 51.63 μm) and from 8.58 μm to 112.2 μm at a quart of usual dose of MTZ (average: 23.01 μm). The bacterial layer seemed to be thinner in presence of 12.5 mg/kg of MTZ but the difference was not significant due to a large variation (Figure 8). In contrast, the mean of thickness of CD17-146 strain had tendency to increase in the group treated with MTZ, from 25.71 μm without MTZ to 43.86 μm with MTZ. However, with this strain, we also found randomly distributed areas either with a high or a low thickness of the *C. difficile* community, from 7.73 µm to 59.73 µm in the group placebo and from 15.05 µm to 113.4 µm in the group treated with 12.5 mg/kg of MTZ. Therefore, there were no statistically significant difference in mean thickness between two groups (Figure 8).

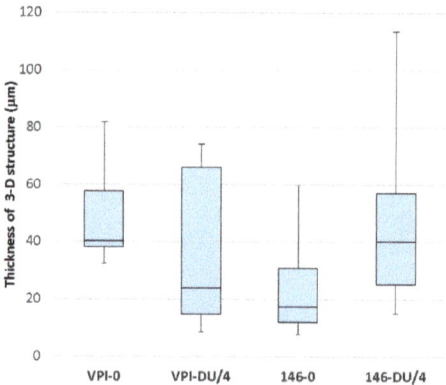

Figure 8. Thickness of bacterial 3-D structure of VPI 10463 (VPI) and CD17-146 (146) in cecum of mono-associated mouse model treated with placebo or with a quarter of usual dose of MTZ. The thickness of the bacterial 3-D structure is defined by the height on which bacteria are distributed. The thickness was determined directly from confocal Z-stack images. At least three mice were used for CLSM analyses for each strain, and at least 8 fields per sample were observed. Data are presented as boxplots with median and minimum-maximum whiskers. No significant difference was observed between strains (Mann-Whitney test).

The levels of intestinal colonization by each strain at day 7 are showed in supplemented data (Figure S2). In this model, no difference in intestinal colonization was observed neither between the two strains for the ability of colonize, nor between the strains in groups treated or not by MTZ.

3. Discussion

The increased antibiotic resistance reported for *C. difficile* clinical isolates and the recurrences of CDI are challenges facing physicians in the treatment of *C. difficile* infection. It has been estimated that approximately 27.3% of CDI treatment failures, as well as 23% of recurrences, are associated to treatment with MTZ [3].

As previously mentioned, the mechanisms of reduced susceptibility to MTZ are complex. Data obtained in recent studies on PCR-ribotype 027 and RT010 strains suggest that the reduced susceptibility is a multifactorial process involving alterations in different metabolic pathways, such as nitroreductase activity, iron uptake, and DNA repair [8,15]. Interestingly, a recent study showed the correlation between resistance to MTZ (MIC = 8 µg·mL^{-1}) and the presence of a plasmid, pCD-METRO, in toxigenic and non-toxigenic strains. One of the plasmidic open reading frames (ORFs) showed homology at the protein level to the *nimB* gene of 5-nitroimidazole reductase described in *Bacteroides fragilis* [16]. Nitroimidazole reductase activity encoded by *nim* genes is supposed to reduce the nitro group of 5-nitroimidazole to an amino group leading to an inactivation of the compound [17]. Another study on chromosomal resistance to MTZ in *C. difficile* demonstrated truncation of the ferrous iron transporter FeoB1 could result in a low-level resistance. Higher-level resistance could be achieved by sequential acquisition of mutations in catalytic domains of pyruvate-ferredoxin/flavodoxin oxidoreductase, a synonymous codon changes to putative xanthine dehydrogenase, and frameshift and point mutations that inactivated the iron-sulfur cluster regulator (IscR). However, resistance involving these genes was observed only in the *feoB1* deletion mutant and not in the isogenic wild-type parent [18]. To go on further the comprehension of the mechanism involved in the bacterial response to MTZ, it could be interesting to study more precisely the nitroreductase or iron transport activities of these two strains, CD17-146 and VPI 10463.

Occasional filamentous forms, accompanied by generalized defects in MTZ transport, have been described in MTZ-resistant mutant of *B. fragilis* [19]. Likewise, *Escherichia coli* that survived high concentration MTZ challenge exhibited an elongated filamentous morphology [20]. Sublethal MTZ concentration also induced elongation of *Fusobacterium nucleatum* and *Porphyromonas gingivalis* [20,21]. In accordance with previous study, we observed a cell elongation in this study with CD17-146 strain with reduced susceptibility to MTZ. Overall, an elongated morphology was associated with MTZ reduced susceptibility in different bacteria. Changes in morphology suggests modifications in cell wall structure which may result in decreased MTZ uptake, one parameter involved in resistance to this drug [22].

Moreover, antibiotic pressure has been shown to enhance biofilm formation in different bacterial species, including *C. difficile* [10,12,23,24]. In accordance with previous studies, we have shown a significant increase of in vitro biofilm formation in strain CD17-146 with reduced susceptibility in presence of MTZ at MIC/2. On the contrary, the ability of the susceptible strain VPI 10463 to produce biofilm in the same conditions did not change when MTZ was added to culture medium. Without MTZ, VPI 10463 was a strong biofilm-producer compared to CD17-146. A previous study has also demonstrated, in the presence of MTZ, a significant increase in biofilm formation in moderate-biofilm forming bacteria, not observable in strongly biofilm-forming strain [9]. Furthermore, Rahmoun et al. compared different susceptible isolates, and a statistically higher percentage of isolates with reduced susceptibility to metronidazole or vancomycin were shown to be biofilm producers [25].

Bacterial flagella are known to influence the adherence step in biofilm formation in motile bacteria. According to our results on biofilm formation, MTZ demonstrated a concentration-dependant inhibition effect on the expression of some flagellar genes (*fliC*, *flgB*, *fliA*) and the motility in both strains. A downregulation of flagellar genes leading to an impaired motility may be a factor for the increased MTZ-induced biofilm production in CD17-146. Differently, a decrease in the expression of flagellar genes and motility by antibiotic pressure did not further increase biofilm production in strain VPI 10463. Previous researches indicate that the precise role of flagella varies between strains. Indeed, strain 630 *C. difficile fliC* and *fliD* mutants were reported to have better adherence on Caco-2 cells, suggesting that flagella and motility may interfere with *C. difficile* adherence to epithelial cell surfaces [26]. In contrast, all flagella mutants (*fliC*, *fliD* and *flgE*) of the epidemic strain R20291 were less effective in adherence to Caco-2 cells than the wild-typein [27].

Our results on Caco-2/TC7 cells- showed that bacterial adherence increased by MTZ at MIC/2 for the CD17-146 strain. As the concentrations of MTZ in watery stools following oral therapy range between 0.8 and 24.2 µg/g [5], it is possible that low concentrations of this antibiotic are present in the gut in some phases of CDI treatment (particularly at the beginning and the end) and that they could stimulate the adherence of *C. difficile* to gut epithelial cell, the first step of colonization. Indeed, our findings demonstrated that weak doses (under doses used usually in the mouse model) of MTZ increased the colonization of CD17-146 strain in cecum of conventional mice, especially the amount of bacteria associated with the cecal mucosa. The same result was not found for strain VPI 10463, which was shown to colonize better than CD17-146 in the cecum of mice, in absence of MTZ. We hypothesized that this could be due to the production of toxins by VPI 10463 while CD17-146 is non-toxigenic. Indeed, a previous study showed that sub-lethal concentrations of *C. difficile* TcdA was able to cause redistribution of plasma membrane components between distinct surface domains and facilitation of bacterial access to BL receptors, leading to a successful colonization of the colonic mucosa [28]. It is also worth noting that there were no significant differences in the level of colonization between the groups treated with usual dose of MTZ and the groups treated with water although MTZ significantly increased the survival rates. This result is in accordance with a previous study on *C. difficile* infection treatments in mice which indicated that MTZ did not reduced the number of spores in feces compared to the infected control group [29].

For several pathogenic bacteria, primary colonization and persistence in the host has been correlated with biofilm formation [30–32]. In addition, we observed in vitro that subinhibitory concentration of MTZ induced biofilm formation of CD17-146. We wondered if there was a link between the increased colonization of this strains and its biofilm production. Therefore, we visualized bacterial distribution in the cecum of monoxenic mice by CLSM. In monoxenic mice infected with CD17-146 strain, the cecal mucosa-associated bacteria formed a 3-D structure, as observed by CLSM analysis. Furthermore, we observed that the median thickness of these structures is increased when mice were treated at a quarter of usual dose of MTZ, although not in a significant manner, suggesting that low doses of MTZ may play a role in the enhancement of persistent structures by strain CD17-146 in this model, but further experiments should be done to confirm this hypothesis. This phenomenon was not observed for the VPI 10463 strain. The persistence of bacterial cells in the human intestine as a protective barrier provided by biofilm could have an important clinical relevance in the treatment failure and/or recurrence of infections associated with *C. difficile* strains. Indeed, *C. difficile* cells in biofilms show specific features that may facilitate the infection, such as spore formation and toxins A and/or B production [33,34] and resistance to antibiotics [10].

Overall, the two strains responded differently to the stress induced by MTZ subinhibitory concentrations except for the decreased motility which occurred in both strains. For CD17-146, strain with reduced susceptibility to MTZ and a moderate biofilm-forming ability without MTZ, we observed under low MTZ concentrations an elongation morphology, increased biofilm production and higher level of colonization in conventional mice and a trend to thicker 3-D bacterial structures at the surface of the cecal mucosa. On the other hand, for VPI 10463, a MTZ sensitive and strong biofilm-forming strain, we did not observe these changes under MTZ pressure. More investigations are now necessary to unravel the different aspects of this complex mechanism.

Our previous proteomic analyzes suggested that the increase of biofilm production could be related to the decrease in production of the protease Cwp84, a cell wall protein, and a higher production of an aminotransferase of the MocR family [35]. Indeed, we previously observed in presence of MTZ at MIC/2 a 3-fold decrease in the amount of Cwp84 in CD17-146. Cwp84 protease cleaves the S-layer protein SlpA on bacterial surface into two subunits. The *cwp84* mutant strain was shown to grow slower and elaborated more robust biofilms compared with the parental *C. difficile* 630Δerm strain. Furthermore, bacterial load of mutant strain in vivo competition assays was maintained over time in the cecum, suggesting there may be stable reservoirs of bacteria and these reservoirs may ultimately transition into the biofilm state [36]. Proteomic analyzes also revealed a 3-fold increased amount of a putative aminotransferase for CD17-146 strain at MIC/2. This protein belonging to MocR family 2 shares 27% identity with PdxR of *Streptococcus mutans*. Interestingly, PdxR is known to have a role in biofilm formation of S. mutans since the pdxR mutant forms significantly fewer biofilm compared to its parental strain [37]. Further research is required to elucidate the mechanism of biofilm induction in CD17-146 strain by MTZ.

Finally, we have mentioned several hypotheses that could explain the greater bacterial persistence with certain strains of *C. difficile*. However, additional experiments should be considered in order to elucidate the exact mechanism involved in this phenomenon. We are aware that these findings on the impact of MTZ on colonization by *C. difficile* were obtained from a limited number of strains and therefore need to be extended to a larger panel of a variety of strains to confirm the relevance of our results to other clinical situations. However, to our knowledge, this report is the first description of the effect of low dose of MTZ on the colonization and cecal distribution of *C. difficile* in vivo.

4. Materials and Methods

4.1. Bacterial Strains and Antibiotic Susceptibility

Two *C. difficile* strains VPI 10463 and CD17-146 were used in this study. The CD17-146 isolate provided by the *C. difficile* French National Center in Saint Antoine hospital (Paris, France) was stored immediately after isolation at −80 °C. This strain has been shown to be a non-toxigenic strain and belonging to the PCR ribotype 596 with reduced susceptibility to MTZ (minimum inhibitory concentration determined by ETEST® on solid agar was 2 µg/mL). The MIC values for MTZ evaluated by broth dilution method in our laboratory were 1 µg/mL for CD17-146 and 0.5 µg/mL for VPI 10463. According to epidemiological cut-off values of the European Committee on Antimicrobial Susceptibility Testing (ECOFF EUCAST2015), resistance to MTZ was defined as MIC > 2µg/mL. Most *C. difficile* susceptible strains have MIC ≤ 0.5 µg/mL (https://mic.eucast.org/Eucast2/regShow.jsp?Id=21294, accessed date: 15 January 2021). Thus, we considered CD17-146 as a strain with reduced susceptibility.

Bacteria were grown at 37 °C under anaerobic conditions (90% N_2, 5% CO_2 and 5% H_2).

4.2. Morphology Observation

Bacteria were grown in BHISG (Brain Heart infusion broth, Difco, Detroit, MI, USA, supplemented with 1.8% Glucose, 0.1% L-Cysteine and 0.5% yeast extract) under subinhibitory concentrations (MIC/4 and MIC/2 for each strain) of MTZ, at 37 °C under anaerobic conditions. When OD600 nm of cultures reaches 0.4, bacteria were observed by optical microscopy after Gram staining.

4.3. In Vitro Biofilm

Biofilm assays were performed in 24-well polystyrene plates (Costar, Washington, DC, USA). Overnight cultures of each *C. difficile* strain in BHISG broth were diluted in fresh BHISG to obtain OD600 nm = 0.05 and 1 mL of diluted pre-culture was added to each well. Plates were incubated at 37 °C under anaerobic conditions for 1 h and the medium was removed to eliminate non-adherent cells. Then, 900 µL of BHISG and 100 µL of a solution of MTZ were added to each well to obtain final concentrations of 0.125, 0.25, 0.5, 1 and 2 µg/mL. For control wells, 100 µL of sterile water was added instead of MTZ. After 48 h of incubation, the supernatant was removed carefully, and wells were gently washed twice with sterile phosphate-buffered saline (PBS). The biofilm was thereafter quantified by crystal violet staining (ACROS OrganicsTM. Somerville, NJ, USA) as previously described [10,38], and by enumeration of viable cells and spores. For viable cell enumeration, 1 mL of sterile pre-reduced PBS was added after washing step to each well, the biofilm formed in the bottom was scraped, the suspension was then diluted and plated on BHI agar supplemented with 3% defibrinated horse blood. For spores, the suspension of biofilm was treated with ethanol 96% in the proportion 1:1 one hour before the enumeration on BHI agar supplemented with 3% defibrinated horse blood and 0.1% taurocholate. The assay was performed in triplicate. Two-tailed, Mann Whitney test with SPSS 20 software was used to evaluate whether the differences observed in the presence or absence of antibiotic were significant for each strain. Differences were considered statistically significant for p values < 0.05.

4.4. Motility Assays

Motility assays were performed using motility agar tubes containing BHI (Brain Heart infusion broth, Difco, USA) medium and 0.3% agar with MTZ at final concentrations of 0.125, 0.25, 0.5 µg/mL. These were stab inoculated and grown anaerobically at 37 °C for 48 h [39]. Control cultures contained no antibiotics. The motile strains *C. difficile* 630 and non-motile mutant strains *C. difficile* 630 ΔfliC were used as control [27].

4.5. RNA Extraction and Quantitative RT-PCR Analysis on Flagellar Genes

C. difficile cultures were grown to an OD600 nm of 0.7 in BHISG, without or with MTZ at MIC/4 or MIC/2, RNAs were extracted using Trizol Reagent (Thermo Fisher Scientific, Waltham, MA, USA). cDNA was synthesized from 1 µg RNA using random primers and SuperScript™ III Reverse Transcriptase (Invitrogen, Waltham, MA, USA) as described by the manufacturer. Real-time PCRs were done with 1 ng of cDNA template using SSo Advanced™ SYBR Green Supermix (Bio-Rad, Hercules, CA, USA). The primers used for the three genes detected *fliC*, *flgB* and *fliA* are listed in Supplementary Table S1, *fliC* coding flagellin in the F1 region of flagellar operon; *flgB*, which is located at the beginning of F3 region; and *fliA*, located near the end of the F3 region which encodes a sigma factor predicted to activate flagellar gene expression in F1 [40]. Reactions were run on a CFX96 Real-time system (Bio-Rad) with the following cycling conditions: 30 s polymerase activation at 95 °C and 40 cycles at 95 °C for 5 s and 60 °C for 10 s. In order to verify the specificity of the real-time PCR reaction for each primer pair, an additional step from a start at 65 °C to 95 °C (0.5 °C/0.5 s) was performed to establish a melting curve. The *gluD* gene was used as reference gene, as described previously [41]. Normalized relative quantities were calculated using the ∆∆CT method. Data were analyzed with Student t test with SPSS 20. Results are expressed as mean ± standard error of mean (SEM).

4.6. Adherence Assays

The enterocyte-like Caco-2/TC7 cell line was used between passages 25 and 35. Cells were grown in DMEM medium (Dulbecco's modified Eagle's minimum, Gibco, Waltham, MA, USA) supplemented with 15% fetal calf serum (Gibco, United States) and 1% non-essential amino acids NEAA (Gibco, USA). The Caco-2/TC7 monolayers were inoculated in 24-well polystyrene culture plates (TPP, Dominique Dutscher SAS, Brumath, France) with 25,000 cells per well and used 14 days after seeding, when cells were differentiated [42].

Prior to adherence assays, cells were washed twice with PBS and 0.5 mL DMEM was added to each well. Overnight cultures of each *C. difficile* strain in BHISG broth, supplemented with subinhibitory concentrations of MTZ, were pelleted (2500 rpm, 5 min) and washed once with PBS. Then, 5×10^7 CFU in 0.5 mL DMEM were added to each well. Bacteria and cells were incubated together for 1 h 30 at 37 °C under anaerobic conditions and wells were washed twice with PBS to discard non-adherent bacteria. After, cells were lysed with 1 mL of 1% saponin per well during 15 min at 4 °C and appropriate dilutions were spread on BHI agar plates supplemented with 3% horse blood (bioMérieux) for enumeration of cell-adherent vegetative bacteria. Bacterial colonies were counted after 48 h of incubation and results were expressed as CFU of cell-adherent bacteria per 100 cells. Assays were carried out in triplicate in three separate experiments. Data were analyzed with Mann-Whitney U test with SPSS 20. Results are expressed as mean ± standard error of mean (SEM).

4.7. Model of Conventional Mice to Study the Impact of MTZ on the Intestinal Colonization of C. difficile

The model used was based on the model developed in previous studies [29,43]. Figure 6 previously presented illustrates the experimental scheme. All animal experiments were performed according to European Union guidelines for the handling of laboratory animals and all procedures were approved by the Ethics Committee CAPSUD (Protocol APAFIS#4617-2016032118119771 vI).

Six to eight weeks-old C57BL/6JOlaHsd female mice, with an initial bodyweight of 16–19 g, were obtained from Charles River. Mice were grouped by 3 animals per cage in ventilated isolators and fed with autoclaved standard chow and water ad libitum throughout the experiment.

In order to disrupt the normal enteric microbiota and established *C. difficile* infection, mice were pretreated with an antibiotic mixture containing kanamycin (40 mg/kg), gentamycin (3.5 mg/kg), colistin (85,000 mg/kg), MTZ (21.5 mg/kg) and vancomycin

(4.5 mg/kg). This cocktail was administered from day 6 to day 3 before infection in the drinking water. The concentrations of antibiotics were calculated based on the average weight of the mice and their expected water consumption. Then, mice were switched back to regular drinking water. One day prior to infection, mice received a single dose of clindamycin (10 mg/kg) by intraperitoneal route. On day 0, mice were challenged by oral gavage with approximately 3×10^5 vegetative cells in 0.3 mL volume. This inoculum was prepared as follows: an overnight culture in BHISG was diluted in BHISG to a final concentration of approximately 1×10^5 vegetative cells per mL, estimated by microscopic cell counting. The bacterial concentration was checked thereafter by enumerating vegetative viable cells. The treatments with MTZ began from 1-day post-infection (Figure 6) by oral gavage with different dose regimes. The mice were divided into 8 groups, 6 mice per group: four groups (A–D) infected with VPI 10463 and four groups (E–H) infected with CD17-146. Two groups (A and E) were treated with placebo (sterile water), six groups were treated with either usual dose of MTZ (B and F, 50 mg/kg), a half (C and G, 25 mg/kg) or a quarter (D and H, 12.5 mg/kg) of usual dose of MTZ twice a day, for 7 days. The usual dose defined in this study was the one used before to treat CDI in a mouse model [29].

Fecal samples were collected from each mouse on day 1 for enumeration of vegetative cells and were processed as previously described [44]. At the end of the 7-day observation period, mice were sacrificed, and the cecum and fecal samples were collected for enumeration of bacteria to assess the colonization rate in the cecum. The cecum contents were collected and used for luminal bacterial count. After three PBS rinses, the mucosal tissues were homogenized for 1 min with Ultra-Turrax T25 (IKA®, Labortechnik, Germany), and tissue-adherent bacteria were enumerated. Both vegetative cells and spores were enumerated in all samples. Vegetative cells were counted by plating serial 10-fold dilutions onto selective cycloserine-cefoxitin blood agar plates (CLO agar; bioMérieux, Marcy l'Etoile, France). Then, samples were mixed with equal volume of 96% alcohol for 1 h and spores were counted as described above. Colonies were counted after incubation anaerobically at 37 °C for 48 h.

Data were collected from two independent experiments and differences between two groups were analyzed with Mann-Whitney U test with SPSS 20. Results are expressed as mean ± standard error of mean (SEM).

4.8. Monoxenic Mouse Model to Visualize C. difficile Intestinal Distribution in the Cecum When Exposed to MTZ

4.8.1. Animal Model

To visualize bacterial distribution over epithelial tissues in the cecum, we used the germ-free mouse model described by Soavelomandrosso et al. [38]. Six to eight weeks old germ-free C3H/HeN female mice were obtained from INRAE (Jouy-en-Josas, France). All animal experiments were performed according to European Union guidelines for the handling of laboratory animals and all procedures were approved by the Ethics Committee CAPSUD (Protocol APAFIS#23414-2019121910116284 v4).

Mice were housed in sterile isolators with ad libitum access to food and water. Before experiments, we checked the germ-free status of each animal as previously described [38]. Mice were challenged by oral gavage with 5×10^5 CFU of *C. difficile*, either VPI 10463 (group A and B) or CD17-146 (group C and D) strain, with inoculum prepared as described for the conventional model. From 1-day post-infection, mice were treated with sterile water (group A and C) or with a quart of usual dose of MTZ: 12.5 mg/kg (group B and D) for 7 days by oral gavage twice a day. We used 3 mice per group. Seven days post-infection, feces were sampled for enumeration of bacteria and mice were euthanized. Data were analyzed with Mann-Whitney U test with SPSS 20. Results are expressed as mean ± standard error of mean (SEM). The caeca were collected for confocal microscopy analyses.

4.8.2. Confocal Laser Scanning Microscopy (CLSM)

The spatial distribution of tissue-associated bacteria was determined by CLSM analysis of mouse mucosa from three mice for each strain. After removal of cecal content, the tissues were washed 3 times in 10 mL of PBS, spread on a glass slide and stained with the LIVE/DEAD® BacLightTM 193 Bacterial Viability Kit (Thermo Fisher Scientific, United States): 20 μL of the diluted mixture (1:1000) was added on the tissues. Samples were visualized with a LSM 510 microscope (Carl Zeiss Inc., Oberkochen Germany). Horizontal plan images were acquired at several different locations for each sample. During the Z overlay, an average of the thickness of the bacterial layer in several places on the tissue sample was calculated. Finally, three-dimensional projections were reconstructed from x-z stacks using Imaris software (Bitplane, Belfast, UK).

Supplementary Materials: The following supporting information can be downloaded at: https://www.mdpi.com/article/10.3390/antibiotics11050624/s1, Figure S1: Heterogeneous distribution of C. difficile over the cecal tissue in a mono-associated mouse model. Confocal laser-scanning microscopy 3-D projection of tissue-associated bacteria obtained from cecum for the CD17-146 without or with treatment of MTZ at 0.125 mg/kg, and the VPI 10463 without or with treatment of MTZ 0.125 mg/kg. Live cells (bacterial [rod] or epithelial) are labeled in green, dead cells are labeled in red. Scale bars (white): 30 μm. Figure S2: Impact of MTZ on cecum colonization of *C. difficile* in monoxenic mice, 7 days post-infection. Germ-free mice were infected by either VPI 10463 (group A and B) or CD17-146 (group C and D) strain with 5×10^5 CFU of *C. difficile*. From 1-day post-infection, mice were treated with sterile water (group A and C) or with a quart of usual dose of MTZ: 12.5 mg/kg (group B and D) for 7 days by oral gavage twice a day. C. difficile shedding was monitored in feces at day 7 post-infection. There were no significant differences in colonization between the group treated with MTZ at usual dose/4 and the group non-treated for both strains. The error bars represent standard error of the mean (SEM). Table S1: Sequences of oligonucleotide primers used in this study.

Author Contributions: Conceptualization, S.P. and M.-F.B.-C.; methodology, S.P. and M.-F.B.-C.; validation, S.P., M.-F.B.-C. and C.J.; formal analysis, T.-H.-D.D.; investigation, T.-H.-D.D. and S.H.; writing—original draft preparation, T.-H.-D.D.; writing—review and editing, S.P., M.-F.B.-C. and C.J.; visualization, T.-H.-D.D.; supervision, S.P. and M.-F.B.-C.; project administration, S.P. and M.-F.B.-C. All authors have read and agreed to the published version of the manuscript.

Funding: This research received no external funding.

Institutional Review Board Statement: The animal study protocol was approved by the Institutional Review Board (or Ethics Committee) of CAPSUD (Protocol APAFIS#4617-2016032118119771 vI for the conventional mouse model (2016) and Protocol APAFIS#23414-2019121910116284 v4 for the monoxenic mouse model (2020)).

Informed Consent Statement: Not applicable.

Acknowledgments: We thank Frédéric Barbut, Saint Antoine hospital (Paris) for kindly providing us CD17-146 strain. The authors would like to thank Transcriptomics platform of Paris-Saclay University, Thomas Candela and Cécile Larrazet for their involvement in qRT-PCR analysis. We also thank Cellular Imaging Platform (MISFIT) for providing their instruments.

Conflicts of Interest: The authors declare no conflict of interest.

References

1. De Roo, A.C.; Regenbogen, S.E. *Clostridium difficile* Infection: An Epidemiology Update. *Clin. Colon Rectal Surg.* **2020**, *33*, 49–57. [CrossRef] [PubMed]
2. McDonald, L.C.; Gerding, D.N.; Johnson, S.; Bakken, J.S.; Carroll, K.C.; Coffin, S.E.; Dubberke, E.R.; Garey, K.W.; Gould, C.V.; Kelly, C.; et al. Clinical Practice Guidelines for *Clostridium difficile* Infection in Adults and Children: 2017 Update by the Infectious Diseases Society of America (IDSA) and Society for Healthcare Epidemiology of America (SHEA). *Clin. Infect. Dis.* **2018**, *66*, e1–e48. [CrossRef] [PubMed]
3. Johnson, S.; Louie, T.J.; Gerding, D.N.; Cornely, O.; Chasan-Taber, S.; Fitts, D.; Gelone, S.P.; Broom, C.; Davidson, D.M. Polymer Alternative for CDI Treatment (PACT) investigators Vancomycin, Metronidazole, or Tolevamer for *Clostridium difficile* Infection: Results from Two Multinational, Randomized, Controlled Trials. *Clin. Infect. Dis.* **2014**, *59*, 345–354. [CrossRef] [PubMed]

4. Lau, A.H.; Lam, N.P.; Piscitelli, S.C.; Wilkes, L.; Danziger, L.H. Clinical Pharmacokinetics of Metronidazole and Other Nitroimidazole Anti-Infectives. *Clin. Pharmacokinet.* **1992**, *23*, 328–364. [CrossRef]
5. Bolton, R.P.; Culshaw, A.M. Faecal Metronidazole Concentrations during Oral and Intravenous Therapy for Antibiotic Associated Colitis Due to Clostridium Difficile. *Gut* **1986**, *27*, 1169–1172. [CrossRef]
6. Peláez, T.; Cercenado, E.; Alcalá, L.; Marín, M.; Martín-López, A.; Martínez-Alarcón, J.; Catalán, P.; Sánchez-Somolinos, M.; Bouza, E. Metronidazole Resistance in *Clostridium difficile* Is Heterogeneous. *J. Clin. Microbiol.* **2008**, *46*, 3028–3032. [CrossRef]
7. Andersson, D.I.; Hughes, D. Microbiological Effects of Sublethal Levels of Antibiotics. *Nat. Rev. Microbiol.* **2014**, *12*, 465–478. [CrossRef]
8. Moura, I.B.; Spigaglia, P.; Barbanti, F.; Mastrantonio, P. Analysis of Metronidazole Susceptibility in Different *Clostridium difficile* PCR Ribotypes. *J. Antimicrob. Chemother.* **2013**, *68*, 362–365. [CrossRef]
9. Vuotto, C.; Moura, I.; Barbanti, F.; Donelli, G.; Spigaglia, P. Subinhibitory Concentrations of Metronidazole Increase Biofilm Formation in *Clostridium difficile* Strains. *Pathog. Dis.* **2016**, *74*, ftv114. [CrossRef]
10. Đapa, T.; Dapa, T.; Leuzzi, R.; Ng, Y.K.; Baban, S.T.; Adamo, R.; Kuehne, S.A.; Scarselli, M.; Minton, N.P.; Serruto, D.; et al. Multiple Factors Modulate Biofilm Formation by the Anaerobic Pathogen *Clostridium difficile*. *J. Bacteriol.* **2013**, *195*, 545–555. [CrossRef]
11. Surawicz, C.M.; Alexander, J. Treatment of Refractory and Recurrent *Clostridium difficile* Infection. *Nat. Rev. Gastroenterol. Hepatol.* **2011**, *8*, 330–339. [CrossRef]
12. Hall-Stoodley, L.; Stoodley, P. Evolving Concepts in Biofilm Infections. *Cell. Microbiol.* **2009**, *11*, 1034–1043. [CrossRef]
13. Li, D.; Renzoni, A.; Estoppey, T.; Bisognano, C.; Francois, P.; Kelley, W.L.; Lew, D.P.; Schrenzel, J.; Vaudaux, P. Induction of Fibronectin Adhesins in Quinolone-Resistant *Staphylococcus aureus* by Subinhibitory Levels of Ciprofloxacin or by Sigma B Transcription Factor Activity Is Mediated by Two Separate Pathways. *Antimicrob. Agents Chemother.* **2005**, *49*, 916–924. [CrossRef]
14. Hoffman, L.R.; D'Argenio, D.A.; MacCoss, M.J.; Zhang, Z.; Jones, R.A.; Miller, S.I. Aminoglycoside Antibiotics Induce Bacterial Biofilm Formation. *Nature* **2005**, *436*, 1171–1175. [CrossRef]
15. Moura, I.; Monot, M.; Tani, C.; Spigaglia, P.; Barbanti, F.; Norais, N.; Dupuy, B.; Bouza, E.; Mastrantonio, P. Multidisciplinary Analysis of a Nontoxigenic *Clostridium difficile* Strain with Stable Resistance to Metronidazole. *Antimicrob. Agents Chemother.* **2014**, *58*, 4957–4960. [CrossRef]
16. Boekhoud, I.M.; Hornung, B.V.H.; Sevilla, E.; Harmanus, C.; Bos-Sanders, I.M.J.G.; Terveer, E.M.; Bolea, R.; Corver, J.; Kuijper, E.J.; Smits, W.K. Plasmid-Mediated Metronidazole Resistance in *Clostridioides difficile*. *Nat. Commun.* **2020**, *11*, 1–12. [CrossRef]
17. Alauzet, C.; Lozniewski, A.; Marchandin, H. Metronidazole Resistance and Nim Genes in Anaerobes: A Review. *Anaerobe* **2019**, *55*, 40–53. [CrossRef]
18. Deshpande, A.; Wu, X.; Huo, W.; Palmer, K.L.; Hurdle, J.G. Chromosomal Resistance to Metronidazole in *Clostridioides difficile* Can Be Mediated by Epistasis between Iron Homeostasis and Oxidoreductases. *Antimicrob. Agents Chemother.* **2020**, *64*, e00415-20. [CrossRef]
19. Britz, M.L.; Wilkinson, R.G. Isolation and Properties of Metronidazole-Resistant Mutants of *Bacteroides fragilis*. *Antimicrob. Agents Chemother.* **1979**, *16*, 19–27. [CrossRef]
20. Jackson, D.; Salem, A.; Coombs, G.H. The In-Vitro Activity of Metronidazole against Strains of *Escherichia coli* with Impaired DNA Repair Systems. *J. Antimicrob. Chemother.* **1984**, *13*, 227–236. [CrossRef]
21. Tally, F.P.; Sutter, V.L.; Finegold, S.M. Treatment of Anaerobic Infections with Metronidazole. *Antimicrob. Agents Chemother.* **1975**, *7*, 672–675. [CrossRef]
22. Kwon, Y.W.; Lee, S.Y. Effect of Sub-Minimal Inhibitory Concentration Antibiotics on Morphology of Periodontal Pathogens. *Int. J. Oral. Biol.* **2014**, *39*, 115–120. [CrossRef]
23. Bedran, T.B.L.; Grignon, L.; Spolidorio, D.P.; Grenier, D. Subinhibitory Concentrations of Triclosan Promote *Streptococcus mutans* Biofilm Formation and Adherence to Oral Epithelial Cells. *PLoS ONE* **2014**, *9*, e89059. [CrossRef]
24. Wu, S.; Li, X.; Gunawardana, M.; Maguire, K.; Guerrero-Given, D.; Schaudinn, C.; Wang, C.; Baum, M.M.; Webster, P. Beta-Lactam Antibiotics Stimulate Biofilm Formation in Non-Typeable *Haemophilus influenzae* by Up-Regulating Carbohydrate Metabolism. *PLoS ONE* **2014**, *9*, e99204. [CrossRef]
25. Abu Rahmoun, L.; Azrad, M.; Peretz, A. Antibiotic Resistance and Biofilm Production Capacity in *Clostridioides difficile*. *Front. Cell. Infect. Microbiol.* **2021**, *11*, 683464. [CrossRef]
26. Dingle, T.C.; Mulvey, G.L.; Armstrong, G.D. Mutagenic Analysis of the *Clostridium difficile* Flagellar Proteins, FliC and FliD, and Their Contribution to Virulence in Hamsters. *Infect. Immun.* **2011**, *79*, 4061–4067. [CrossRef]
27. Baban, S.T.; Kuehne, S.A.; Barketi-Klai, A.; Cartman, S.T.; Kelly, M.L.; Hardie, K.R.; Kansau, I.; Collignon, A.; Minton, N.P. The Role of Flagella in *Clostridium difficile* Pathogenesis: Comparison between a Non-Epidemic and an Epidemic Strain. *PLoS ONE* **2013**, *8*, e73026. [CrossRef]
28. Kasendra, M.; Barrile, R.; Leuzzi, R.; Soriani, M. *Clostridium difficile* Toxins Facilitate Bacterial Colonization by Modulating the Fence and Gate Function of Colonic Epithelium. *J. Infect. Dis.* **2014**, *209*, 1095–1104. [CrossRef]
29. Erikstrup, L.T.; Aarup, M.; Hagemann-Madsen, R.; Dagnaes-Hansen, F.; Kristensen, B.; Olsen, K.E.P.; Fuursted, K. Treatment of *Clostridium difficile* Infection in Mice with Vancomycin Alone Is as Effective as Treatment with Vancomycin and Metronidazole in Combination. *BMJ Open Gastroenterol.* **2015**, *2*, e000038. [CrossRef]

30. Cooper, R.; Bjarnsholt, T.; Alhede, M. Biofilms in Wounds: A Review of Present Knowledge. *J. Wound Care* **2014**, *23*, 570–580. [CrossRef]
31. Mihai, M.M.; Holban, A.M.; Giurcaneanu, C.; Popa, L.G.; Oanea, R.M.; Lazar, V.; Chifiriuc, M.C.; Popa, M.; Popa, M.I. Microbial Biofilms: Impact on the Pathogenesis of Periodontitis, Cystic Fibrosis, Chronic Wounds and Medical Device-Related Infections. *Curr. Top. Med. Chem.* **2015**, *15*, 1552–1576. [CrossRef] [PubMed]
32. Lund-Palau, H.; Turnbull, A.R.; Bush, A.; Bardin, E.; Cameron, L.; Soren, O.; Wierre-Gore, N.; Alton, E.W.F.W.; Bundy, J.G.; Connett, G.; et al. *Pseudomonas aeruginosa* Infection in Cystic Fibrosis: Pathophysiological Mechanisms and Therapeutic Approaches. *Expert Rev. Respir. Med.* **2016**, *10*, 685–697. [CrossRef] [PubMed]
33. Semenyuk, E.G.; Laning, M.L.; Foley, J.; Johnston, P.F.; Knight, K.L.; Gerding, D.N.; Driks, A. Spore Formation and Toxin Production in *Clostridium difficile* Biofilms. *PLoS ONE* **2014**, *9*, e87757. [CrossRef] [PubMed]
34. Crowther, G.S.; Chilton, C.H.; Todhunter, S.L.; Nicholson, S.; Freeman, J.; Baines, S.D.; Wilcox, M.H. Comparison of Planktonic and Biofilm-Associated Communities of *Clostridium difficile* and Indigenous Gut Microbiota in a Triple-Stage Chemostat Gut Model. *J. Antimicrob. Chemother.* **2014**, *69*, 2137–2147. [CrossRef]
35. Doan, T.-H.-D.; Yen-Nicolaÿ, S.; Bernet-Camard, M.-F.; Martin-Verstraete, I.; Péchiné, S. Impact of Subinhibitory Concentrations of Metronidazole on Proteome of *Clostridioides difficile* Strains with Different Levels of Susceptibility. *PLoS ONE* **2020**, *15*, e0241903. [CrossRef]
36. Pantaléon, V.; Soavelomandroso, A.P.; Bouttier, S.; Briandet, R.; Roxas, B.; Chu, M.; Collignon, A.; Janoir, C.; Vedantam, G.; Candela, T. The *Clostridium difficile* Protease Cwp84 Modulates Both Biofilm Formation and Cell-Surface Properties. *PLoS ONE* **2015**, *10*, e0124971. [CrossRef]
37. Liao, S.; Bitoun, J.; Nguyen, A.; Bozner, D.; Yao, X.; Wen, Z.T. Deficiency of PdxR in *Streptococcus mutans* Affects Vitamin B6 Metabolism, Acid Tolerance Response and Biofilm Formation. *Mol. Oral Microbiol.* **2015**, *30*, 255–268. [CrossRef]
38. Soavelomandroso, A.P.; Gaudin, F.; Hoys, S.; Nicolas, V.; Vedantam, G.; Janoir, C.; Bouttier, S. Biofilm Structures in a Mono-Associated Mouse Model of *Clostridium difficile* Infection. *Front. Microbiol.* **2017**, *8*, 2086. [CrossRef]
39. Pantaléon, V.; Monot, M.; Eckert, C.; Hoys, S.; Collignon, A.; Janoir, C.; Candela, T. *Clostridium difficile* Forms Variable Biofilms on Abiotic Surface. *Anaerobe* **2018**, *53*, 34–37. [CrossRef]
40. Purcell, E.B.; McKee, R.W.; McBride, S.M.; Waters, C.M.; Tamayo, R. Cyclic Diguanylate Inversely Regulates Motility and Aggregation in *Clostridium difficile*. *J. Bacteriol.* **2012**, *194*, 3307–3316. [CrossRef]
41. Metcalf, D.; Sharif, S.; Weese, J.S. Evaluation of Candidate Reference Genes in *Clostridium difficile* for Gene Expression Normalization. *Anaerobe* **2010**, *16*, 439–443. [CrossRef]
42. Denève, C.; Deloménie, C.; Barc, M.-C.; Collignon, A.; Janoir, C. Antibiotics Involved in *Clostridium difficile*-Associated Disease Increase Colonization Factor Gene Expression. *J. Med. Microbiol.* **2008**, *57*, 732–738. [CrossRef]
43. Chen, X.; Katchar, K.; Goldsmith, J.D.; Nanthakumar, N.; Cheknis, A.; Gerding, D.N.; Kelly, C.P. A Mouse Model of *Clostridium difficile*—Associated Disease. *Gastroenterology* **2008**, *135*, 1984–1992. [CrossRef]
44. Péchiné, S.; Janoir, C.; Boureau, H.; Gleizes, A.; Tsapis, N.; Hoys, S.; Fattal, E.; Collignon, A. Diminished Intestinal Colonization by *Clostridium difficile* and Immune Response in Mice after Mucosal Immunization with Surface Proteins of Clostridium Difficile. *Vaccine* **2007**, *25*, 3946–3954. [CrossRef]

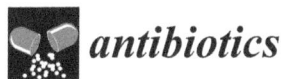

Article

Clostridioides difficile Toxin B PCR Cycle Threshold as a Predictor of Toxin Testing in Stool Specimens from Hospitalized Adults

Sean Lee [1], Neha Nanda [2], Kenichiro Yamaguchi [1], Yelim Lee [3] and Rosemary C. She [1,*]

[1] Department of Pathology, Keck School of Medicine of the University of Southern California, Los Angeles, CA 90033, USA; seanshlee41@gmail.com (S.L.); ky91789@gmail.com (K.Y.)
[2] Department of Medicine, Division of Infectious Diseases, Keck School of Medicine of the University of Southern California, Los Angeles, CA 90033, USA; neha.nanda@med.usc.edu
[3] Department of Biology and Biological Sciences, California Institute of Technology, Pasadena, CA 91125, USA; ylee9912@gmail.com
* Correspondence: rosemary.she@med.usc.edu

Abstract: Rapid, accurate detection of *Clostridioides difficile* toxin may potentially be predicted by toxin B PCR cycle threshold (*tcdB* C_t). We investigated the validity of this approach in an inpatient adult population. Patients who tested positive by *C. difficile* PCR (Cepheid GeneXpert) from December 2016 to October 2020 (*n* = 368) at a tertiary medical center were included. All stool samples were further tested by rapid glutamate dehydrogenase (GDH)/toxin B EIA and cell cytotoxin neutralization assay (CCNA). Receiver operating characteristic curves were analyzed. The area under the curve for *tcdB* C_t predicting toxin result by EIA was 0.795 (95% confidence interval (CI) 0.747–0.843) and by CCNA was 0.771 (95% CI 0.720–0.822). The Youden C_t cutoff for CCNA was ≤27.8 cycles (sensitivity 65.0%, specificity 77.2%). For specimens with C_t ≤ 25.0 cycles (*n* = 115), CCNA toxin was positive in >90%. The negative predictive value of *tcdB* C_t for CCNA was no greater than 80% regardless of cutoff chosen. In summary, very low C_t values (≤25.0) could have limited value as a rapid indicator of positive toxin status by CCNA in our patient population. A broad distribution of C_t values for toxin-negative and toxin-positive specimens precluded more robust prediction. Additional data are needed before broader application of C_t values from qualitatively designed assays to clinical laboratory reporting.

Keywords: neutralization assay; toxin immunoassay; receiver operating characteristic curve

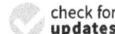

Citation: Lee, S.; Nanda, N.; Yamaguchi, K.; Lee, Y.; She, R.C. *Clostridioides difficile* Toxin B PCR Cycle Threshold as a Predictor of Toxin Testing in Stool Specimens from Hospitalized Adults. *Antibiotics* 2022, *11*, 576. https://doi.org/10.3390/antibiotics11050576

Academic Editor: Guido Granata

Received: 1 April 2022
Accepted: 20 April 2022
Published: 26 April 2022

Publisher's Note: MDPI stays neutral with regard to jurisdictional claims in published maps and institutional affiliations.

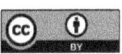

Copyright: © 2022 by the authors. Licensee MDPI, Basel, Switzerland. This article is an open access article distributed under the terms and conditions of the Creative Commons Attribution (CC BY) license (https:// creativecommons.org/licenses/by/ 4.0/).

1. Introduction

Clostridioides difficile is an anaerobic, spore-forming Gram-positive bacillus and one of the most commonly reported pathogens in health care-associated infections [1]. In the context of a perturbed fecal microbiota, *C. difficile* causes disease via toxin production, leading to intestinal mucosal damage. Major risk factors for disease include prior antibiotic usage, older age, and healthcare exposure. The spectrum of disease ranges from diarrhea to pseudomembranous colitis and toxic megacolon. Both toxins A and B are produced by most pathogenic strains, but toxin B is detected in nearly all cases of *C. difficile* disease. Diagnosis is based upon the clinical suspicion and detection of toxigenic *C. difficile* or its toxins in stool [2].

The rapid, accurate diagnosis of *C. difficile* infection (CDI) is not yet fully optimized, but toxin detection may be considered the strongest correlate with clinical outcomes [3]. Methods to detect toxin B in stool include enzyme immunoassay (EIA), which has variable levels of performance [2,4], and cell culture cytotoxicity neutralization assay (CCNA). The detection of toxins correlates with disease severity [5], and CCNA results have been shown to correlate most closely with CDI compared to EIA-based toxin assays and toxigenic culture [3]. However, as CCNA is a time-consuming, with a manual method that requires up to 72 h for final results, surrogate methods have been put forth to hasten the time to an accurate toxicology result.

It has been demonstrated that the bacterial load of toxigenic *C. difficile* in stool correlates with the detection of toxins, with higher bacterial loads observed in specimens that test toxin-positive than those that test toxin-negative [6,7]. Several studies have therefore evaluated the cycle threshold (C_t) from real-time PCR amplification of *C. difficile tcdB* from stool as a potentially rapid predictor of toxin status [6–9]. In our clinical experience, toxin EIA has performed poorly compared to CCNA [10], and we have not observed an obvious correlation between *tcdB* C_t and toxin status. It was therefore suspected that the predictive ability of *tcdB* C_t values may not be broadly applicable to different toxin assays or patient populations. The objective of this study was to investigate the potential use of *tcdB* C_t values in a hospitalized adult population for predicting toxin status by either toxin EIA or CCNA.

2. Results

2.1. Patient Demographics

Of 370 PCR-positive samples from hospitalized inpatients, 2 were excluded because CCNA was not performed due to lab error. The remaining 368 samples were from 191 (51.9%) male and 177 (48.1%) female patients (Table S1). Mean and median ages were 58.7 and 62.0 years, respectively. Reasons for admission were largely related to patient history of solid organ transplant (n = 64 (17.4%)), hematopoietic stem cell transplant (n = 23 (6.3%)), malignancy (n = 105 (28.5%)), and surgical procedures (n = 97 (20.4%)). Underlying conditions of all patients are summarized in Table 1.

Table 1. Underlying medical conditions of hospitalized adult patients with positive *C. difficile* PCR included in this study.

Medical Condition	*n* (%)
Malignancy	105 (28.5)
Hematologic	15 (4.1)
Non-hematologic	90 (24.5)
Solid organ transplant	64 (17.4)
Hematopoietic stem cell transplant	23 (6.3)
Surgical procedure	97 (20.4)
Neurosurgery	22 (6.0)
Abdominal	29 (7.9)
Cardiovascular	26 (7.1)
Orthopedic	8 (1.6)
Urologic	4 (1.1)
Other	8 (2.2)
Cardiovascular disease	20 (5.4)
Hepatic failure	17 (4.6)
Inflammatory bowel disease	15 (4.1)
Gastrointestinal disease (non-surgical)	9 (2.4)
Non-cancerous neoplasm	5 (1.4)
Other conditions	13 (3.5)
Total	368 (100)

2.2. Summary Statistics

Out of the 368 toxigenic *C. difficile* PCR-positive specimens, 326 (88.6%) tested positive by GDH EIA, 127 (34.5%) by toxin EIA, and 254 (69.0%) by CCNA. Compared to CCNA as the reference standard, toxin EIA had a sensitivity of 48.4% (123/254; 95% confidence interval (CI) 42.1–54.8%) and specificity of 96.5% (110/114; 95% CI 91.3–99.0%). The *tcdB* C_t values of the toxin EIA-positive, CCNA-negative specimens ranged from 26.1 to 35.0. Distribution of results demonstrated CCNA toxin-positive specimens to have a more gradual decline in numbers as C_t values increased, compared to toxin EIA-positive samples which demonstrated a denser clustering at lower C_t values (Figure 1).

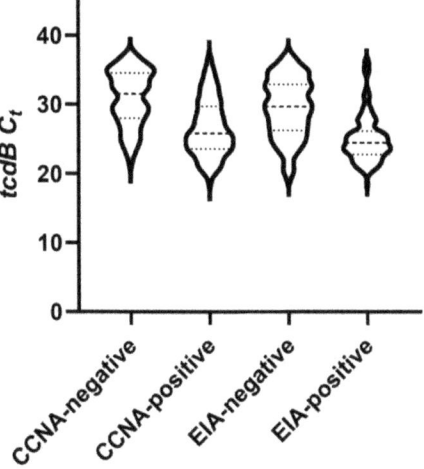

Figure 1. Box and violin plot shows distributions of *tcdB* C_t values according to toxin test results. Minimum, maximum, median (large dashed line), and 25th and 75th percentiles (small dashed lines) are indicated. Observed frequencies of values are represented by width of the plot interval.

2.3. Cycle Threshold Value and GDH, Toxin EIA, and CCNA Results

The *tcdB* C_t values were significantly higher for GDH-negative than GDH-positive samples, toxin EIA-negative than toxin EIA-positive samples, CCNA-negative than CCNA-positive samples, and EIA-positive than CCNA-positive samples. There was no statistically significant difference between NAP1-negative and NAP1-presumptive positive samples (Table 2, Figure 2). However, NAP1-presumptive positive specimens were significantly more frequently EIA-positive (31/53; 58.5%) than NAP1-presumptive negative specimens (95/315; 30.2%) ($p = 0.0001$); and more frequently CCNA-positive (44/53; 83.0%) than NAP-1 presumptive negative specimens (210/315; 66.7%) ($p = 0.016$).

Table 2. Summary statistics of C_t values for *tcdB* by GDH EIA, toxin EIA, CCNA, and PCR NAP1 results.

	n	Median (Mean) C_t	*p*-Value [a]
GDH-positive	326	27.5 (27.3)	<0.001
GDH-negative	42	32.9 (32.7)	
Toxin EIA-positive	127	25.0 (24.5) [b]	<0.001
Toxin EIA-negative	241	29.5 (29.7)	
CCNA-positive	254	25.8 (26.6) [b]	<0.001
CCNA-negative	114	31.5 (30.9)	
NAP1-presumptive positive	53	25.3 (26.9)	0.056
NAP1-negative	315	27.7 (28.1)	
All samples	368	27.5 (27.9)	NA

[a] Mann–Whitney U test. [b] $p = 0.002$ for comparison by Mann–Whitney U test. Abbreviations: C_t, threshold cycle; GDH, glutamate dehydrogenase; EIA, enzyme immunoassay; CCNA, cell culture cytotoxicity neutralization assay; NAP1, North American PFGE type 1; NA, not applicable.

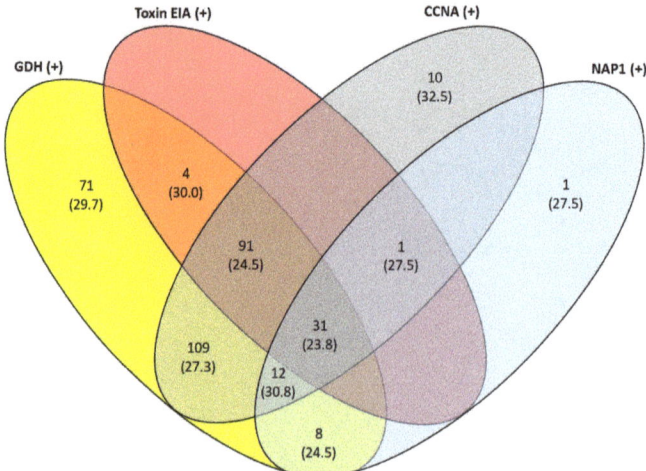

Figure 2. Venn diagram illustrates the number of specimens with each different test result combination, given as *n* (median tcdB C_t value). Abbreviations: C_t, threshold cycle; GDH, glutamate dehydrogenase; EIA, enzyme immunoassay; CCNA, cell culture cytotoxicity neutralization assay; NAP1, North American PFGE type 1.

2.4. Use of tcdB C_t Value as an Indicator of Toxin Results

An ROC curve analysis of tcdB C_t values to predict toxin EIA results yielded an AUC of 0.795 (95% CI 0.747–0.843) (Figure 3). The Youden C_t cutoff of ≤26.2 cycles had a sensitivity of 75.6% (95% CI 67.4–82.2%) and specificity of 75.1% (95% CI 69.2–80.1%). The ROC curve for tcdB C_t values to predict CCNA toxin result yielded an AUC of 0.771 (95% CI 0.720–0.822) (Figure 3). The Youden C_t cutoff of ≤27.8 cycles had a sensitivity of 65.0% (95% CI 58.9–70.6%) and specificity of 77.2% (95% CI 68.7–83.9%). To account for the rapid turnaround time and accuracy of toxin EIA-positive results, we performed a subset analysis on toxin EIA-negative specimens, for which CCNA toxin results were potentially more applicable. In toxin EIA-negative specimens, the AUC was 0.677 (95% CI 0.610–0.745).

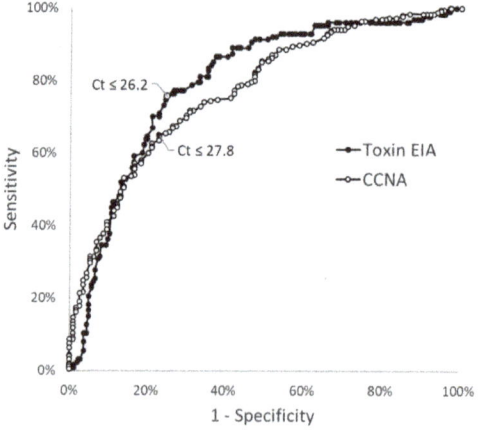

Figure 3. Receiver operating characteristic (ROC) curve for *tcdB* C_t value predicting EIA toxin status (AUC = 0.795), or CCNA toxin status (AUC = 0.771). Youden cutoffs are indicated on each curve with their corresponding C_t value cutoffs.

When examining the positive predictive value of tcdB C_t for CCNA toxin results by C_t value, we found that tcdB $C_t \leq 21.3$ cycles was the highest cutoff at which positive toxin detection by CCNA could be predicted with 100% accuracy ($n = 22$). A cutoff of $C_t \leq 25.0$ cycles was the highest at which >90.0% (104/115) of such specimens tested positive for toxin by CCNA. No meaningful $\geq C_t$ cutoff could predict negative CCNA toxin results beyond 80% accuracy. Even at a cutoff of ≥ 35.4 cycles, 4 of 19 (21.1%) specimens still tested CCNA-positive.

3. Discussion

Our analysis of data from a recent four-year period sought to characterize the predictive value of the tcdB C_t value for *C. difficile* toxin status in PCR-positive fecal specimens in an adult inpatient population. Our findings could be relevant to institutions considering the use of algorithmic or combination testing for *C. difficile* by toxin assays and PCR, particularly as we correlated PCR C_t values with CCNA, a reference standard toxin assay [11,12]. The rapid toxin EIA test used here can provide results within minutes, negating much of the benefit of using for C_t value from PCR to predict its results. Conversely, the low sensitivity for *C. difficile* toxin B by EIA compared to CCNA (48.4% in this study) limits its utility as a rapid toxin assay. Furthermore, use of the tcdB C_t value to predict toxin results obtained by CCNA could be considered more impactful given that CCNA toxin results have been shown to correspond with *C. difficile* disease severity [2,5], and that tcdB C_t values are obtained at the time of real-time PCR but CCNA requires 1 to 3 days.

In this study, *tcdB* C_t values yielded similar AUCs for toxin results by EIA and CCNA, and it was shown that using *tcdB* C_t value as predictor of toxin results yielded suboptimal sensitivity and specificity (~75%) at the optimal cutoffs. Selecting a separate cutoff *tcdB* C_t value for positive and negative toxin results by CCNA offered some advantages, albeit limited. Although a cutoff of $C_t \leq 25.0$ cycles could predict positive CCNA results for a specimen with >90% accuracy, more than half of CCNA-positive specimens actually had Ct numbers >25.0. In our analysis, there no practical *tcdB* C_t cutoff value was found that reliably corresponded to CCNA-negative results given the wide and even distribution of CCNA-positive specimens across C_t values.

Of note, other studies evaluating the ability of tcdB C_t results to predict toxin status showed better performance than found here. An AUC as high as 0.921 for predicting combined results of toxin testing by EIA and CCNA using the Xpert assay, quantitatively calibrated to tcdB target concentrations, has been demonstrated (7). A sensitivity of 99.0% for rapid EIA toxin detection was attained with a tcdB C_t cutoff of <27.55 (Xpert), although the corresponding specificity was 58.8% [8]. It is noteworthy that in these two aforementioned studies, toxigenic bacterial load clustered tightly according to toxin test result, in contrast to our tcdB C_t results, which were much more broadly distributed. Similar to our study, another study evaluating Xpert PCR results from a 6-year period described significant overlap of C_t values between EIA toxin-positive and -negative specimens [13]. We can only speculate that differences in C_t value distribution seen between studies could have resulted from studies of longer study periods capturing more variation in test operators and assay lot-to-lot differences. Discrepancies in performance characteristics for the same *C. difficile* toxin and PCR assays have furthermore been observed to occur between different geographic sites and strain types [2,14,15], potentially contributing to our observed results. The low sensitivity of the rapid GDH/toxin combination at our institution is described in other studies, though it contrasts with the performance found by others [10,16–19], a trend which remained consistent throughout this four-year study period. Our results were similar to those described in a cancer center patient population, in which an AUC of 0.83 was obtained with a Youden cutoff of ≤ 28.0 cycles (vs. our Youden cutoff of ≤ 27.8 cycles) for the prediction of CCNA toxin results. Overlapping distributions of Ct values of 25.0–28.0 were also noted between CCNA-negative and CCNA-positive cases in another comparison [20]. Although others have not found adverse outcomes associated with the implementation of

Informed Consent Statement: Patient consent was waived due to the study involving no more than minimal risk to subjects and the determination that the waiver would not adversely affect the rights and welfare of subjects.

Data Availability Statement: The data presented in this study are available in the Supplementary Materials.

Conflicts of Interest: The authors declare no conflict of interest.

References

1. Magill, S.S.; Edwards, J.R.; Bamberg, W.; Beldavs, Z.G.; Dumyati, G.; Kainer, M.A.; Lynfield, R.; Maloney, M.; McAllister-Hollod, L.; Nadle, J.; et al. Multistate point-prevalence survey of health care-associated infections. *N. Engl. J. Med.* **2014**, *370*, 1198–1208. [CrossRef] [PubMed]
2. Van Prehn, J.; Reigadas, E.; Vogelzang, E.H.; Bouza, E.; Hristea, A.; Guery, B.; Krutova, M.; Norén, T.; Allerberger, F.; Coia, J.; et al. European Society of Clinical Microbiology and Infectious Diseases: 2021 update on the treatment guidance document for *Clostridioides difficile* infection in adults. *Clin. Microbiol. Infect.* **2021**, *27* (Suppl. S2), S1–S21. [CrossRef] [PubMed]
3. Planche, T.D.; Davies, K.A.; Coen, P.G.; Finney, J.M.; Monahan, I.M.; Morris, K.A.; O'Connor, L.; Oakley, S.J.; Pope, C.F.; Wren, M.W.; et al. Differences in outcome according to *Clostridium difficile* testing method: A prospective multicentre diagnostic validation study of *C difficile* infection. *Lancet Infect. Dis.* **2013**, *13*, 936–945. [CrossRef]
4. Planche, T.; Aghaizu, A.; Holliman, R.; Riley, P.; Poloniecki, J.; Breathnach, A.; Krishna, S. Diagnosis of *Clostridium difficile* in-fection by toxin detection kits: A systematic review. *Lancet Infect. Dis.* **2008**, *8*, 777–784. [CrossRef]
5. Longtin, Y.; Trottier, S.; Brochu, G.; Paquet-Bolduc, B.; Garenc, C.; Loungnarath, V.; Beaulieu, C.; Goulet, D.; Longtin, J. Impact of the Type of Diagnostic Assay on *Clostridium difficile* Infection and Complication Rates in a Mandatory Reporting Program. *Clin. Infect. Dis.* **2012**, *56*, 67–73. [CrossRef]
6. Dionne, L.L.; Raymond, F.; Corbeil, J.; Longtin, J.; Gervais, P.; Longtin, Y. Correlation between *Clostridium difficile* bacterial load, commercial real-time PCR cycle thresholds, and results of diagnostic tests based on enzyme immunoassay and cell culture cytotoxicity assay. *J. Clin. Microbiol.* **2013**, *51*, 3624–3630. [CrossRef]
7. Leslie, J.L.; Cohen, S.H.; Solnick, J.V.; Polage, C.R. Role of fecal *Clostridium difficile* load in discrepancies between toxin tests and PCR: Is quantitation the next step in *C. difficile* testing? *Eur. J. Clin. Microbiol. Infect. Dis.* **2012**, *31*, 3295–3299. [CrossRef]
8. Senchyna, F.; Gaur, R.L.; Gombar, S.; Truong, C.Y.; Schroeder, L.F.; Banaei, N. *Clostridium difficile* PCR Cycle Threshold Predicts Free Toxin. *J. Clin. Microbiol.* **2017**, *55*, 2651–2660. [CrossRef]
9. Kamboj, M.; Brite, J.; McMillen, T.; Robilotti, E.; Herrera, A.; Sepkowitz, K.; Babady, N.E. Potential of real-time PCR threshold cycle (C(T)) to predict presence of free toxin and clinically relevant *C. difficile* infection (CDI) in patients with cancer. *J. Infect.* **2018**, *76*, 369–375. [CrossRef]
10. Ashraf, Z.; Rahmati, E.; Bender, J.M.; Nanda, N.; She, R.C. GDH and toxin immunoassay for the diagnosis of Clostridioides (Clostridium) difficile infection is not a 'one size fit all' screening test. *Diagn. Microbiol. Infect. Dis.* **2018**, *94*, 109–112. [CrossRef]
11. Centers for Disease Control and Prevention. Short Summary: Testing for *C. difficile* and Standardized Infection Ratios, National Healthcare Safety Network. 2019. Available online: https://www.cdc.gov/nhsn/pdfs/ps-analysis-resources/Cdiff-testing-sir-508.pdf (accessed on 24 February 2022).
12. Bagdasarian, N.; Rao, K.; Malani, P.N. Diagnosis and treatment of *Clostridium difficile* in adults: A systematic review. *JAMA* **2015**, *313*, 398–408. [CrossRef] [PubMed]
13. Wilmore, S.; Goldenberg, S.D. Potential of real-time PCR threshold cycle (CT) to predict presence of free toxin and clinically relevant *C. difficile* infection (CDI) in patients with cancer: A reply. *J. Infect.* **2018**, *76*, 424–426. [CrossRef] [PubMed]
14. Tenover, F.C.; Novak-Weekley, S.; Woods, C.W.; Peterson, L.R.; Davis, T.; Schreckenberger, P.; Fang, F.C.; Dascal, A.; Gerding, D.N.; Nomura, J.H.; et al. Impact of Strain Type on Detection of Toxigenic *Clostridium difficile*: Comparison of Molecular Diagnostic and Enzyme Immunoassay Approaches. *J. Clin. Microbiol.* **2010**, *48*, 3719–3724. [CrossRef] [PubMed]
15. Rizzardi, K.; Åkerlund, T.; Norén, T.; Matussek, A. Impact of ribotype on *Clostridioides difficile* diagnostics. *Eur. J. Clin. Microbiol.* **2020**, *39*, 847–853. [CrossRef] [PubMed]
16. Quinn, C.D.; Sefers, S.E.; Babiker, W.; He, Y.; Alcabasa, R.; Stratton, C.W.; Carroll, K.C.; Tang, Y.-W.C. Diff Quik Chek Complete Enzyme Immunoassay Provides a Reliable First-Line Method for Detection of *Clostridium difficile* in Stool Specimens. *J. Clin. Microbiol.* **2010**, *48*, 603–605. [CrossRef] [PubMed]
17. Chung, H.-S.; Lee, M. Evaluation of the performance of C. DIFF QUIK CHEK COMPLETE and its usefulness in a hospital setting with a high prevalence of *Clostridium difficile* infection. *J. Investig. Med.* **2017**, *65*, 88–92. [CrossRef]
18. Larson, A.M.; Fung, A.M.; Fang, F.C. Evaluation of *tcdB* Real-Time PCR in a Three-Step Diagnostic Algorithm for Detection of Toxigenic *Clostridium difficile*. *J. Clin. Microbiol.* **2010**, *48*, 124–130. [CrossRef]
19. Gomez, E.J.; Montgomery, S.; Alby, K.; Robinson, D.P.; Roundtree, S.S.; Blecker-Shelly, D.; Sullivan, K.V. Poor yield of *Clostridium difficile* testing algorithms using glutamate dehydrogenase antigen and *C. difficile* toxin enzyme immunoassays in a pediatric population with declining prevalence of *clostridium difficile* strain BI/NAP1/027. *Diagn. Microbiol. Infect. Dis.* **2018**, *91*, 229–232. [CrossRef]

20. Shah, M.D.; Balada-Llasat, J.-M.; Coe, K.; Reed, E.; Sandlund, J.; Pancholi, P. Evaluation of Cycle Threshold, Toxin Concentration, and Clinical Characteristics of *Clostridioides difficile* Infection in Patients with Discordant Diagnostic Test Results. *J. Clin. Microbiol.* **2020**, *58*, e01681-19. [CrossRef]
21. Hitchcock, M.M.; Holubar, M.; Hogan, C.A.; Tompkins, L.S.; Banaei, N. Dual Reporting of *Clostridioides difficile* PCR and Pre-dicted Toxin Result Based on PCR Cycle Threshold Reduces Treatment of Toxin-Negative Patients without Increases in Ad-verse Outcomes. *J. Clin. Microbiol.* **2019**, *57*, e01288-19. [CrossRef]
22. Bai, Y.; Sun, X.; Jin, Y.; Wang, Y.; Li, J. Accuracy of Xpert *Clostridium difficile* assay for the diagnosis of *Clostridium difficile* infection: A meta analysis. *PLoS ONE* **2017**, *12*, e0185891. [CrossRef] [PubMed]
23. Deshpande, A.; Pasupuleti, V.; Rolston, D.D.; Jain, A.; Deshpande, N.; Pant, C.; Hernandez, A.V. Diagnostic accuracy of re-al-time polymerase chain reaction in detection of *Clostridium difficile* in the stool samples of patients with suspected *Clostridium difficile* Infection: A meta-analysis. *Clin. Infect. Dis.* **2011**, *53*, e81–e90. [CrossRef] [PubMed]
24. Reigadas, E.; Alcalá, L.; Valerio, M.; Marín, M.; Martin, A.; Bouza, E. Toxin B PCR cycle threshold as a predictor of poor out-come of *Clostridium difficile* infection: A derivation and validation cohort study. *J. Antimicrob. Chemother.* **2016**, *71*, 1380–1385. [CrossRef]
25. De Francesco, M.A.; Lorenzin, G.; Piccinelli, G.; Corbellini, S.; Bonfanti, C.; Caruso, A. Correlation between tcdB gene PCR cycle threshold and severe *Clostridium difficile* disease. *Anaerobe* **2019**, *59*, 141–144. [CrossRef] [PubMed]
26. Origüen, J.; Orellana, M.Á.; Fernández-Ruiz, M.; Corbella, L.; San Juan, R.; Ruiz-Ruigómez, M.; López-Medrano, F.; Lizasoain, M.; Ruiz-Merlo, T.; Maestro-de la Calle, G.; et al. Toxin B PCR Amplification Cycle Thresh-old Adds Little to Clinical Variables for Predicting Outcomes in *Clostridium difficile* Infection: A Retrospective Cohort Study. *J. Clin. Microbiol.* **2019**, *57*, e01125-18. [CrossRef]
27. Garvey, M.I.; Bradley, C.W.; Wilkinson, M.A.; Holden, E. Can a toxin gene NAAT be used to predict toxin EIA and the severity of *Clostridium difficile* infection? *Antimicrob. Resist Infect. Control* **2017**, *6*, 127. [CrossRef]
28. Doolan, C.P.; Louie, T.; Lata, C.; Larios, O.E.; Stokes, W.; Kim, J.; Brown, K.; Beck, P.; Deardon, R.; Pillai, D.R. Latent Class Analysis for the Diagnosis of *Clostridioides difficile* Infection. *Clin. Infect. Dis.* **2020**, *73*, e2673–e2679. [CrossRef]
29. Scardina, T.; Labuszewski, L.; Pacheco, S.; Adams, W.; Schreckenberger, P.; Johnson, S. *Clostridium difficile* Infection (CDI) Severity and Outcome among Patients Infected with the NAP1/BI/027 Strain in a Non-Epidemic Setting. *Infect. Control Hosp. Epidemiol.* **2015**, *36*, 280–286. [CrossRef]
30. Katz, K.C.; Golding, G.R.; Choi, K.B.; Pelude, L.; Amaratunga, K.R.; Taljaard, M.; Alexandre, S.; Collet, J.C.; Davis, I.; Du, T.; et al. The evolving epidemiology of *Clostridium difficile* infection in Canadian hospitals during a postepidemic period (2009–2015). *Can. Med Assoc. J.* **2018**, *190*, E758–E765. [CrossRef]
31. Sirard, S.; Valiquette, L.; Fortier, L.-C. Lack of Association between Clinical Outcome of *Clostridium difficile* Infections, Strain Type, and Virulence-Associated Phenotypes. *J. Clin. Microbiol.* **2011**, *49*, 4040–4046. [CrossRef]
32. Warny, M.; Pepin, J.; Fang, A.; Killgore, G.; Thompson, A.; Brazier, J.; Frost, E.; McDonald, L.C. Toxin production by an emerging strain of *Clostridium difficile* associated with outbreaks of severe disease in North America and Europe. *Lancet* **2005**, *366*, 1079–1084. [CrossRef]
33. Kwon, J.H.; Reske, K.A.; Hink, T.; Burnham, C.-A.D.; Dubberke, E.R. Evaluation of Correlation between Pretest Probability for *Clostridium difficile* Infection and *Clostridium difficile* Enzyme Immunoassay Results. *J. Clin. Microbiol.* **2017**, *55*, 596–605. [CrossRef] [PubMed]
34. Caroff, D.A.; Edelstein, P.H.; Hamilton, K.; Pegues, D.A.; CDC Prevention Epicenters Program. The Bristol Stool Scale and Its Relationship to *Clostridium difficile* Infection. *J. Clin. Microbiol.* **2014**, *52*, 3437–3439. [CrossRef] [PubMed]

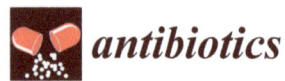

Review

Fidaxomicin for the Treatment of *Clostridioides difficile* Infection in Adult Patients: An Update on Results from Randomized Controlled Trials

Daniele Roberto Giacobbe [1,2,*], Antonio Vena [1,2], Marco Falcone [3], Francesco Menichetti [3] and Matteo Bassetti [1,2]

1. Department of Health Sciences (DISSAL), University of Genoa, 16132 Genoa, Italy
2. Infectious Diseases Unit, IRCCS Ospedale Policlinico San Martino, 16132 Genoa, Italy
3. Infectious Diseases Unit, Department of Clinical and Experimental Medicine, Azienda Ospedaliera Universitaria Pisana, University of Pisa, 56126 Pisa, Italy
* Correspondence: danieleroberto.giacobbe@unige.it; Tel.: +39-010-555-4654; Fax: +39-010-555-6712

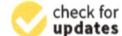

Citation: Giacobbe, D.R.; Vena, A.; Falcone, M.; Menichetti, F.; Bassetti, M. Fidaxomicin for the Treatment of *Clostridioides difficile* Infection in Adult Patients: An Update on Results from Randomized Controlled Trials. *Antibiotics* 2022, 11, 1365. https://doi.org/10.3390/antibiotics11101365

Academic Editor: Kevin W. Garey

Received: 22 September 2022
Accepted: 4 October 2022
Published: 6 October 2022

Publisher's Note: MDPI stays neutral with regard to jurisdictional claims in published maps and institutional affiliations.

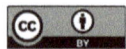

Copyright: © 2022 by the authors. Licensee MDPI, Basel, Switzerland. This article is an open access article distributed under the terms and conditions of the Creative Commons Attribution (CC BY) license (https://creativecommons.org/licenses/by/4.0/).

Abstract: In recently updated international guidelines, fidaxomicin is preferentially recommended as first-line treatment over vancomycin both for the first episode of CDI and for rCDI, based on the results of different randomized controlled trials (RCTs). Although noninferiority was the rule in phase-3 RCTs with regard to the primary endpoint of clinical cure, for shaping these recommendations, particular attention was devoted to the improved global cure and reduced risk of recurrent CDI (rCDI) observed with fidaxomicin compared to vancomycin in RCTs. Overall, while the major driver of choice should remain the global benefit for the patient, consideration of available resources should be necessarily weighed in the balance, since fidaxomicin still remains more costly than vancomycin. Against this background, precisely stratifying risk groups for rCDI will represent a crucial research trajectory of future real-life studies on the treatment of first CDI episodes. In the current narrative review, we discuss the updated evidence from RCTs on the efficacy of fidaxomicin for the treatment of either the first CDI episode or rCDI, which eventually supports its positioning within current treatment algorithms and guidelines.

Keywords: fidaxomicin; CDI; rCDI; *Clostridioides difficile*; randomized clinical trials; RCT

1. Introduction

Clostridioides difficile is the most common causative agent of infectious diarrhea in hospitalized patients; although, community-acquired *C. difficile* infection (CDI) has also become epidemiologically and clinically relevant during the last decade [1–6].

In the treatment approach to CDI, clinicians aim both to cure the index episode and to reduce the risk of recurrences. Indeed, recurrent CDI (rCDI) develops in 10–30% of cases after the first CDI episode, with the risk further increasing with each successive episode [7–10]. In the recently released updates of guidelines/guidance documents from the Infectious Diseases Society of America/Society for Healthcare Epidemiology of America (IDSA/SHEA) and from the European Society of Clinical Microbiology and Infectious Diseases (ESCMID), there have been changes in the recommendations pertaining to the use of fidaxomicin, a macrocyclic antibiotic approved both in the US and in Europe for the treatment of CDI [11,12].

In the present narrative review, we discuss the updated evidence from randomized controlled trials (RCTs) on the efficacy of fidaxomicin for the treatment of either the first CDI episode or rCDI, which eventually supports its positioning within current treatment algorithms and guidelines.

2. Methods

In August 2022, we performed a PubMed search using the keyword "fidaxomicin". After title and abstract screening of the retrieved 657 records, 227 of them were selected for initial full-text assessment. In line with the narrative nature of the present review, relevant articles pertaining to the topic were further selected by the authors and organized in the following structure: (i) an introductory section on the characteristics, mechanism of action, and antimicrobial activity of fidaxomicin; (ii) a main section on the results from phase-3/4 RCTs; (iii) a conclusions section.

3. Characteristics, Mechanism of Action, and Antimicrobial Activity of Fidaxomicin

Fidaxomicin, administered orally, is the first member of the macrocycles class of antibiotics, and it shows bactericidal activity against *C. difficile* [13,14]. In addition, fidaxomicin has negligible activity against other bacteria constituting the gut microbiota [15,16]. This selective activity relies on the fact that the *C. difficile* RNA polymerase (inhibited by fidaxomicin [17]) has a specific residue (lysine 84) that is bound by fidaxomicin and acts as a crucial sensitizer allowing fidaxomicin killing activity [18]. This specific residue is absent in gut bacteria belonging to the phyla Bacteroides and Proteobacteria [18,19]. In line with the largely reported more favorable effect than other CDI treatments in terms of microbiota disruption [16,20–23], combined with its modest activity (although inhibitory at the achieved stool concentrations) against vancomycin-resistant enterococci (VRE) [24], fidaxomicin treatment resulted in a reduced frequency of novel stool culture positivity for vancomycin-resistant enterococci (VRE) and *Candida* spp. compared to vancomycin among patients with negative pre-treatment stool cultures enrolled in a phase-3 RCT (7% vs. 31% for VRE acquisition among 247 patients, $p < 0.001$; 19% vs. 29% for *Candida* spp. acquisition among 252 patients, $p = 0.03$) [25]. In patients with pre-treatment VRE colonization, a larger decrease in the mean stool concentration of VRE was observed with fidaxomicin therapy than with vancomycin therapy; although, selection of some subpopulations of VRE with high fidaxomicin minimum inhibitory concentration (MIC) was observed during fidaxomicin treatment [25]. Of note, in patients receiving vancomycin, the risk of colonization and subsequent bloodstream infections by *Candida* spp. or enterococci may be possibly higher among those receiving high vancomycin dosages (>500 mg/day) [26].

Another peculiar characteristic of fidaxomicin, not shared by other anti-*C. difficile* agents such as vancomycin and metronidazole, is its long post-antibiotic effect, which might be relevant considering the hastened intestinal transit and drug elimination in patients with diarrhea [14,27]. Following oral administration, fidaxomicin is poorly absorbed, reaching high intracolonic concentrations [28,29]. Together with the lack of cytochrome P450 metabolism, the very low bioavailability of fidaxomicin may explain its low potential for systemic adverse events and drug interactions [14,30,31]. The main metabolite of fidaxomicin, OP-1118, is produced in vivo by the action of an esterase, and retains antimicrobial activity against *C. difficile* [13,32,33].

The activity of fidaxomicin against *C. difficile* has been assessed in several in vitro studies. Among 403 non duplicate *C. difficile* isolates from Taiwan, fidaxomicin showed potent in vitro activity, with MIC_{90} of 0.5 mg/L (range $\leq$ 0.015 to 0.5 mg/L) [34]. An even lower MIC_{90} of 0.125 mg/L was measured among 188 *C. difficile* isolates from Hungary, with only four isolates displaying a MIC value of 0.5 mg/L [35]. In another surveillance study on 925 *C. difficile* isolates from the US, MIC_{90} for fidaxomicin was 0.5 mg/L, with a range from 0.004 to 4 mg/L [36]. The same MIC_{90} of 0.5 mg/L, with a range from 0.004 to 1 mg/L, was observed in a subsequent update on a larger sample of 1889 *C. difficile* isolates [37]. In a surveillance study from Japan, MIC_{90} for fidaxomicin was 0.25 mg/L among 100 *C. difficile* isolates (range 0.03 to 0.5 mg/L) [38]. A MIC_{90} of 0.25 mg/L for fidaxomicin was also observed in a surveillance study on 105 *C. difficile* isolates from Thailand (range 0.004 to 0.25 mg/L) [39]. Among 101 *C. difficile* isolates from China, MIC_{90} for fidaxomicin was 0.5 mg/L (range 0.032 to 1 mg/L), whereas it was 0.03 mg/L among 100 *C. difficile* isolates from the US in another study (range $\leq$ 0.008 to 8 mg/L) [40,41]. In a small study on 64 *C. difficile* isolates from the Czech Republic, MIC_{90} for fidaxomicin was 0.125 mg/L (range 0.06 to 0.25 mg/L) [42]. Fidaxomicin showed the greatest in vitro potency compared to the other seven antimicrobial agents tested against 1310 *C. difficile* isolates from Canada (with 027 being the most frequent ribotype, 24.5%), showing a MIC_{90} of 0.25 mg/L (range 0.055 to 2 mg/L) [43]. In a large pan-European surveillance study of 953 *C. difficile* isolates, MIC_{90} for fidaxomicin was 0.125 mg/L (range ≤ 0.002 to 0.25 mg/L), and all strains were considered susceptible according to an epidemiological cut-off of 1 mg/L [44]. In subsequent updates of the same surveillance study including up to 3499 *C. difficile* isolates, a fidaxomicin MIC ≥ 4 mg/L was observed only in a single case [45,46]. Low MIC_{90} values for fidaxomicin were also displayed by *C. difficile* isolates from phase-2 (38 isolates, MIC_{90} of 0.125 mg/L, range ≤ 0.008 to 0.25 mg/L) and phase-3 (719 isolates, MIC_{90} of 0.25 mg/L, range 0.03 to 1 mg/L) studies of fidaxomicin, with only one strain isolated from a patient from a phase-3 study who developed rCDI showing a fidaxomicin MIC of 16 mg/L at the time of rCDI [47,48].

According to the in vitro studies reported above, reduced susceptibility to fidaxomicin is very rare; although, it has seldom been described [49]. In vitro, reduced susceptibility to fidaxomicin was selected through serial passages in a medium over a range of drug concentrations [50]. *C. difficile* isolates with reduced fidaxomicin susceptibility selected through serial passages harbored mutations in *rpoB*, encoding the β-subunit of RNA polymerase, or in *CD22120*, encoding a homolog of the family of transcriptional regulators MarR [50,51]. In a subsequent study, three *C. difficile* mutants with reduced susceptibility to fidaxomicin (MIC of 2, 8, and >32 mg/L, respectively) after the introduction of non-synonymous single-nucleotide polymorphisms in *rpoB* by allelic exchange also showed attenuated growth and reduced sporulation capacity, toxin A/B production, and cytotoxicity compared with the parental strain [52]. In a hamster model, the three mutants had impaired virulence in comparison to the parental strain; although, caecum colonization capacity was similar to the parental strain [52]. In a more recent study, a V1143D mutation was characterized in the *rpoB* gene of a clinical *C. difficile* isolate with fidaxomicin MIC > 64 mg/L and was associated with a less marked fitness defect than previously reported [53].

Regarding other particular characteristics, fidaxomicin and its metabolite OP-1118, differently from vancomycin, are able to inhibit sporulation (spore formation) of *C. difficile*, a fact which is thought to contribute to the observed increased rates of sustained response and reduced risk of recurrence in comparisons with other treatments (see the following section), since spores may persist after completion of a successful treatment course and subsequently germinate and proliferate, leading to a novel CDI episode [54–56]. After spores are formed, fidaxomicin, like vancomycin, is unable to inhibit germination, but both agents are able to counteract the outgrowth of vegetative cells from germinating spores [57]. However, fidaxomicin, but not vancomycin, has been demonstrated to persist on *C. difficile* spores after washing in saline and fecal filtrate, with consequent higher inhibitory effect on the outgrowth of vegetative cells and toxin production [58,59]. A substantial direct inhibitory effect of fidaxomicin and OP-1118 on toxin production may also explain the less frequent detection of post-treatment toxin production in fidaxomicin-treated patients than in vancomycin-treated patients [56,60,61]. A reduction in toxin A- and toxin B-mediated inflammatory responses and colonic tissue damage has also been described following exposure to fidaxomicin [62,63]. Another effect of fidaxomicin reported in in vitro studies, not observed with vancomycin, is the inhibition of biofilm formation, which could have implications for reducing the risk of both *C. difficile* colonization and CDI [64–67]. Finally, reduced shedding and environmental contamination by *C. difficile* have been described with fidaxomicin treatment more than with metronidazole or, although to a lesser extent, vancomycin [68–71].

4. Results of Phase-3/4 Randomized Controlled Trials

A summary of the main results of phase-3/4 RCTs assessing the efficacy of fidaxomicin for the treatment of CDI in adult patients is available in Table 1.

The first two large phase-3 randomized controlled trials (RCTs) assessing the efficacy of fidaxomicin for the treatment of CDI were the OPT-80-003 and OPT-80-004 studies [72,73]. Of note, patients with life-threatening or fulminant CDI were excluded from these studies [72,73].

In the non-inferiority, double-blind OPT-80-003 RCT, fidaxomicin (200 mg orally twice daily for 10 days) was compared to vancomycin (125 mg orally four times daily for 10 days) for the treatment of CDI [73]. The primary endpoint was clinical cure (defined as resolution of the symptoms and no need for further CDI treatment), assessed on the second day after the end of treatment. The secondary endpoints were rCDI (defined as diarrhea plus toxin test positivity on stool within 4 weeks after treatment of the previous episodes) and global cure (defined as clinical cure plus lack of rCDI). The primary study populations were the modified intention to treat (mITT) population (patients with documented CDI who received at least one dose of the study drug) and the per-protocol population (patients of the mITT population who received at least 3 days of treatment in the case of failure and at least 8 days of treatment in the case of clinical cure). Regarding the primary endpoint, fidaxomicin was found to be noninferior to vancomycin in terms of clinical cure both in the mITT population (88.2% (253/287) vs. 85.8% (265/309) in the fidaxomicin and vancomycin arms, respectively; lower margin of the 97.5% confidence interval [CI] for difference equal to -3.1%) and in the per-protocol population (92.1% (244/265) vs. 89.8% (254/283) in the fidaxomicin and vancomycin arms, respectively; lower margin of the 97.5% CI for difference equal to -2.6%). Regarding secondary endpoints, a lower frequency of rCDI was observed in fidaxomicin-treated than vancomycin-treated patients, both in the mITT population (15.4% (39/253) vs. 25.3% (67/265) in the fidaxomicin and vancomycin arms, respectively, with 95% CI for the difference from -16.6% to -2.9%) and in the per-protocol population (13.3% (28/211) vs. 24.0% (53/221) in the fidaxomicin and vancomycin arms, respectively, with 95% CI for the difference from -17.9% to -3.3%). A reduced frequency of rCDI in fidaxomicin-treated than in vancomycin-treated patients was retained in most subgroups; although, not in the subgroup of patients with CDI due to the 027 ribotype (27.1% (16/59) vs. 20.9% (14/67) in the fidaxomicin and vancomycin arms, respectively, in the mITT population). Finally, a higher frequency of global cure was registered in fidaxomicin-treated than in vancomycin-treated patients, both in the mITT population (74.6% (214/287) vs. 64.1% (198/309) in the fidaxomicin and vancomycin arms, respectively, with 95% CI from 3.1% to 17.7%) and in the per-protocol population (77.7% (206/265) vs. 67.1% (190/283) in the fidaxomicin and vancomycin arms, respectively, with 95% CI for the difference from 3.1% to 17.9%) [73]. Dosing schedules, endpoints, and primary study populations of the OPT-80-004 study were defined as in the OPT-80-003 study [72,73]. With regard to clinical cure (primary endpoint), fidaxomicin achieved noninferiority to vancomycin also in the OPT-80-004 study, both in the mITT population (87.7% (221/252) vs. 86.8% (223/257) in the fidaxomicin and vancomycin arms, respectively; lower margin of the 97.5% CI for difference equal to -4.9%) and in the per-protocol population (91.7% (198/216) vs. 90.6% (213/235) in the fidaxomicin and vancomycin arms, respectively; lower margin of the 97.5% CI for difference equal to -4.3%). A lower frequency of rCDI was observed in fidaxomicin-treated than in vancomycin-treated patients also in the OPT-80-004 study, both in the mITT population (12.7% (28/221) vs. 26.9% (60/223) in the fidaxomicin and vancomycin arms, respectively, with 95% CI for the difference from -21.4% to -6.8%) and in the per-protocol population (12.8% (23/180) vs. 25.3% (46/182) in the fidaxomicin and vancomycin arms, respectively, with 95% CI for the difference from -20.3% to -4.4%). Differently from the OTP-80-003 study, in the OTP-80-004 study, a lower frequency of rCDI in the fidaxomicin arm was also registered in the subgroup of patients with CDI due to the 027 ribotype (22.2% (12/54) vs. 38.0% (19/50) in the fidaxomicin and vancomycin arms, respectively, in the mITT population). As in the OPT-80-003 study, a higher frequency of global cure (also defined as a sustained response) was registered in fidaxomicin-treated than in vancomycin-treated patients, both in the mITT population (76.6% (193/252) vs. 63.4% (163/257) in the fidaxomicin and vancomycin arms, respectively, with 95% CI from 5.2% to 20.9%) and in the per-protocol population (79.6% (172/216) vs. 65.5% (154/235) in the fidaxomicin and vancomycin arms, respectively, with 95% CI for the difference from 5.9% to 22.1%) [72].

Different meta-analyses were conducted by pooling data from OTP-80-003 and OTP-80-004 after the two RCTs were released. In one of them, an exploratory, post hoc time-to-event analysis was conducted by means of fixed-effect meta-analysis and Cox regression [74]. Overall, the analysis included 1164 patients (ITT population) from the two RCTs and showed a reduction of persistent diarrhea, rCDI, or death (composite endpoint) of 40% (95% CI from 26% to 51%) through day 40 in fidaxomicin-treated patients vs. vancomycin-treated patients [74]. In another meta-analysis pooling data from the two RCTs, the odds ratio (OR) for clinical cure was 1.17 for fidaxomicin vs. vancomycin as reference (95% CI from 0.82 to 1.66) [75]. In subgroup analyses, the OR for clinical cure was 1.45 (95% CI from 0.63 to 3.36) and 0.86 (95% CI from 0.50 to 1.47) in patients with non-severe CDI and severe CDI, respectively. The OR for rCDI was 0.47 for fidaxomicin vs. vancomycin as a reference (95% CI from 0.34 to 0.65). In subgroup analyses, the OR for rCDI was 0.49 (95% CI from 0.32 to 0.74) and 0.46 (95% CI from 0.26 to 0.79) in patients with non-severe CDI and severe CDI, respectively. The OR for global cure was 1.75 for fidaxomicin vs. vancomycin as a reference (95% CI from 1.35 to 2.27). In subgroup analyses, the pooled OR for global cure was 1.92 (95% CI from 1.37 to 2.69) and 1.49 (95% CI from 0.99 to 2.26) in patients with non-severe CDI and severe CDI, respectively [75]. In another meta-analysis with pooled data from OTP-80-003 and OTP-80-004, the OR for symptomatic cure (defined as initial resolution of diarrhea and no evidence of recurrence up to 4 weeks) was 1.17 for fidaxomicin vs. vancomycin as reference (95% CI from 1.07 to 1.27) [76].

Combining data from the OTP-80-003 and OTP-80-004 studies, the efficacy of fidaxomicin vs. vancomycin for the treatment of CDI was evaluated in the following subgroups of patients with CDI: (i) patients who were concomitantly receiving other antibiotics for concomitant infections; and (ii) patients who were not receiving other concomitant antibiotics [77]. In presence of other concomitant antibiotic treatments, the clinical cure was higher in fidaxomicin-treated than in vancomycin-treated patients (90.0% (81/90) vs. 79.4% (81/102) in the fidaxomicin and vancomycin arms, respectively, with 95% CI for the difference from 0.2% to 20.4%), whereas clinical cure was similar between the two arms in the absence of other concomitant antibiotic treatments (92.3% (361/391) vs. 92.8% (386/416) in the fidaxomicin and vancomycin arms, respectively, with 95% CI for the difference from −4.1% to 3.2%). With regard to secondary endpoints, rates of rCDI and global cure were lower and higher, respectively, in fidaxomicin-treated than in vancomycin-treated patients both in patients receiving concomitant antibiotics and in patients not receiving concomitant antibiotics, in line with the main results of OTP-80-003 and OTP-80-004 [77]. Another exploratory post hoc analysis of combined data from OTP-80-003 and OTP-80-004 was conducted in the subgroups of CDI patients with and without cancer [78]. In patients with cancer, the clinical cure was 85.1% (74/87) and 74.0% (71/96) in patients treated with fidaxomicin and in patients treated with vancomycin, respectively (OR 2.00, with 95% CI from 0.95 to 4.22). In patients without cancer, the clinical cure was 88.5% (400/452) and 88.7% (417/470) in patients treated with fidaxomicin and in patients treated with vancomycin, respectively (odds ratio (OR) 0.98, with 95% CI from 0.65 to 1.47). The rates of rCDI and global cure were lower and higher, respectively, in fidaxomicin-treated than in vancomycin-treated patients both in patients with cancer and in patients without cancer, again in line with the main results of OTP-80-003 and OTP-80-004. Of note, the median time to resolution of diarrhea was longer in patients with cancer than in those without cancer in the vancomycin arm (123 h vs. 58 h, log-rank $p < 0.001$), but not in the fidaxomicin arm (74 h vs. 54 h, log-rank $p = 0.145$) [78]. Another study combining data from OTP-80-003 and OTP-80-004 employed restriction endonuclease analysis (REA) typing on paired isolates from the index episode and recurrence (available from 90/146 patients with rCDI), to differentiate between relapse (identical REA type strain) and reinfection (different REA type strain) [79]. There was no comparison between fidaxomicin and vancomycin in terms of the study endpoints of the original RCTs, whereas a comparison between the two agents was made in terms of mean time to relapse and reinfection. The mean time to relapse in fidaxomicin-treated and in vancomycin-treated patients was 11.2 days (standard deviation (SD) ±6.1) and 14.3 days (SD ±6.2), respectively (t test, $p = 0.044$). The mean time to reinfection in fidaxomicin-treated and in vancomycin-treated patients was 13.9 days (SD ±7.5) and 16.8 days (SD ±4.6), respectively (t test, $p = 0.497$) [79]. In a further study combining data from OTP-80-003 and

OTP-80-004 and employing whole-genome sequencing for distinguishing relapse (paired samples from CDI and rCDI ≤ 2 single-nucleotide variants apart) from reinfection (paired samples from CDI and rCDI > 2 single-nucleotide variants apart), the reduction in the risks of relapse and reinfection in fidaxomicin-treated vs. vancomycin-treated patients was explored using competing risk models (subdistribution hazard ratio (sHR) 0.40 for relapse, with 95% CI from 0.25 to 0.66; sHR 0.33 for reinfection, with 95% CI from 0.11 to 1.01) [80]. Regarding patients with rCDI, their possible differential risk of developing further recurrences based on fidaxomicin vs. vancomycin treatment was explored in a subset analysis of combined data from the OTP-80-003 and OTP-80-004 studies, including 128 patients who had a recent CDI episode before the index episode leading to enrollment [81]. In this analysis, the frequency of clinical cure was similar in fidaxomicin-treated and vancomycin-treated patients (93.7% (74/79) vs. 91.6% (76/83) in the fidaxomicin and vancomycin arms, respectively), whereas the frequency of rCDI (in this subgroup representing a second occurrence of rCDI) was lower in fidaxomicin-treated than in vancomycin-treated patients (19.7% (13/66) vs. 35.5% (22/62) in the fidaxomicin and vancomycin arms, respectively, with 95% CI for the difference from −30.4% to −0.3%) [81]. Finally, treatment with fidaxomicin was associated with a 60% reduced risk of recurrence in comparison with vancomycin in a logistic regression model adjusted for *C. difficile* strain, age, and concomitant antibiotics in 567 patients from OTP-80-003 and OTP-80-004 studies [82].

Subsequently, a phase-3 study was also conducted in Japan to assess the efficacy of fidaxomicin vs. vancomycin for the treatment of CDI. The drugs were administered at the same dosages of OTP-80-003 and OTP-80-004 [83]. The primary endpoint was global cure, which was assessed in the full analysis set (FAS) population and achieved in 67.3% (70/104) and 65.7% (71/108) of fidaxomicin-treated and vancomycin-treated patients, respectively (95% CI for the difference from −11.3 to 13.7, thereby not allowing demonstration of noninferiority). In a post hoc analysis of FAS patients who received at least 3 days of treatment, the global cure was 72.2% (70/97) and 67.0% (71/106) in fidaxomicin-treated and vancomycin-treated patients, respectively (95% CI for the difference from −7.9% to 17.1%). The frequency of rCDI in the FAS for recurrence (FAS-R) population, composed of FAS patients who achieved clinical cure during the index episode, was 19.5% (17/87) and 25.3% (24/95) in fidaxomicin-treated and vancomycin-treated patients, respectively (95% CI for the difference from −16.7% to 7.0%) [83]. In a network meta-analysis including pooled data from the RCT conducted in Japan, the OTP-80-003 RCT, and the OTP-80-004 RCT, the clinical cure was found to be similar between fidaxomicin and vancomycin (OR 1.17 with vancomycin as a reference, with 95% credible intervals from 0.78 to 1.48), whereas fidaxomicin showed a favorable association both with rCDI (OR 0.50 with vancomycin as a reference, with 95% credible intervals from 0.37 to 0.68) and global cure (OR 1.61 with vancomycin as a reference, with 95% credible intervals from 1.27 to 2.05) [84].

Three other small RCTs assessing the efficacy of fidaxomicin at standard dosage (200 mg twice daily for 10 days) for the treatment of CDI were recently published [61,85,86]. In one of them, the standard dosage of fidaxomicin was compared with vancomycin (125 mg four times daily for 10 days) for the treatment of first CDI episodes [85]. The primary endpoint was the percentage of subjects achieving a reduction of at least 2 $\log_{10}$ colony-forming units (CFU)/g of spores in stools from screening to the end of therapy, and was achieved more frequently in fidaxomicin-treated than vancomycin-treated patients (67% (8/12) vs. 14% (1/7)) [85]. In another small, pilot RCT of 12 patients, the standard dosage of fidaxomicin was compared with vancomycin (125 mg four times daily for 10 days) with respect to the reduction in toxin concentrations in stools from baseline, with results suggesting a favorable association between fidaxomicin and a sustained reduction in toxins A and B up to day 30 after therapy [61]. Finally, 64 patients with rCDI were randomized into three arms (standard dosage fidaxomicin, standard dosage vancomycin, and fecal microbiota transplant (FMT)) in a third small RCT [86]. The primary endpoint was a combination of clinical resolution and a negative toxin polymerase chain reaction at 8 weeks after allocation, and was achieved in 33% (8/24), 19% (3/16), and 71% (17/24) of patients receiving fidaxomicin, vancomycin, and FMT, respectively [86]. A recent meta-analysis pooling data also from these three small RCTs in addition to OTP-80-003, OTP-80-004, and the RCT conducted in Japan, showed a comparable clinical cure between fidaxomicin and vancomycin (risk ratio (RR) 1.02, with 95% CI from 0.98 to 1.06), and favorable associations between fidaxomicin and reduced risk of rCDI (RR 0.59, with 95% CI from 0.47 to 0.75) and improved global cure (RR 1.18, with 95% CI from 1.09 to 1.26) [87].

Table 1. Main efficacy data from phase-3/4 randomized controlled trials of fidaxomicin for the treatment of CDI in adult patients.

Author, Year Study Name [Ref]	Fidaxomicin Regimen (Dosage)	Comparator/s (Dosage)	Study Population Endpoint (Primary/Secondary)	Frequency (Events/Treated)	% Difference [a] (95% CI)
Louie et al., 2011 OTP-80-003 [73]	Standard regimen (200 mg orally twice daily for 10 days)	Vancomycin (125 mg orally four times daily for 10 days)	*mITT population* [b] *Clinical cure (primary)* Fidaxomicin Vancomycin *rCDI (secondary)* Fidaxomicin Vancomycin *Global cure (secondary)* Fidaxomicin Vancomycin *Per-protocol population* [c] *Clinical cure (primary)* Fidaxomicin Vancomycin *rCDI (secondary)* Fidaxomicin Vancomycin *Global cure (secondary)* Fidaxomicin Vancomycin	88.2% (253/287) 85.8% (265/309) 15.4% (39/253) 25.3% (67/265) 74.6% (214/287) 64.1% (198/309) 92.1% (244/265) 89.8% (254/283) 13.3% (28/211) 24.0% (53/221) 77.7% (206/265) 67.1% (190/283)	2.4 (−3.1 [d]) Reference −9.9 (−16.6 to −2.9) Reference 10.5 (3.1 to 17.7) Reference 2.3 (−2.6 [d]) Reference −10.7 (−17.9 to −3.3) Reference 10.6 (3.1 to 17.9) Reference
Cornely et al., 2012 OTP-80-004 [72]	Standard regimen (200 mg orally twice daily for 10 days)	Vancomycin (125 mg orally four times daily for 10 days)	*mITT population* [b] *Clinical cure (primary)* Fidaxomicin Vancomycin *rCDI (secondary)* Fidaxomicin Vancomycin *Sustained response (secondary)* Fidaxomicin Vancomycin *Per-protocol population* [c] *Clinical cure (primary)* Fidaxomicin Vancomycin *rCDI (secondary)* Fidaxomicin Vancomycin *Global cure (secondary)* Fidaxomicin Vancomycin	87.7% (221/252) 86.8% (223/257) 12.7% (28/221) 26.9% (60/223) 76.6% (193/252) 63.4% (163/257) 91.7% (198/216) 90.6% (213/235) 12.8% (23/180) 25.3% (46/182) 79.6% (172/216) 65.5% (154/235)	0.9 (−4.9 [d]) Reference −14.2 (−21.4 to −6.8) Reference 13.2 (5.3 to 21.0) Reference 1.1 (−4.3 [d]) Reference −12.5 (−20.5 to −4.5) Reference 14.1 (6.0 to 22.2) Reference
Mikamo et al., 2018 [83]	Standard regimen (200 mg orally twice daily for 10 days)	Vancomycin (125 mg orally four times daily for 10 days)	*FAS population Global cure (primary)* Fidaxomicin Vancomycin *FAS-R population* [e] *rCDI (secondary)* Fidaxomicin Vancomycin	67.3% (70/104) 65.7% (71/108) 19.5% (17/87) 25.3% (24/95)	1.2 (−11.3 to 13.7) Reference −4.9 (−16.7 to 7.0) Reference

Table 1. Cont.

Author, Year Study Name [Ref]	Fidaxomicin Regimen (Dosage)	Comparator/s (Dosage)	Study Population Endpoint (Primary/Secondary)	Frequency (Events/Treated)	% Difference [a] (95% CI)
Housman et al., 2016 [85]	Standard regimen (200 mg orally twice daily for 10 days)	Vancomycin (125 mg orally four times daily for 10 days)	Patients with CDI Reduction of spores (primary) [f] Fidaxomicin Vancomycin	66.7% (8/12) 14.3% (1/7)	52.4 (NA) Reference
Hvas et al., 2019 [86]	Standard regimen (200 mg orally twice daily for 10 days)	Vancomycin (125 mg orally four times daily for 10 days) or FMT	Patients with rCDI Clinical resolution (primary) [g] Fidaxomicin FMT Vancomycin	33.3% (8/24) 70.8% (17/24) 18.8% (3/16)	14.5% (NA) 52.0% NA) Reference
Guery et al., 2018 EXTEND [88]	Extended-pulsed regimen (200 mg twice daily on days 1–5, and then only once daily on alternate days from day 7 to day 25)	Vancomycin (125 mg orally four times daily for 10 days)	Modified FAS population [h] Sustained clinical cure (primary) Fidaxomicin Vancomycin Per-protocol population rCDI at day 40 (secondary) Fidaxomicin Vancomycin rCDI at day 55 (secondary) Fidaxomicin Vancomycin rCDI at day 90 (secondary) Fidaxomicin Vancomycin	70.1% (124/177) 59.2% (106/179) 2.4% (3/124) 17.6% (22/125) 5.6% (7/124) 18.4% (23/125) 8.8% (11/124) 18.4% (23/125)	OR 1.62 (1.04 to 2.54) Reference OR 0.12 (0.04 to 0.41) Reference OR 0.31 (0.13 to 0.73) Reference OR 0.49 (0.23 to 1.04) Reference

CDI, *Clostridioides difficile* infection; CI, confidence interval; FAS, full analysis set; FMT, fecal microbiota transplant; mITT, modified intention-to-treat; NA, not available; OR, odds ratio; rCDI, recurrent CDI. [a] Unless otherwise indicated. [b] Including patients with documented CDI who received at least one dose of study drug. [c] Including patients of the mITT population who received at least 3 days of treatment in the case of failure and at least 8 days of treatment in the case of clinical cure. [d] One-sided 97.5% CI. [e] FAS patients who achieved clinical cure during the index episode. [f] Defined as percentage of subjects achieving a reduction of at least 2 $\log_{10}$ colony-forming units (CFU)/g of spores in stools from screening to the end of therapy. [g] Defined as combination of clinical resolution and a negative toxin polymerase chain reaction at 8 weeks after allocation. [h] Including all randomized patients who received at least one dose of study drug.

The results of the EXTEND RCT were published in 2018 [88]. EXTEND was an open-label phase-3b/4 RCT comparing extended-pulsed fidaxomicin (administered orally at 200 mg twice daily on days 1–5, and then only once daily on alternate days from day 7 to day 25) vs. vancomycin (at the standard dosage of 125 mg four times daily for 10 days) in inpatients aged 60 years or older. The primary endpoint was sustained clinical cure at 30 days after the end of treatment in the modified FAS population (all randomized patients who received at least one dose of the study drug), and was achieved in 70% (124/177) and 59% (106/179) of patients in extended-pulsed fidaxomicin and vancomycin arms, respectively (95% CI for the difference from 1.0% to 20.7%), thereby demonstrating superiority (a fact which is in line with the enhanced suppression of *C. difficile* by a pulsed fidaxomicin regimen in preclinical studies [89]; although, the limitations of the lack of comparison vs. the standard fidaxomicin dosage and an extended-pulsed vancomycin regimen were acknowledged in the EXTEND study). With regard to rCDI (one of the study's secondary endpoints), lower rates of recurrences were registered in the extended-pulsed fidaxomicin arm than in the vancomycin arm at day 40 (3/124 (2.4%) vs. 22/125 (17.6%)), day55 (7/124 (5.6%) vs. 23/125 (18.4%)), and day 90 (11/124 (8.8%) vs. 23/125 (18.4%)) [88]. Of note, pharmacokinetic/pharmacodynamic data from patients enrolled in EXTEND revealed that fidaxomicin concentrations in stools were above the MIC$_{90}$ of *C. difficile* isolates (inferred from in vitro studies) until day 26 ± 1 [90]. The subgroup analyses of the EXTEND study showed higher clinical cure rates in the extended-pulsed fidaxomicin arm independent of age, prior CDI, infection with PCR-ribotype 027, CDI severity, or presence of cancer [91]. A post hoc analysis of the EXTEND study conducted after testing stools of enrolled patients at screening, also with the BioFire FilmArray Gastrointestinal Panel (BioMérieux, Basingstoke, UK), suggested that co-infection with other pathogens could possibly explain clinical failures [92]. In a meta-analysis pooling data from five of the RCTs discussed above plus the EXTEND study, fidaxomicin was associated with improved sustained symptomatic cure compared to vancomycin (OR 0.67, with 95% CI from 0.55 to 0.82) [93].

In hematopoietic stem cell transplantation (HSCT) recipients, the development of CDI is more frequent than in the general population of hospitalized patients, and it has been associated with an increased risk of bloodstream infections, new-onset graft versus host disease, and non-relapse mortality [94–97]. In the double-blind DEFLECT-1 RCT, fidaxomicin was compared to a placebo for the prophylaxis of CDI in HSCT recipients (either allo-HSCT or auto-HSCT) undergoing fluoroquinolone prophylaxis [98]. The primary composite endpoint, assessed in the mITT population (subjects receiving at least one dose of study drug/placebo) was prophylaxis failure, defined as confirmed CDI, receipt of anti-C. *difficile* drugs for any indication, or missed assessment of CDI for any reason. Fidaxomicin was administered at the dosage of 200 mg daily, starting from 2 days after conditioning or initiation of prophylaxis with fluoroquinolones, and continuing until 7 days after neutrophil engraftment or completion of prophylaxis with fluoroquinolones/treatment with other antimicrobials, for up to 40 days. Prophylaxis failure was similar in patients receiving fidaxomicin and in patients receiving placebo (28.6% (86/301) vs. 30.8% (92/299), respectively, with 95% CI for the difference from −5.1% to 9.5%); although, it is of note that most failures occurred because of non-CDI events and confirmed CDI was less frequent in the fidaxomicin arm than in the placebo arm in a sensitivity analysis (4.3% (13/301) vs. 10.7% (32/299), with 95% CI for the difference from 2.2% to 10.6%) [98].

Among currently ongoing RCT comparing fidaxomicin vs. other treatments for CDI is OpTION, a double-blind study that is being conducted in patients with rCDI and is comparing the efficacy of three different treatment regimens: (i) 200 mg of fidaxomicin twice daily, for 10 days; (ii) 125 mg of vancomycin four times daily, for 10 days; and (iii) 125 mg of vancomycin four times daily, for 10 days, followed by a taper/pulse regimen of vancomycin for 3 weeks [99]. Other ongoing phase-3/4 RCTs are comparing fidaxomicin vs. FMT in patients with rCDI (NCT05266807, NCT05201079). The results of an open-label RCT comparing standard dosage fidaxomicin vs. standard dosage vancomycin in patients with CDI receiving concurrent antibiotics for other infections have been recently released, with the primary endpoint of clinical cure having been registered in 73% (54/74) and 62.9% (44/70) of patients in the fidaxomicin and vancomycin arms, respectively [100]. Among secondary endpoints, rCDI developed in 3.3% (2/60) and 4.0% (2/50) of patients in the fidaxomicin and vancomycin arms, respectively [100].

In RCTs, fidaxomicin was overall well tolerated. In the OPT-80-003 and OPT-80-004 studies, its safety profile was similar to oral vancomycin, and there were no differences between the two drugs in the frequency of death or serious adverse events [101]. The only numerical imbalances in these studies were related to gastrointestinal hemorrhage (4.1% vs. 3.1% in fidaxomicin-treated and vancomycin-treated patients, respectively) and leukopenia (4.1% vs. 1.7% in fidaxomicin-treated and vancomycin-treated patients, respectively); although, there was no evidence of a causal relationship between fidaxomicin administration and the occurrence of these events [101]. Similar tolerability profiles of fidaxomicin and vancomycin were observed in the phase-3 study conducted in Japan [83]. The incidence of treatment-emergent adverse events was similar in the extended-pulsed fidaxomicin arm and in the vancomycin arm in the EXTEND study [88]. One death in the vancomycin arm was deemed as being related to the study drug by the investigators [88]. The registered drug-related adverse events were 15% and 20% in the fidaxomicin and placebo arms in the DEFLECT-1 RCT [98].

5. Conclusions

In both the recently updated IDSA/SHEA guidelines and the updated ESCMID guidance document, fidaxomicin is preferentially recommended as first-line treatment over vancomycin both for the first episode of CDI and for rCDI (see Table 2 for more details) [11,12]. Although vancomycin remains a suitable alternative to fidaxomicin (non-inferiority was indeed the rule in phase-3 RCTs with regard to the primary endpoint of clinical response), for shaping these recommendations particular attention was devoted to the improved global cure and reduced risk of rCDI observed with fidaxomicin compared to vancomycin in RCTs. The overall scenario is thus shifting from "administer vancomycin first, because of reduced cost and similar efficacy" to "consider fidaxomicin first, in view of the global benefits for the patient, if feasible". With regard to feasibility, fidaxomicin still remains more costly than vancomycin, and, while the major driver of choice should solidly remain the global benefit for the patient, consideration of available resources should also be necessarily weighed in the balance. Against this background, a clear mistake would be that of continuing to administer vancomycin for any first CDI episode only because of reduced costs, thereby ignoring the evidence arising from RCTs about the improved global benefits following fidaxomicin treatment. Rather, risk models for rCDI should be used for selecting patients to preferentially receive fidaxomicin (i.e., to clearly identify those patients for whom fidaxomicin-driven global benefits are relevant). In our opinion, precisely stratifying risk groups for rCDI will represent a crucial research trajectory of future real-life studies on the treatment of initial CDI episodes. In addition, after reviewing the results of existing RCTs summarized in the previous sections, we also consider some other remaining grey areas as relevant fields for current and future research: (i) the exact positioning of the extended-pulsed fidaxomicin regimen, and its comparative efficacy with an extended-pulsed vancomycin regimen; (ii) the comparative efficacy of fidaxomicin vs. vancomycin in severe and severe-complicated CDI; (iii) the efficacy of fidaxomicin plus bezlotoxumab in preventing rCDI in comparison to other bezlotoxumab-including regimens; and (iv) when to precisely consider FMT instead of treatment with oral drugs, including fidaxomicin. Elucidating all of these remaining areas could further optimize the current positioning of fidaxomicin within CDI and rCDI treatment algorithms and, in turn, patients' health.

Table 2. Current IDSA/SHEA and ESCMID recommendations regarding fidaxomicin for the treatment of CDI and rCDI.

Guidelines/Guidance Document	Recommended Treatment for First CDI Episode *	Recommended Treatment for rCDI *
ESCMID guidance document [12]	• The use of a standard regimen of fidaxomicin is suggested over vancomycin *(Strong recommendation, with moderate level of evidence)* • Risk stratification should be considered when access to fidaxomicin is limited (e.g., older age >65 years plus one or more of the following: healthcare-associated CDI; hospitalization; in the previous 3 months, administration of concomitant antibiotics, initiation of PPIs during or after diagnosis of CDI; previous CDI episode) *(Good practice statement)* • When fidaxomicin is unavailable or unfeasible, vancomycin is a suitable alternative *(Strong recommendation, with high level of evidence)* • An extended-pulsed regiment of fidaxomicin could be considered in case of risk of rCDI, especially in old inpatients *(Weak recommendation, with low level of evidence)* • For severe or severe-complicated CDI, a standard regimen of fidaxomicin or vancomycin is suggested *(good practice statement)*	• If the initial CDI episode was treated with metronidazole or vancomycin, the use of a standard regimen of fidaxomicin is preferentially recommended *(Strong recommendation, with low level of evidence)* • If the initial CDI episode was treated with fidaxomicin, considered bezlotoxumab in addition to fidaxomicin *(Weak recommendation, with moderate level of evidence; "addition to fidaxomicin" as a good practice statement)* • When fidaxomicin and bezlotoxumab are unavailable or unfeasible, consider a tapered/pulsed regimen of vancomycin *(Weak recommendation, with very low level of evidence)* • For multiple recurrences, FMT or bezlotoxumab in addition to standard of care is suggested *(Weak recommendation, with moderate level of evidence for FMT and low level of evidence for bezlotoxumab)*

Table 2. *Cont.*

Guidelines/Guidance Document	Recommended Treatment for First CDI Episode *	Recommended Treatment for rCDI *
IDSA/SHEA guidelines [11]	• The use of a standard regimen of fidaxomicin is suggested over a standard course of vancomycin. A high value is placed on the beneficial effects and the safety of fidaxomicin, with implementations depending on available resources and with vancomycin remaining an acceptable alternative *(Conditional recommendation with moderate certainty of evidence)*	• The use of a standard or extended-pulsed regimen of fidaxomicin is suggested over a standard regimen of vancomycin. For a first rCDI episode, vancomycin in a standard or tapered/pulsed regimen is an acceptable alternative. For multiple recurrences, possible options are fidaxomicin (standard or extended-pulsed regimen), vancomycin in a tapered/pulsed regimen, vancomycin followed by rifaximin, and FMT *(Conditional recommendation with low certainty of evidence)*

CDI, *Clostridioides difficile* infection; ESCMID, European Society of Clinical Microbiology and Infectious Diseases; FMT, fecal microbiota transplant; IDSA, Infectious Diseases Society of America; PPIs, proton pump inhibitors; rCDI, recurrent CDI; SHEA, Society for Healthcare Epidemiology of America. * For other recommendations about the use of other agents (e.g., bezlotoxumab) or FMT and not directly involving a decision about fidaxomicin please refer to the original guidelines/guidance documents [11,12]. For a fulminant CDI episode (hypotension or shock, ileus, or megacolon), IDSA/SHEA guidelines recommend oral/nasogastric tube vancomycin 500 mg four times daily plus intravenous metronidazole 500 mg thrice daily plus rectal instillation of vancomycin if ileus.

Author Contributions: Conceptualization, D.R.G., A.V. and M.B.; methodology, D.R.G.; writing—original draft preparation, D.R.G.; writing—review and editing, D.R.G., A.V., M.F., F.M. and M.B. All authors have read and agreed to the published version of the manuscript.

Funding: This research received no external funding.

Data Availability Statement: Not applicable.

Conflicts of Interest: Outside the submitted work, Daniele Roberto Giacobbe reports investigator-initiated grants from Pfizer, Shionogi, and Gilead Italia, and speaker fees and/or advisory board fees from Pfizer and Tillotts Pharma. Outside the submitted work, Matteo Bassetti reports research grants and/or personal fees for advisor/consultant and/or speaker/chairman from Bayer, BioMérieux, Cidara, Cipla, Gilead, Menarini, MSD, Pfizer, and Shionogi. The other authors have no conflict of interest to disclose.

References

1. Guh, A.Y.; Mu, Y.; Winston, L.G.; Johnston, H.; Olson, D.; Farley, M.M.; Wilson, L.E.; Holzbauer, S.M.; Phipps, E.C.; Dumyati, G.K.; et al. Trends in U.S. Burden of *Clostridioides difficile* Infection and Outcomes. *N. Engl. J. Med.* **2020**, *382*, 1320–1330. [CrossRef] [PubMed]
2. Khanna, S. My Treatment Approach to *Clostridioides difficile* Infection. *Mayo Clin. Proc.* **2021**, *96*, 2192–2204. [CrossRef] [PubMed]
3. Khanna, S.; Pardi, D.S.; Aronson, S.L.; Kammer, P.P.; Orenstein, R.; St Sauver, J.L.; Harmsen, W.S.; Zinsmeister, A.R. The epidemiology of community-acquired *Clostridium difficile* infection: A population-based study. *Am. J. Gastroenterol.* **2012**, *107*, 89–95. [CrossRef]
4. Lessa, F.C. Community-associated *Clostridium difficile* infection: How real is it? *Anaerobe* **2013**, *24*, 121–123. [CrossRef]
5. Alicino, C.; Giacobbe, D.R.; Durando, P.; Bellina, D.; AM, D.I.B.; Paganino, C.; Del Bono, V.; Viscoli, C.; Icardi, G.; Orsi, A. Increasing incidence of *Clostridium difficile* infections: Results from a 5-year retrospective study in a large teaching hospital in the Italian region with the oldest population. *Epidemiol. Infect.* **2016**, *144*, 2517–2526. [CrossRef]
6. Finn, E.; Andersson, F.L.; Madin-Warburton, M. Burden of *Clostridioides difficile* infection (CDI)—A systematic review of the epidemiology of primary and recurrent CDI. *BMC Infect. Dis.* **2021**, *21*, 456. [CrossRef]
7. Fekety, R.; McFarland, L.V.; Surawicz, C.M.; Greenberg, R.N.; Elmer, G.W.; Mulligan, M.E. Recurrent *Clostridium difficile* diarrhea: Characteristics of and risk factors for patients enrolled in a prospective, randomized, double-blinded trial. *Clin. Infect. Dis.* **1997**, *24*, 324–333. [CrossRef] [PubMed]
8. Granata, G.; Petrosillo, N.; Adamoli, L.; Bartoletti, M.; Bartoloni, A.; Basile, G.; Bassetti, M.; Bonfanti, P.; Borromeo, R.; Ceccarelli, G.; et al. Prospective Study on Incidence, Risk Factors and Outcome of Recurrent *Clostridioides difficile* Infections. *J. Clin. Med.* **2021**, *10*, 1127. [CrossRef]
9. McFarland, L.V.; Surawicz, C.M.; Rubin, M.; Fekety, R.; Elmer, G.W.; Greenberg, R.N. Recurrent *Clostridium difficile* disease: Epidemiology and clinical characteristics. *Infect. Control Hosp. Epidemiol.* **1999**, *20*, 43–50. [CrossRef]

10. Falcone, M.; Tiseo, G.; Iraci, F.; Raponi, G.; Goldoni, P.; Delle Rose, D.; Santino, I.; Carfagna, P.; Murri, R.; Fantoni, M.; et al. Risk factors for recurrence in patients with *Clostridium difficile* infection due to 027 and non-027 ribotypes. *Clin. Microbiol. Infect.* **2019**, *25*, 474–480. [CrossRef]
11. Johnson, S.; Lavergne, V.; Skinner, A.M.; Gonzales-Luna, A.J.; Garey, K.W.; Kelly, C.P.; Wilcox, M.H. Clinical Practice Guideline by the Infectious Diseases Society of America (IDSA) and Society for Healthcare Epidemiology of America (SHEA): 2021 Focused Update Guidelines on Management of *Clostridioides difficile* Infection in Adults. *Clin. Infect. Dis.* **2021**, *73*, 755–757. [CrossRef] [PubMed]
12. van Prehn, J.; Reigadas, E.; Vogelzang, E.H.; Bouza, E.; Hristea, A.; Guery, B.; Krutova, M.; Noren, T.; Allerberger, F.; Coia, J.E.; et al. European Society of Clinical Microbiology and Infectious Diseases: 2021 update on the treatment guidance document for *Clostridioides difficile* infection in adults. *Clin. Microbiol. Infect.* **2021**, *27* (Suppl. S2), S1–S21. [CrossRef] [PubMed]
13. Babakhani, F.; Gomez, A.; Robert, N.; Sears, P. Killing kinetics of fidaxomicin and its major metabolite, OP-1118, against *Clostridium difficile*. *J. Med. Microbiol.* **2011**, *60*, 1213–1217. [CrossRef] [PubMed]
14. Cornely, O.A. Current and emerging management options for *Clostridium difficile* infection: What is the role of fidaxomicin? *Clin. Microbiol. Infect.* **2012**, *18* (Suppl. S6), 28–35. [CrossRef] [PubMed]
15. Louie, T.J.; Emery, J.; Krulicki, W.; Byrne, B.; Mah, M. OPT-80 eliminates *Clostridium difficile* and is sparing of bacteroides species during treatment of *C. difficile* infection. *Antimicrob. Agents Chemother.* **2009**, *53*, 261–263. [CrossRef] [PubMed]
16. Tannock, G.W.; Munro, K.; Taylor, C.; Lawley, B.; Young, W.; Byrne, B.; Emery, J.; Louie, T. A new macrocyclic antibiotic, fidaxomicin (OPT-80), causes less alteration to the bowel microbiota of *Clostridium difficile*-infected patients than does vancomycin. *Microbiology* **2010**, *156*, 3354–3359. [CrossRef] [PubMed]
17. Artsimovitch, I.; Seddon, J.; Sears, P. Fidaxomicin is an inhibitor of the initiation of bacterial RNA synthesis. *Clin. Infect. Dis.* **2012**, *55* (Suppl. S2), S127–S131. [CrossRef]
18. Cao, X.; Boyaci, H.; Chen, J.; Bao, Y.; Landick, R.; Campbell, E.A. Basis of narrow-spectrum activity of fidaxomicin on *Clostridioides difficile*. *Nature* **2022**, *604*, 541–545. [CrossRef]
19. How the antibiotic fidaxomicin targets an intestinal pathogen. *Nature* **2022**, *online ahead of print*. [CrossRef]
20. Ajami, N.J.; Cope, J.L.; Wong, M.C.; Petrosino, J.F.; Chesnel, L. Impact of Oral Fidaxomicin Administration on the Intestinal Microbiota and Susceptibility to *Clostridium difficile* Colonization in Mice. *Antimicrob. Agents Chemother.* **2018**, *62*, e02112-17. [CrossRef]
21. Yamaguchi, T.; Konishi, H.; Aoki, K.; Ishii, Y.; Chono, K.; Tateda, K. The gut microbiome diversity of *Clostridioides difficile*-inoculated mice treated with vancomycin and fidaxomicin. *J. Infect. Chemother.* **2020**, *26*, 483–491. [CrossRef] [PubMed]
22. Deshpande, A.; Hurless, K.; Cadnum, J.L.; Chesnel, L.; Gao, L.; Chan, L.; Kundrapu, S.; Polinkovsky, A.; Donskey, C.J. Effect of Fidaxomicin versus Vancomycin on Susceptibility to Intestinal Colonization with Vancomycin-Resistant Enterococci and Klebsiella pneumoniae in Mice. *Antimicrob. Agents Chemother.* **2016**, *60*, 3988–3993. [CrossRef] [PubMed]
23. Louie, T.J.; Cannon, K.; Byrne, B.; Emery, J.; Ward, L.; Eyben, M.; Krulicki, W. Fidaxomicin preserves the intestinal microbiome during and after treatment of *Clostridium difficile* infection (CDI) and reduces both toxin reexpression and recurrence of CDI. *Clin. Infect. Dis.* **2012**, *55* (Suppl. S2), S132–S142. [CrossRef] [PubMed]
24. Biedenbach, D.J.; Ross, J.E.; Putnam, S.D.; Jones, R.N. In vitro activity of fidaxomicin (OPT-80) tested against contemporary clinical isolates of Staphylococcus spp. and Enterococcus spp. *Antimicrob. Agents Chemother.* **2010**, *54*, 2273–2275. [CrossRef] [PubMed]
25. Nerandzic, M.M.; Mullane, K.; Miller, M.A.; Babakhani, F.; Donskey, C.J. Reduced acquisition and overgrowth of vancomycin-resistant enterococci and Candida species in patients treated with fidaxomicin versus vancomycin for *Clostridium difficile* infection. *Clin. Infect. Dis.* **2012**, *55* (Suppl. S2), S121–S126. [CrossRef]
26. Falcone, M.; Russo, A.; Iraci, F.; Carfagna, P.; Goldoni, P.; Vullo, V.; Venditti, M. Risk Factors and Outcomes for Bloodstream Infections Secondary to *Clostridium difficile* Infection. *Antimicrob. Agents Chemother.* **2016**, *60*, 252–257. [CrossRef]
27. Babakhani, F.; Gomez, A.; Robert, N.; Sears, P. Postantibiotic effect of fidaxomicin and its major metabolite, OP-1118, against *Clostridium difficile*. *Antimicrob. Agents Chemother.* **2011**, *55*, 4427–4429. [CrossRef]
28. Sears, P.; Crook, D.W.; Louie, T.J.; Miller, M.A.; Weiss, K. Fidaxomicin attains high fecal concentrations with minimal plasma concentrations following oral administration in patients with *Clostridium difficile* infection. *Clin. Infect. Dis.* **2012**, *55* (Suppl. S2), S116–S120. [CrossRef]
29. Soriano, M.M.; Liao, S.; Danziger, L.H. Fidaxomicin: A minimally absorbed macrocyclic antibiotic for the treatment of *Clostridium difficile* infections. *Expert Rev. Anti-Infect. Ther.* **2013**, *11*, 767–776. [CrossRef]
30. Mullane, K.M.; Gorbach, S. Fidaxomicin: First-in-class macrocyclic antibiotic. *Expert Rev. Anti-Infect. Ther.* **2011**, *9*, 767–777. [CrossRef]
31. Shue, Y.K.; Sears, P.S.; Shangle, S.; Walsh, R.B.; Lee, C.; Gorbach, S.L.; Okumu, F.; Preston, R.A. Safety, tolerance, and pharmacokinetic studies of OPT-80 in healthy volunteers following single and multiple oral doses. *Antimicrob. Agents Chemother.* **2008**, *52*, 1391–1395. [CrossRef] [PubMed]
32. Zhanel, G.G.; Walkty, A.J.; Karlowsky, J.A. Fidaxomicin: A novel agent for the treatment of *Clostridium difficile* infection. *Can. J. Infect. Dis. Med. Microbiol.* **2015**, *26*, 305–312. [CrossRef]
33. Goldstein, E.J.; Babakhani, F.; Citron, D.M. Antimicrobial activities of fidaxomicin. *Clin. Infect. Dis.* **2012**, *55* (Suppl. S2), S143–S148. [CrossRef]

34. Liao, C.H.; Ko, W.C.; Lu, J.J.; Hsueh, P.R. Characterizations of clinical isolates of *Clostridium difficile* by toxin genotypes and by susceptibility to 12 antimicrobial agents, including fidaxomicin (OPT-80) and rifaximin: A multicenter study in Taiwan. *Antimicrob. Agents Chemother.* **2012**, *56*, 3943–3949. [CrossRef] [PubMed]
35. Eitel, Z.; Terhes, G.; Soki, J.; Nagy, E.; Urban, E. Investigation of the MICs of fidaxomicin and other antibiotics against Hungarian *Clostridium difficile* isolates. *Anaerobe* **2015**, *31*, 47–49. [CrossRef] [PubMed]
36. Snydman, D.R.; McDermott, L.A.; Jacobus, N.V.; Thorpe, C.; Stone, S.; Jenkins, S.G.; Goldstein, E.J.; Patel, R.; Forbes, B.A.; Mirrett, S.; et al. U.S.-Based National Sentinel Surveillance Study for the Epidemiology of *Clostridium difficile*-Associated Diarrheal Isolates and Their Susceptibility to Fidaxomicin. *Antimicrob. Agents Chemother.* **2015**, *59*, 6437–6443. [CrossRef]
37. Thorpe, C.M.; McDermott, L.A.; Tran, M.K.; Chang, J.; Jenkins, S.G.; Goldstein, E.J.C.; Patel, R.; Forbes, B.A.; Johnson, S.; Gerding, D.N.; et al. U.S.-Based National Surveillance for Fidaxomicin Susceptibility of *Clostridioides difficile*-Associated Diarrheal Isolates from 2013 to 2016. *Antimicrob. Agents Chemother.* **2019**, *63*, e00391-19. [CrossRef] [PubMed]
38. Yamagishi, Y.; Nishiyama, N.; Koizumi, Y.; Matsukawa, Y.; Suematsu, H.; Hagihara, M.; Katsumata, K.; Mikamo, H. Antimicrobial activity of fidaxomicin against *Clostridium difficile* clinical isolates in Aichi area in Japan. *J. Infect. Chemother.* **2017**, *23*, 724–726. [CrossRef] [PubMed]
39. Putsathit, P.; Maneerattanaporn, M.; Piewngam, P.; Knight, D.R.; Kiratisin, P.; Riley, T.V. Antimicrobial susceptibility of *Clostridium difficile* isolated in Thailand. *Antimicrob. Resist. Infect. Control.* **2017**, *6*, 58. [CrossRef] [PubMed]
40. Cheng, J.W.; Yang, Q.W.; Xiao, M.; Yu, S.Y.; Zhou, M.L.; Kudinha, T.; Kong, F.; Liao, J.W.; Xu, Y.C. High in vitro activity of fidaxomicin against *Clostridium difficile* isolates from a university teaching hospital in China. *J. Microbiol. Immunol. Infect.* **2018**, *51*, 411–416. [CrossRef]
41. Wolfe, C.; Pagano, P.; Pillar, C.M.; Shinabarger, D.L.; Boulos, R.A. Comparison of the in vitro antibacterial activity of Ramizol, fidaxomicin, vancomycin, and metronidazole against 100 clinical isolates of *Clostridium difficile* by broth microdilution. *Diagn. Microbiol. Infect. Dis.* **2018**, *92*, 250–252. [CrossRef]
42. Beran, V.; Kuijper, E.J.; Harmanus, C.; Sanders, I.M.; van Dorp, S.M.; Knetsch, C.W.; Janeckova, J.; Seidelova, A.; Barekova, L.; Tvrdik, J.; et al. Molecular typing and antimicrobial susceptibility testing to six antimicrobials of *Clostridium difficile* isolates from three Czech hospitals in Eastern Bohemia in 2011-2012. *Folia Microbiol.* **2017**, *62*, 445–451. [CrossRef]
43. Karlowsky, J.A.; Adam, H.J.; Kosowan, T.; Baxter, M.R.; Nichol, K.A.; Laing, N.M.; Golding, G.; Zhanel, G.G. PCR ribotyping and antimicrobial susceptibility testing of isolates of *Clostridium difficile* cultured from toxin-positive diarrheal stools of patients receiving medical care in Canadian hospitals: The Canadian *Clostridium difficile* Surveillance Study (CAN-DIFF) 2013-2015. *Diagn. Microbiol. Infect. Dis.* **2018**, *91*, 105–111. [CrossRef]
44. Freeman, J.; Vernon, J.; Morris, K.; Nicholson, S.; Todhunter, S.; Longshaw, C.; Wilcox, M.H.; Pan-European Longitudinal Surveillance of Antibiotic Resistance among Prevalent *Clostridium difficile* Ribotypes' Study Group. Pan-European longitudinal surveillance of antibiotic resistance among prevalent *Clostridium difficile* ribotypes. *Clin. Microbiol. Infect.* **2015**, *21*, 248.E9–248.E16. [CrossRef]
45. Freeman, J.; Vernon, J.; Pilling, S.; Morris, K.; Nicholson, S.; Shearman, S.; Longshaw, C.; Wilcox, M.H.; Pan-European Longitudinal Surveillance of Antibiotic Resistance among Prevalent *Clostridium difficile* Ribotypes Study Group. The ClosER study: Results from a three-year pan-European longitudinal surveillance of antibiotic resistance among prevalent *Clostridium difficile* ribotypes, 2011–2014. *Clin. Microbiol. Infect.* **2018**, *24*, 724–731. [CrossRef] [PubMed]
46. Freeman, J.; Vernon, J.; Pilling, S.; Morris, K.; Nicolson, S.; Shearman, S.; Clark, E.; Palacios-Fabrega, J.A.; Wilcox, M.; Pan-European Longitudinal Surveillance of Antibiotic Resistance among Prevalent *Clostridium difficile* Ribotypes' Study Group. Five-year Pan-European, longitudinal surveillance of *Clostridium difficile* ribotype prevalence and antimicrobial resistance: The extended ClosER study. *Eur. J. Clin. Microbiol. Infect. Dis.* **2020**, *39*, 169–177. [CrossRef]
47. Citron, D.M.; Babakhani, F.; Goldstein, E.J.; Nagaro, K.; Sambol, S.; Sears, P.; Shue, Y.K.; Gerding, D.N. Typing and susceptibility of bacterial isolates from the fidaxomicin (OPT-80) phase II study for *C. difficile* infection. *Anaerobe* **2009**, *15*, 234–236. [CrossRef]
48. Goldstein, E.J.; Citron, D.M.; Sears, P.; Babakhani, F.; Sambol, S.P.; Gerding, D.N. Comparative susceptibilities to fidaxomicin (OPT-80) of isolates collected at baseline, recurrence, and failure from patients in two phase III trials of fidaxomicin against *Clostridium difficile* infection. *Antimicrob. Agents Chemother.* **2011**, *55*, 5194–5199. [CrossRef]
49. Peng, Z.; Jin, D.; Kim, H.B.; Stratton, C.W.; Wu, B.; Tang, Y.W.; Sun, X. Update on Antimicrobial Resistance in *Clostridium difficile*: Resistance Mechanisms and Antimicrobial Susceptibility Testing. *J. Clin. Microbiol.* **2017**, *55*, 1998–2008. [CrossRef] [PubMed]
50. Leeds, J.A.; Sachdeva, M.; Mullin, S.; Barnes, S.W.; Ruzin, A. In vitro selection, via serial passage, of *Clostridium difficile* mutants with reduced susceptibility to fidaxomicin or vancomycin. *J. Antimicrob. Chemother.* **2014**, *69*, 41–44. [CrossRef] [PubMed]
51. Leeds, J.A. Antibacterials Developed to Target a Single Organism: Mechanisms and Frequencies of Reduced Susceptibility to the Novel Anti-*Clostridium difficile* Compounds Fidaxomicin and LFF571. *Cold Spring Harb. Perspect. Med.* **2016**, *6*, a025445. [CrossRef]
52. Kuehne, S.A.; Dempster, A.W.; Collery, M.M.; Joshi, N.; Jowett, J.; Kelly, M.L.; Cave, R.; Longshaw, C.M.; Minton, N.P. Characterization of the impact of rpoB mutations on the in vitro and in vivo competitive fitness of *Clostridium difficile* and susceptibility to fidaxomicin. *J. Antimicrob. Chemother.* **2018**, *73*, 973–980. [CrossRef]
53. Schwanbeck, J.; Riedel, T.; Laukien, F.; Schober, I.; Oehmig, I.; Zimmermann, O.; Overmann, J.; Gross, U.; Zautner, A.E.; Bohne, W. Characterization of a clinical *Clostridioides difficile* isolate with markedly reduced fidaxomicin susceptibility and a V1143D mutation in rpoB. *J. Antimicrob. Chemother.* **2019**, *74*, 6–10. [CrossRef] [PubMed]

54. Babakhani, F.; Bouillaut, L.; Gomez, A.; Sears, P.; Nguyen, L.; Sonenshein, A.L. Fidaxomicin inhibits spore production in *Clostridium difficile*. *Clin. Infect. Dis.* **2012**, *55* (Suppl. S2), S162–S169. [CrossRef]
55. Chilton, C.H.; Crowther, G.S.; Freeman, J.; Todhunter, S.L.; Nicholson, S.; Longshaw, C.M.; Wilcox, M.H. Successful treatment of simulated *Clostridium difficile* infection in a human gut model by fidaxomicin first line and after vancomycin or metronidazole failure. *J. Antimicrob. Chemother.* **2014**, *69*, 451–462. [CrossRef]
56. Aldape, M.J.; Packham, A.E.; Heeney, D.D.; Rice, S.N.; Bryant, A.E.; Stevens, D.L. Fidaxomicin reduces early toxin A and B production and sporulation in *Clostridium difficile* in vitro. *J. Med. Microbiol.* **2017**, *66*, 1393–1399. [CrossRef]
57. Allen, C.A.; Babakhani, F.; Sears, P.; Nguyen, L.; Sorg, J.A. Both fidaxomicin and vancomycin inhibit outgrowth of *Clostridium difficile* spores. *Antimicrob. Agents Chemother.* **2013**, *57*, 664–667. [CrossRef] [PubMed]
58. Chilton, C.H.; Crowther, G.S.; Ashwin, H.; Longshaw, C.M.; Wilcox, M.H. Association of Fidaxomicin with *C. difficile* Spores: Effects of Persistence on Subsequent Spore Recovery, Outgrowth and Toxin Production. *PLoS ONE* **2016**, *11*, e0161200. [CrossRef]
59. Basseres, E.; Endres, B.T.; Montes-Bravo, N.; Perez-Soto, N.; Rashid, T.; Lancaster, C.; Begum, K.; Alam, M.J.; Paredes-Sabja, D.; Garey, K.W. Visualization of fidaxomicin association with the exosporium layer of *Clostridioides difficile* spores. *Anaerobe* **2021**, *69*, 102352. [CrossRef] [PubMed]
60. Babakhani, F.; Bouillaut, L.; Sears, P.; Sims, C.; Gomez, A.; Sonenshein, A.L. Fidaxomicin inhibits toxin production in *Clostridium difficile*. *J. Antimicrob. Chemother.* **2013**, *68*, 515–522. [CrossRef] [PubMed]
61. Thabit, A.K.; Alam, M.J.; Khaleduzzaman, M.; Garey, K.W.; Nicolau, D.P. A pilot study to assess bacterial and toxin reduction in patients with *Clostridium difficile* infection given fidaxomicin or vancomycin. *Ann. Clin. Microbiol. Antimicrob.* **2016**, *15*, 22. [CrossRef]
62. Koon, H.W.; Wang, J.; Mussatto, C.C.; Ortiz, C.; Lee, E.C.; Tran, D.H.; Chen, X.; Kelly, C.P.; Pothoulakis, C. Fidaxomicin and OP-1118 Inhibit *Clostridium difficile* Toxin A- and B-Mediated Inflammatory Responses via Inhibition of NF-kappaB Activity. *Antimicrob. Agents Chemother.* **2018**, *62*, e01513-17. [CrossRef] [PubMed]
63. Koon, H.W.; Ho, S.; Hing, T.C.; Cheng, M.; Chen, X.; Ichikawa, Y.; Kelly, C.P.; Pothoulakis, C. Fidaxomicin inhibits *Clostridium difficile* toxin A-mediated enteritis in the mouse ileum. *Antimicrob. Agents Chemother.* **2014**, *58*, 4642–4650. [CrossRef] [PubMed]
64. Dapa, T.; Unnikrishnan, M. Biofilm formation by *Clostridium difficile*. *Gut Microbes* **2013**, *4*, 397–402. [CrossRef]
65. Hamada, M.; Yamaguchi, T.; Ishii, Y.; Chono, K.; Tateda, K. Inhibitory effect of fidaxomicin on biofilm formation in *Clostridioides difficile*. *J. Infect. Chemother.* **2020**, *26*, 685–692. [CrossRef] [PubMed]
66. James, G.A.; Chesnel, L.; Boegli, L.; deLancey Pulcini, E.; Fisher, S.; Stewart, P.S. Analysis of *Clostridium difficile* biofilms: Imaging and antimicrobial treatment. *J. Antimicrob. Chemother.* **2018**, *73*, 102–108. [CrossRef] [PubMed]
67. Pantaleon, V.; Bouttier, S.; Soavelomandroso, A.P.; Janoir, C.; Candela, T. Biofilms of Clostridium species. *Anaerobe* **2014**, *30*, 193–198. [CrossRef] [PubMed]
68. Biswas, J.S.; Patel, A.; Otter, J.A.; Wade, P.; Newsholme, W.; van Kleef, E.; Goldenberg, S.D. Reduction in *Clostridium difficile* environmental contamination by hospitalized patients treated with fidaxomicin. *J. Hosp. Infect.* **2015**, *90*, 267–270. [CrossRef]
69. Davies, K.; Mawer, D.; Walker, A.S.; Berry, C.; Planche, T.; Stanley, P.; Goldenberg, S.; Sandoe, J.; Wilcox, M.H. An Analysis of *Clostridium difficile* Environmental Contamination During and After Treatment for C difficile Infection. *Open Forum Infect. Dis.* **2020**, *7*, ofaa362. [CrossRef]
70. Turner, N.A.; Warren, B.G.; Gergen-Teague, M.F.; Addison, R.M.; Addison, B.; Rutala, W.A.; Weber, D.J.; Sexton, D.J.; Anderson, D.J. Impact of Oral Metronidazole, Vancomycin, and Fidaxomicin on Host Shedding and Environmental Contamination with *Clostridioides difficile*. *Clin. Infect. Dis.* **2022**, *74*, 648–656. [CrossRef]
71. Cataldo, M.A.; Granata, G.; Petrosillo, N. *Clostridium difficile* infection: New approaches to prevention, non-antimicrobial treatment, and stewardship. *Expert Rev. Anti-Infect. Ther.* **2017**, *15*, 1027–1040. [CrossRef]
72. Cornely, O.A.; Crook, D.W.; Esposito, R.; Poirier, A.; Somero, M.S.; Weiss, K.; Sears, P.; Gorbach, S.; Group, O.P.T.C.S. Fidaxomicin versus vancomycin for infection with *Clostridium difficile* in Europe, Canada, and the USA: A double-blind, non-inferiority, randomised controlled trial. *Lancet Infect. Dis.* **2012**, *12*, 281–289. [CrossRef]
73. Louie, T.J.; Miller, M.A.; Mullane, K.M.; Weiss, K.; Lentnek, A.; Golan, Y.; Gorbach, S.; Sears, P.; Shue, Y.K.; OPT-80-003 Clinical Study Group. Fidaxomicin versus vancomycin for *Clostridium difficile* infection. *N. Engl. J. Med.* **2011**, *364*, 422–431. [CrossRef]
74. Crook, D.W.; Walker, A.S.; Kean, Y.; Weiss, K.; Cornely, O.A.; Miller, M.A.; Esposito, R.; Louie, T.J.; Stoesser, N.E.; Young, B.C.; et al. Fidaxomicin versus vancomycin for *Clostridium difficile* infection: Meta-analysis of pivotal randomized controlled trials. *Clin. Infect. Dis.* **2012**, *55* (Suppl. S2), S93–S103. [CrossRef]
75. Cornely, O.A.; Nathwani, D.; Ivanescu, C.; Odufowora-Sita, O.; Retsa, P.; Odeyemi, I.A. Clinical efficacy of fidaxomicin compared with vancomycin and metronidazole in *Clostridium difficile* infections: A meta-analysis and indirect treatment comparison. *J. Antimicrob. Chemother.* **2014**, *69*, 2892–2900. [CrossRef]
76. Nelson, R.L.; Suda, K.J.; Evans, C.T. Antibiotic treatment for *Clostridium difficile*-associated diarrhoea in adults. *Cochrane Database Syst. Rev.* **2017**, *3*, CD004610. [CrossRef]
77. Mullane, K.M.; Miller, M.A.; Weiss, K.; Lentnek, A.; Golan, Y.; Sears, P.S.; Shue, Y.K.; Louie, T.J.; Gorbach, S.L. Efficacy of fidaxomicin versus vancomycin as therapy for *Clostridium difficile* infection in individuals taking concomitant antibiotics for other concurrent infections. *Clin. Infect. Dis.* **2011**, *53*, 440–447. [CrossRef]
78. Cornely, O.A.; Miller, M.A.; Fantin, B.; Mullane, K.; Kean, Y.; Gorbach, S. Resolution of *Clostridium difficile*-associated diarrhea in patients with cancer treated with fidaxomicin or vancomycin. *J. Clin. Oncol.* **2013**, *31*, 2493–2499. [CrossRef]

79. Figueroa, I.; Johnson, S.; Sambol, S.P.; Goldstein, E.J.; Citron, D.M.; Gerding, D.N. Relapse versus reinfection: Recurrent *Clostridium difficile* infection following treatment with fidaxomicin or vancomycin. *Clin. Infect. Dis.* **2012**, *55* (Suppl. S2), S104–S109. [CrossRef]
80. Eyre, D.W.; Babakhani, F.; Griffiths, D.; Seddon, J.; Del Ojo Elias, C.; Gorbach, S.L.; Peto, T.E.; Crook, D.W.; Walker, A.S. Whole-genome sequencing demonstrates that fidaxomicin is superior to vancomycin for preventing reinfection and relapse of infection with *Clostridium difficile*. *J. Infect. Dis.* **2014**, *209*, 1446–1451. [CrossRef]
81. Cornely, O.A.; Miller, M.A.; Louie, T.J.; Crook, D.W.; Gorbach, S.L. Treatment of first recurrence of *Clostridium difficile* infection: Fidaxomicin versus vancomycin. *Clin. Infect. Dis.* **2012**, *55* (Suppl. S2), S154–S161. [CrossRef] [PubMed]
82. Louie, T.J.; Miller, M.A.; Crook, D.W.; Lentnek, A.; Bernard, L.; High, K.P.; Shue, Y.K.; Gorbach, S.L. Effect of age on treatment outcomes in *Clostridium difficile* infection. *J. Am. Geriatr. Soc.* **2013**, *61*, 222–230. [CrossRef] [PubMed]
83. Mikamo, H.; Tateda, K.; Yanagihara, K.; Kusachi, S.; Takesue, Y.; Miki, T.; Oizumi, Y.; Gamo, K.; Hashimoto, A.; Toyoshima, J.; et al. Efficacy and safety of fidaxomicin for the treatment of Clostridioides (Clostridium) difficile infection in a randomized, double-blind, comparative Phase III study in Japan. *J. Infect. Chemother.* **2018**, *24*, 744–752. [CrossRef]
84. Okumura, H.; Fukushima, A.; Taieb, V.; Shoji, S.; English, M. Fidaxomicin compared with vancomycin and metronidazole for the treatment of *Clostridioides* (*Clostridium*) *difficile* infection: A network meta-analysis. *J. Infect. Chemother.* **2020**, *26*, 43–50. [CrossRef]
85. Housman, S.T.; Thabit, A.K.; Kuti, J.L.; Quintiliani, R.; Nicolau, D.P. Assessment of *Clostridium difficile* Burden in Patients Over Time with First Episode Infection Following Fidaxomicin or Vancomycin. *Infect. Control Hosp. Epidemiol.* **2016**, *37*, 215–218. [CrossRef] [PubMed]
86. Hvas, C.L.; Dahl Jorgensen, S.M.; Jorgensen, S.P.; Storgaard, M.; Lemming, L.; Hansen, M.M.; Erikstrup, C.; Dahlerup, J.F. Fecal Microbiota Transplantation Is Superior to Fidaxomicin for Treatment of Recurrent *Clostridium difficile* Infection. *Gastroenterology* **2019**, *156*, 1324–1332. [CrossRef] [PubMed]
87. Tashiro, S.; Mihara, T.; Sasaki, M.; Shimamura, C.; Shimamura, R.; Suzuki, S.; Yoshikawa, M.; Hasegawa, T.; Enoki, Y.; Taguchi, K.; et al. Oral fidaxomicin versus vancomycin for the treatment of *Clostridioides difficile* infection: A systematic review and meta-analysis of randomized controlled trials. *J. Infect. Chemother.* **2022**, *28*, 1536–1545. [CrossRef]
88. Guery, B.; Menichetti, F.; Anttila, V.J.; Adomakoh, N.; Aguado, J.M.; Bisnauthsing, K.; Georgopali, A.; Goldenberg, S.D.; Karas, A.; Kazeem, G.; et al. Extended-pulsed fidaxomicin versus vancomycin for *Clostridium difficile* infection in patients 60 years and older (EXTEND): A randomised, controlled, open-label, phase 3b/4 trial. *Lancet Infect. Dis.* **2018**, *18*, 296–307. [CrossRef]
89. Chilton, C.H.; Crowther, G.S.; Todhunter, S.L.; Ashwin, H.; Longshaw, C.M.; Karas, A.; Wilcox, M.H. Efficacy of alternative fidaxomicin dosing regimens for treatment of simulated *Clostridium difficile* infection in an in vitro human gut model. *J. Antimicrob. Chemother.* **2015**, *70*, 2598–2607. [CrossRef]
90. Guery, B.; Georgopali, A.; Karas, A.; Kazeem, G.; Michon, I.; Wilcox, M.H.; Cornely, O.A. Pharmacokinetic analysis of an extended-pulsed fidaxomicin regimen for the treatment of *Clostridioides* (*Clostridium*) *difficile* infection in patients aged 60 years and older in the EXTEND randomized controlled trial. *J. Antimicrob. Chemother.* **2020**, *75*, 1014–1018. [CrossRef]
91. Cornely, O.A.; Vehreschild, M.; Adomakoh, N.; Georgopali, A.; Karas, A.; Kazeem, G.; Guery, B. Extended-pulsed fidaxomicin versus vancomycin for *Clostridium difficile* infection: EXTEND study subgroup analyses. *Eur. J. Clin. Microbiol. Infect. Dis.* **2019**, *38*, 1187–1194. [CrossRef]
92. Wilcox, M.H.; Cornely, O.A.; Guery, B.; Longshaw, C.; Georgopali, A.; Karas, A.; Kazeem, G.; Palacios-Fabrega, J.A.; Vehreschild, M. Microbiological Characterization and Clinical Outcomes After Extended-Pulsed Fidaxomicin Treatment for *Clostridioides difficile* Infection in the EXTEND Study. *Open Forum Infect. Dis.* **2019**, *6*, ofz436. [CrossRef]
93. Beinortas, T.; Burr, N.E.; Wilcox, M.H.; Subramanian, V. Comparative efficacy of treatments for *Clostridium difficile* infection: A systematic review and network meta-analysis. *Lancet Infect. Dis.* **2018**, *18*, 1035–1044. [CrossRef]
94. Vehreschild, M.J.; Weitershagen, D.; Biehl, L.M.; Tacke, D.; Waldschmidt, D.; Tox, U.; Wisplinghoff, H.; Von Bergwelt-Baildon, M.; Cornely, O.A.; Vehreschild, J.J. *Clostridium difficile* infection in patients with acute myelogenous leukemia and in patients undergoing allogeneic stem cell transplantation: Epidemiology and risk factor analysis. *Biol. Blood Marrow Transplant.* **2014**, *20*, 823–828. [CrossRef]
95. Trifilio, S.M.; Pi, J.; Mehta, J. Changing epidemiology of *Clostridium difficile*-associated disease during stem cell transplantation. *Biol. Blood Marrow Transplant.* **2013**, *19*, 405–409. [CrossRef]
96. Dubberke, E.R.; Reske, K.A.; Srivastava, A.; Sadhu, J.; Gatti, R.; Young, R.M.; Rakes, L.C.; Dieckgraefe, B.; DiPersio, J.; Fraser, V.J. *Clostridium difficile*-associated disease in allogeneic hematopoietic stem-cell transplant recipients: Risk associations, protective associations, and outcomes. *Clin. Transplant.* **2010**, *24*, 192–198. [CrossRef]
97. Alonso, C.D.; Treadway, S.B.; Hanna, D.B.; Huff, C.A.; Neofytos, D.; Carroll, K.C.; Marr, K.A. Epidemiology and outcomes of *Clostridium difficile* infections in hematopoietic stem cell transplant recipients. *Clin. Infect. Dis.* **2012**, *54*, 1053–1063. [CrossRef] [PubMed]
98. Mullane, K.M.; Winston, D.J.; Nooka, A.; Morris, M.I.; Stiff, P.; Dugan, M.J.; Holland, H.; Gregg, K.; Adachi, J.A.; Pergam, S.A.; et al. A Randomized, Placebo-controlled Trial of Fidaxomicin for Prophylaxis of *Clostridium difficile*-associated Diarrhea in Adults Undergoing Hematopoietic Stem Cell Transplantation. *Clin. Infect. Dis.* **2019**, *68*, 196–203. [CrossRef] [PubMed]
99. Johnson, S.; Gerding, D.N.; Li, X.; Reda, D.J.; Donskey, C.J.; Gupta, K.; Goetz, M.B.; Climo, M.W.; Gordin, F.M.; Ringer, R.; et al. Defining optimal treatment for recurrent *Clostridioides difficile* infection (OpTION study): A randomized, double-blind comparison of three antibiotic regimens for patients with a first or second recurrence. *Contemp. Clin. Trials* **2022**, *116*, 106756. [CrossRef] [PubMed]

100. A Comparison of Fidaxomicin and Vancomycin in Patients with CDI Receiving Antibiotics for Concurrent. Available online: https://clinicaltrials.gov/ct2/show/study/NCT02692651 (accessed on 9 September 2022).
101. Weiss, K.; Allgren, R.L.; Sellers, S. Safety analysis of fidaxomicin in comparison with oral vancomycin for *Clostridium difficile* infections. *Clin. Infect. Dis.* **2012**, *55* (Suppl. S2), S110–S115. [CrossRef] [PubMed]

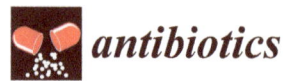

Perspective

Bezlotoxumab in Patients with a Primary *Clostridioides difficile* Infection: A Literature Review

Guido Granata [1,*], Francesco Schiavone [2] and Giuseppe Pipitone [3]

1. Clinical and Research Department for Infectious Diseases, National Institute for Infectious Diseases L. Spallanzani, IRCCS, 00149 Rome, Italy
2. Divers and Raiders Group Command "Teseo Tesei" COMSUBIN, Medical Service, Italian Navy, 19025 Portovenere, Italy
3. Infectious Disease Unit, ARNAS Civico-Di Cristina, Piazza Leotta, 5, 90100 Palermo, Italy
* Correspondence: guido.granata@inmi.it; Tel.: +39-06-55170264

Abstract: Background: Nowadays, one of the main issues in the management of *Clostridioides difficile* infection (CDI) is the high rate of recurrences (rCDI), causing increased mortality and higher health care costs. Objectives: To assess the available evidence on the use of bezlotoxumab for the prevention of rCDI during a first CDI episode. Methods: Published articles on bezlotoxumab during a primary CDI episode were identified through computerized literature searches with the search terms [(bezlotoxumab) AND (CDI) OR (*Clostridioides difficile* infection)] using PubMed and by reviewing the references of retrieved articles. PubMed was searched until 31 August 2022. Results: Eighty-eight studies were identified as published from December 2014 to June 2022. Five studies were included in this study, one was a phase III clinical trial and four were sub-analyses or extensions of the previous phase III clinical trial. In the phase III clinical trial, the subgroup analysis on the included primary CDI patients showed that 13.5% of patients receiving bezlotoxumab had an rCDI, whilst 20.9% of patients in the placebo group had an rCDI at the twelve weeks follow-up (absolute difference: −7.4). Conclusions: Bezlotoxumab administration during the standard of care antibiotic therapy is effective and safe in reducing the rate of rCDI. Despite its high cost, evidence suggests considering bezlotoxumab in patients with a primary CDI episode. Further studies are needed to assess the benefit in specific subgroups of primary CDI patients and to define the risk factors to guide bezlotoxumab use.

Keywords: primary CDI; *Clostridioides difficile*; TcdB; toxin; bezlotoxumab; recurrence of CDI; CDI recurrence prevention; cost-effectiveness; prevention; health care cost

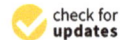

Citation: Granata, G.; Schiavone, F.; Pipitone, G. Bezlotoxumab in Patients with a Primary *Clostridioides difficile* Infection: A Literature Review. *Antibiotics* **2022**, *11*, 1495. https://doi.org/10.3390/antibiotics11111495

Academic Editor: Kevin W. Garey

Received: 9 October 2022
Accepted: 25 October 2022
Published: 28 October 2022

Publisher's Note: MDPI stays neutral with regard to jurisdictional claims in published maps and institutional affiliations.

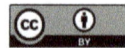

Copyright: © 2022 by the authors. Licensee MDPI, Basel, Switzerland. This article is an open access article distributed under the terms and conditions of the Creative Commons Attribution (CC BY) license (https://creativecommons.org/licenses/by/4.0/).

1. Introduction

The Gram-positive anaerobic bacterium *Clostridioides difficile* is among the main pathogens responsible for nosocomial diarrhea, causing significant morbidity, mortality, prolonged hospital stay and high healthcare costs worldwide [1–7]. A relevant issue during CDI is its high rate of recurrences (rCDI). Clinical studies show wide-ranging rCDI rates after the primary CDI, between 10% and 30% [8–11]. rCDI is associated with a higher risk of death and higher hospitalization costs [1–7]. Currently, the main approaches to treat a primary CDI are the oral anti-*Clostridioides difficile* antibiotics vancomycin or fidaxomicin, while oral metronidazole should be used only when vancomycin and fidaxomicin are not available or feasible. For rCDI, additional non-antimicrobial approaches may be considered, i.e., fecal microbiota transplant or bezlotoxumab. Bezlotoxumab is a monoclonal antibody directed against *Clostridioides difficile* toxin B, effective in reducing the rate of further rCDI. One of the main drawbacks of bezlotoxumab is its high cost.

In the recently released updates of guidelines/guidance documents from the Infectious Diseases Society of America/Society for Healthcare Epidemiology of America (IDSA/SHEA) and from the European Society of Clinical Microbiology and Infectious

Diseases (ESCMID), there have been changes in the recommendations pertaining to the use of bezlotoxumab [12,13]. The IDSA/SHEA guidelines recommend that in settings where logistics is not an issue, patients with a primary CDI episode and other risk factors for rCDI and severe CDI on presentation may particularly benefit from receiving bezlotoxumab. The ESCMID guidelines recommend considering bezlotoxumab in addition to standard-of-care antibiotics for the treatment of a second or further rCDI.

We performed a literature review with the main aim of summarizing available evidence on the use of bezlotoxumab during a first CDI episode to prevent rCDI.

2. Materials and Methods

Search strategy and Article Identification

Published articles (from June 2017 to November 2020) assessing the efficacy and safety of bezlotoxumab for the prevention of rCDI after a first CDI episode were identified through computerized literature searches using PubMed until 31 August 2022. A combination of the following search terms was used: [(Bezlotoxumab) AND (*Clostridioides difficile*) OR (CDI)]. English language restriction was applied.

Randomized clinical trials and original research articles reporting original data on the use of bezlotoxumab during a first CDI episode were included in this study. Studies published only in abstract form, correction articles, reviews, case reports, editorials, guidance articles or guidelines and clinical trial protocols were not included.

Quantitative and qualitative information from the included studies was summarized by means of textual descriptions.

3. Results

Studies Description

Figure 1 shows the selection process of the included studies. Through a PubMed search with the search terms "bezlotoxumab" and "*Clostridioides difficile*" or "CDI", we identified 88 studies published from December 2014 to June 2022. Of the 22 full-text articles assessed for eligibility, fifteen studies were excluded because they did not report data on bezlotoxumab for a first CDI episode, one study was excluded because it was a "review article" and one study was excluded because it was a "correction article". The remaining five studies were included in this study (Figure 1) [14–18]. Of the five studies, one was a phase III clinical trial study on the efficacy and safety of bezlotoxumab for the prevention of rCDI, and four studies were sub-analysis or extensions of the previous phase III clinical trial. A summary description of the five included studies is reported in Table 1.

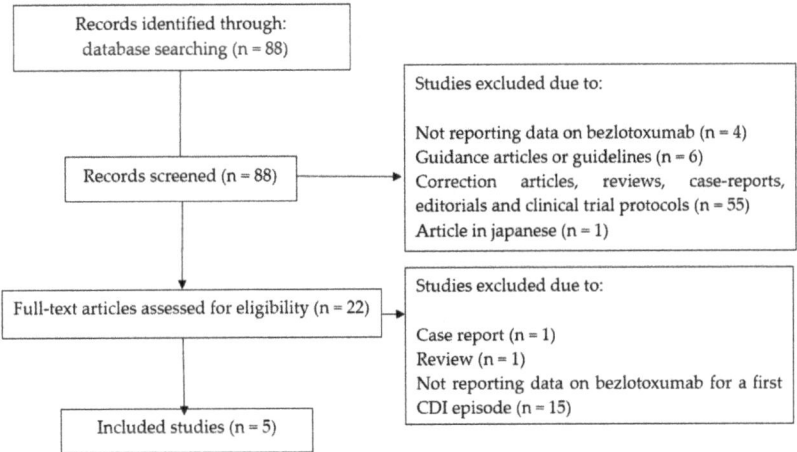

Figure 1. Flowchart depicting the selection process of studies included in this study.

Table 1. Summary description of the 5 studies providing data on the use of bezlotoxumab for the prevention of rCDI after a first CDI episode.

Author	Country	Study Design	Study Aim	Methods	Study Results
Wilcox M et al., 2017 [14]	30 different Countries	Placebo-controlled, double-blind, single-infusion, phase III clinical trial	To evaluate the efficacy and safety of bezlotoxumab (alone and in combination with actoxumab) for the prevention of rCDI	2655 adult patients with primary or rCDI were randomized 1:1:1 to receive 60 min intravenous infusion of bezlotoxumab (10 mg/kg), actoxumab plus bezlotoxumab (10 mg/kg each) or placebo during the standard of care antibiotic therapy Primary endpoint was the proportion of participants with rCDI during 12 weeks of follow-up in the modified intention-to-treat population	Rate of rCDI was lower with bezlotoxumab than with placebo (MODIFY II: 16% vs. 26%, $p < 0.001$) The subgroup analysis providing the rCDI rate among primary CDI patients showed that 75/556 (13.5%) patients receiving bezlotoxumab plus standard-of-care treatment had an rCDI, whilst 114/545 (20.9%) patients in the placebo group had rCDI at the twelve weeks follow-up (absolute difference: −7.4)
Goldstein EJC et al., 2020 [15]	30 different Countries	Extension of MODIFY II clinical trial	To assess the long-term rates of rCDI and *Clostridioides difficile* colonization following bezlotoxumab infusion	The study included 293 participants of MODIFY II who provided stool samples at 6, 9 and 12 months. *Clostridioides difficile* colonization at months 6, 9 and 12 was assessed based on whether a toxigenic *Clostridioides difficile* strain was isolated in samples	At 12 months, the incidence of rCDI in the bezlotoxumab and placebo groups was 18.8% and 51.5% respectively. *Clostridioides difficile* colonization rates were 16–24% in the bezlotoxumab group and 19–32% in the placebo groups
Gerding DN et al., 2018 [16]	30 different Countries	Sub-analysis of the MODIFY I-II clinical trials	To evaluate the efficacy of bezlotoxumab in reducing rCDI among patients with characteristics associated with increased risk factors for rCDI	Patients treated with bezlotoxumab vs. placebo were stratified by risk factors The efficacy was evaluated as: a) achieving initial clinical cure rate, b) reducing the rate of rCDI and c) reducing the rate of FMT	Bezlotoxumab did not affect initial clinical cure rate; bezlotoxumab reduced the rate of rCDI compared to the low-risk group Among primary CDI patients, 69/424 (16.3%) patients treated with bezlotoxumab versus 106/400 (26.5%) controls had rCDI at 12 weeks (absolute difference: −10.1%)

Table 1. Cont.

Author	Country	Study Design	Study Aim	Methods	Study Results
Mikamo H et al., 2018 [17]	Japan	Sub-analysis of the MODIFY I-II clinical trial	To evaluate the efficacy of bezlotoxumab and actoxumab in reducing rCDI rate at week 12	95 Japanese patients were randomized to bezlotoxumab, actoxumab plus bezlotoxumab or placebo in a 1:1:1 ratio Vancomycin, metronidazole and fidaxomicin were administered as standard-of-care antibiotic treatment	The rCDI rate was lower in the bezlotoxumab group (21%) compared to placebo (46%), p: 0.0197
Prabhu VS et al., 2018 [18]	30 different Countries	Sub-analysis of MODIFY I-II clinical trial	To assess the cost-effectiveness of bezlotoxumab in subgroups of patients at risk of rCDI	The computer simulation followed the cohort over a lifetime, and healthcare services costs were compared to estimate the incremental cost-effectiveness ratios	In the subgroup of patients with no previous CDI episodes in the past six months, the cost-effectiveness model showed that, compared with placebo, bezlotoxumab could reduce rCDI by 10.1% (26.6% versus 16.5%), and the 180-day mortality by 1.1% Bezlotoxumab was associated with a gain in quality-adjusted life-years and was cost-effective

rCDI: recurrence of CDI; FMT: fecal microbiota transplant.

The large randomized, placebo-controlled, phase III trials on bezlotoxumab MODIFY I and MODIFY II showed a substantially lower rate of rCDI than placebo with a comparable safety profile [14]. The primary endpoint of the MODIFY II trial was the proportion of participants with rCDI through 12 weeks of follow-up. The subgroup analysis provided the rCDI rate of the primary CDI patients included in this trial (namely, no CDI episodes in the past six months). Furthermore, 75 out of 556 (13.5%) primary CDI patients receiving bezlotoxumab plus standard of care treatment had an rCDI, whilst 114/545 (20.9%) primary CDI patients in the placebo group had rCDI at the twelve weeks follow-up (absolute difference: −7.4) [14].

A study extending the MODIFY II trial follow-up to twelve months was performed to assess the long-term rates of rCDI and *Clostridioides difficile* colonization following bezlotoxumab infusion. At the end of the twelve-month follow-up of this study, no participants who achieved sustained clinical cure following bezlotoxumab infusion experienced rCDI, whilst only one patient in the placebo group experienced rCDI [15].

A post-hoc analysis of the MODIFY I and II trials was performed to assess bezlotoxumab efficacy in participants with characteristics associated with increased risk for rCDI [16]. In this study, patients enrolled in the MODIFY trials were grouped according to their risk factors for rCDI, including age ≥ 65 years, history of CDI, compromised immunity, severe CDI, and ribotype 027/078/244. Data showed that 424 primary CDI patients were treated with bezlotoxumab and 400 primary CDI patients received placebo. Moreover, 69/424 (16.3%) versus 106/400 (26.5%) had rCDI in 12 weeks, with an absolute difference of −10.1%, significantly favoring bezlotoxumab [16].

A subgroup analysis was performed on the data from the Japanese patients included in the MODIFY trials. In comparison to the general population included in the MODIFY trials, Japanese patients were older (Japanese older than 65 years: 91% versus overall MODIFY patients: 53%) and the proportion of Japanese patients with severe CDI was higher (Japanese: 24%, overall MODIFY patients: 16%). In addition, the proportion of subjects with a prior history of CDI was lower (Japanese: 19/93, 20%, overall MODIFY patients: 28%). Among the 95 Japanese patients, the observed rCDI rate was 46% in the placebo arm versus 21% in the bezlotoxumab arm (p: 0.0197) [17].

A study was performed to assess the cost-effectiveness of bezlotoxumab, compared with standard of care alone, in subgroups of CDI patients included in the MODIFY trials [18]. This study adopted a computer-based Markov health state transition model to track the natural history of patients infected with CDI. The simulation followed the cohort over a lifetime horizon, and costs and utilities for the various health states were used to estimate incremental cost-effectiveness ratios. Regarding the subgroup of CDI patients with no previous CDI episodes in the past six months, the cost-effectiveness model showed that, compared with placebo, bezlotoxumab could reduce rCDI by 10.1% (26.6% versus 16.5%), and the 180-day mortality by 1.1%. In this model, bezlotoxumab was also cost-effective in preventing rCDI recurrences [18].

4. Discussion

Nowadays, CDI and rCDI remain associated with a reduction in patient quality of life and with increased healthcare costs. Bezlotoxumab is a promising option to reduce the burden of rCDI. The randomized, placebo-controlled phase III trial MODIFY II showed a substantially lower rate of rCDI in patients treated with bezlotoxumab [14]. Nonetheless, experiences outside randomized controlled trials remain scant. The MODIFY trial has the limitation that the target population was a selected sample of participants with a low prevalence of multiple risk factors for recurrence.

Currently, the most recent international guidelines differ in the recommendations regarding the use of bezlotoxumab for the first episode of CDI and rate the certainty of the evidence as only moderate [12,13]. The IDSA/SHEA guidelines recommend that in settings where logistics are not an issue, patients with a primary CDI episode and other risk factors for rCDI or severe CDI may receive bezlotoxumab despite its high cost [12]. Differently, the ESCMID guidelines recommend considering bezlotoxumab in addition to standard-of-care antibiotics only for the treatment of a second or further rCDI.

Importantly, it has to be kept in mind that in patients with a history of congestive heart failure, bezlotoxumab should be reserved for use when the benefits outweigh the risk [12,13].

Nevertheless, it is promising that in the MODIFY II trial, the estimated number needed to treat to prevent one episode of rCDI after a primary CDI episode with bezlotoxumab was 10 [14]. Interestingly, available data suggest that the efficacy of bezlotoxumab is due to rCDI prevention rather than a delay in rCDI onset after antibody concentrations were diminished [15]. Moreover, in post-hoc analyses of the MODIFY trials, bezlotoxumab reduced the rate of rCDI even in the group of patients with a primary CDI and no risk factors for rCDI [16,17].

Despite the growing data evidence supporting the use of bezlotoxumab to prevent rCDI, its use in many European countries is still limited and restricted to participants who experienced previous CDI episodes. This might be mainly explained by the direct drug cost of bezlotoxumab. However, studies adopting cost-effectiveness models show that for preventing rCDI recurrences, bezlotoxumab may be cost-effective [18].

It is likely that the overall future scenario may change from "administer bezlotoxumab only in high-risk patients, because of the high cost of this compound" to "if feasible, consider bezlotoxumab even for a primary CDI episode, in view of the global benefits for the patient and the cost-effectiveness provided by the reduction of the rate of the expensive rCDI episodes". In our opinion, future studies are needed to clarify some remaining unanswered questions: First, the efficacy of fidaxomicin plus bezlotoxumab in preventing rCDI in comparison to vancomycin plus bezlotoxumab. Second, the use of bezlotoxumab in specific, high-risk subgroups of patients experiencing a primary CDI, i.e., hematologic patients, hematopoietic cell transplantation patients, patients receiving immunosuppression after solid organ transplantation, patients with impairment of humoral immunity. Third, bezlotoxumab use in patients with severe CDI.

5. Conclusions

Data coming from the first available research studies show that bezlotoxumab administration during the standard of care antibiotic therapy is effective and safe in reducing the rate of further rCDI. Despite its high cost, this evidence suggests considering bezlotoxumab not only among patients with multiple CDI episodes, but also in patients with a primary CDI episode.

Further studies are needed to assess the exact benefit associated with bezlotoxumab in specific subgroups of primary CDI patients and to define the risk factors to guide bezlotoxumab use.

Author Contributions: Conceptualization, G.G.; methodology, G.G.; software, F.S., G.P. and G.G.; validation, G.G.; formal analysis, G.G. and G.P.; investigation, F.S., G.P. and G.G.; resources, G.G.; data curation, G.P. and G.G.; writing—original draft preparation, G.G; writing—review and editing, G.P. and G.P.; visualization, G.G.; supervision, G.G.; All authors have read and agreed to the published version of the manuscript.

Funding: This research received no external funding.

Institutional Review Board Statement: Not applicable.

Informed Consent Statement: Not applicable.

Data Availability Statement: The data presented in this study are openly available in the MEDLINE database.

Conflicts of Interest: The authors declare no conflict of interest. The authors declare that they have no known competing financial interests or personal relationships that could have appeared to influence the work reported in this paper.

References

1. Evans, C.T.; Safdar, N. Current trends in the epidemiology and outcomes of *Clostridium difficile* infection. *Clin. Inf. Dis.* **2015**, *60*, S66–S71. [CrossRef] [PubMed]
2. Guh, A.Y.; Mu, Y.; Winston, L.G.; Johnston, H.; Olson, D.; Farley, M.M.; Wilson, L.E.; Holzbauer, S.M.; Phipps, E.C.; Dumyati, G.K.; et al. Trends in U.S. Burden of *Clostridioides difficile* Infection and Outcomes. *N. Engl. J. Med.* **2020**, *382*, 1320–1330. [CrossRef] [PubMed]
3. Khanna, S. My Treatment Approach to *Clostridioides difficile* Infection. *Mayo Clin. Proc.* **2021**, *96*, 2192–2204. [CrossRef] [PubMed]
4. Khanna, S.; Pardi, D.S.; Aronson, S.L.; Kammer, P.P.; Orenstein, R.; St Sauver, J.L.; Harmsen, W.S.; Zinsmeister, A.R. The epidemiology of community-acquired Clostridium difficile infection: A population-based study. *Am. J. Gastroenterol.* **2012**, *107*, 89–95. [CrossRef] [PubMed]
5. Lessa, F.C. Community-associated *Clostridium difficile* infection: How real is it? *Anaerobe* **2013**, *24*, 121–123. [CrossRef]
6. Alicino, C.; Giacobbe, D.R.; Durando, P.; Bellina, D.; AM, D.I.B.; Paganino, C.; Del Bono, V.; Viscoli, C.; Icardi, G.; Orsi, A. Increasing incidence of *Clostridium difficile* infections: Results from a 5-year retrospective study in a large teaching hospital in the Italian region with the oldest population. *Epidemiol. Infect.* **2016**, *144*, 2517–2526. [CrossRef]
7. Finn, E.; Andersson, F.L.; Madin-Warburton, M. Burden of *Clostridioides difficile* infection (CDI)—A systematic review of the epidemiology of primary and recurrent CDI. *BMC Infect. Dis.* **2021**, *21*, 456. [CrossRef] [PubMed]
8. Fekety, R.; McFarland, L.V.; Surawicz, C.M.; Greenberg, R.N.; Elmer, G.W.; Mulligan, M.E. Recurrent *Clostridium difficile* diarrhea: Characteristics of and risk factors for patients enrolled in a prospective, randomized, double-blinded trial. *Clin. Infect. Dis.* **1997**, *24*, 324–333. [CrossRef] [PubMed]
9. Granata, G.; Petrosillo, N.; Adamoli, L.; Bartoletti, M.; Bartoloni, A.; Basile, G.; Bassetti, M.; Bonfanti, P.; Borromeo, R.; Ceccarelli, G.; et al. Prospective Study on Incidence, Risk Factors and Outcome of Recurrent *Clostridioides difficile* Infections. *J. Clin. Med.* **2021**, *10*, 1127. [CrossRef] [PubMed]
10. McFarland, L.V.; Surawicz, C.M.; Rubin, M.; Fekety, R.; Elmer, G.W.; Greenberg, R.N. Recurrent *Clostridium difficile* disease: Epidemiology and clinical characteristics. *Infect. Control Hosp. Epidemiol.* **1999**, *20*, 43–50. [CrossRef] [PubMed]

11. Falcone, M.; Tiseo, G.; Iraci, F.; Raponi, G.; Goldoni, P.; Delle Rose, D.; Santino, I.; Carfagna, P.; Murri, R.; Fantoni, M.; et al. Risk factors for recurrence in patients with *Clostridium difficile* infection due to 027 and non-027 ribotypes. *Clin. Microbiol. Infect.* **2019**, *25*, 474–480. [CrossRef] [PubMed]
12. Johnson, S.; Lavergne, V.; Skinner, A.M.; Gonzales-Luna, A.J.; Garey, K.W.; Kelly, C.P.; Wilcox, M.H. Clinical Practice Guideline by the Infectious Diseases Society of America (IDSA) and Society for Healthcare Epidemiology of America (SHEA): 2021 Focused Update Guidelines on Management of Clostridioides difficile Infection in Adults. *Clin. Infect. Dis.* **2021**, *73*, 755–757. [CrossRef] [PubMed]
13. van Prehn, J.; Reigadas, E.; Vogelzang, E.H.; Bouza, E.; Hristea, A.; Guery, B.; Krutova, M.; Noren, T.; Allerberger, F.; Coia, J.E.; et al. European Society of Clinical Microbiology and Infectious Diseases: 2021 update on the treatment guidance document for Clostridioides difficile infection in adults. *Clin. Microbiol. Infect.* **2021**, *27* (Suppl. 2), S1–S21. [CrossRef]
14. Wilcox, M.H.; Gerding, D.N.; Poxton, I.R.; Kelly, C.; Nathan, R.; Birch, T.; Cornely, O.A.; Rahav, G.; Bouza, E.; Lee, C.; et al. MODIFY I and MODIFY II Investigators. Bezlotoxumab for Prevention of Recurrent *Clostridium difficile* Infection. *N. Engl. J. Med.* **2017**, *376*, 305–317. [CrossRef] [PubMed]
15. Goldstein, E.J.C.; Citron, D.M.; Gerding, D.N.; Wilcox, M.H.; Gabryelski, L.; Pedley, A.; Zeng, Z.; Dorr, M.B. Bezlotoxumab for the Prevention of Recurrent *Clostridioides difficile* Infection: 12-Month Observational Data From the Randomized Phase III Trial, MODIFY II. *Clin. Infect. Dis.* **2020**, *71*, 1102–1105. [CrossRef] [PubMed]
16. Gerding, D.N.; Kelly, C.P.; Rahav, G.; Lee, C.; Dubberke, E.R.; Kumar, P.N.; Yacyshyn, B.; Kao, D.; Eves, K.; Ellison, M.C.; et al. Bezlotoxumab for Prevention of Recurrent *Clostridium difficile* Infection in Patients at Increased Risk for Recurrence. *Clin. Infect. Dis.* **2018**, *67*, 649–656. [CrossRef] [PubMed]
17. Mikamo, H.; Aoyama, N.; Sawata, M.; Fujimoto, G.; Dorr, M.B.; Yoshinari, T. The effect of bezlotoxumab for prevention of recurrent *Clostridium difficile* infection (CDI) in Japanese patients. *J. Infect. Chemother.* **2018**, *24*, 123–129. [CrossRef]
18. Prabhu, V.S.; Dubberke, E.R.; Dorr, M.B.; Elbasha, E.; Cossrow, N.; Jiang, Y.; Marcella, S. Cost-effectiveness of Bezlotoxumab Compared With Placebo for the Prevention of Recurrent *Clostridium difficile* Infection. *Clin. Infect. Dis.* **2018**, *66*, 355–362. [CrossRef]

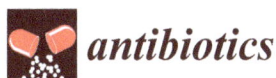

Communication

The Regulatory Approach for Faecal Microbiota Transplantation as Treatment for *Clostridioides difficile* Infection in Italy

Maria Chiara de Stefano *, Benedetta Mazzanti, Francesca Vespasiano, Letizia Lombardini and Massimo Cardillo

Italian National Transplant Centre, Istituto Superiore di Sanità, 00161 Rome, Italy; benedetta.mazzanti@iss.it (B.M.); francesca.vespasiano@iss.it (F.V.); letizia.lombardini@iss.it (L.L.); massimo.cardillo@iss.it (M.C.)
* Correspondence: mariachiara.destefano@iss.it

Abstract: Faecal microbiota transplantation (FMT) is regarded as an efficacious treatment for recurrent *C. difficile* infection. Unfortunately, widespread patient access is hindered by regulatory hurdles, which are the primary barriers to incorporating FMT into clinical practice. At the European and International level, there is no uniform perspective on FMT classification, and a coordinated effort is desirable to solve this regulatory puzzle. In this communication, we report the regulatory principles and the implementation approach for FMT application in Italy. Our experience suggests that the EU Tissue and Cell Directives are suited to ensure safe and efficient FMT for *C. difficile* management, especially through extensive high-quality donor selection and full traceability maintenance.

Keywords: *Clostridioides difficile* (*C. difficile*); faecal microbiota transplantation; FMT; FMT regulation; regulatory framework; EU Tissue and Cell Directive

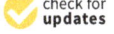

Citation: de Stefano, M.C.; Mazzanti, B.; Vespasiano, F.; Lombardini, L.; Cardillo, M. The Regulatory Approach for Faecal Microbiota Transplantation as Treatment for *Clostridioides difficile* Infection in Italy. *Antibiotics* 2022, 11, 480. https://doi.org/10.3390/antibiotics11040480

Academic Editor: Guido Granata

Received: 15 March 2022
Accepted: 3 April 2022
Published: 5 April 2022

Publisher's Note: MDPI stays neutral with regard to jurisdictional claims in published maps and institutional affiliations.

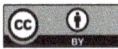

Copyright: © 2022 by the authors. Licensee MDPI, Basel, Switzerland. This article is an open access article distributed under the terms and conditions of the Creative Commons Attribution (CC BY) license (https://creativecommons.org/licenses/by/4.0/).

1. Regulatory Approaches for Faecal Microbiota Transplantation in *Clostridioides difficile* Infection (CDI) Management

Disease recurrence is a relevant issue in CDI management, as up to 25% of patients experience at least one recurrence within 8 weeks of successful antibiotic therapy for the initial episode, and a first recurrence, in turn, increases the risk of subsequent recurrences [1,2]. This scenario can negatively impact the rate of hospitalization and patient survival as well as the clinical and healthcare burden [1,3,4]. In addition to risk factors such as advanced age, immune status, comorbidities, and continued antibiotics use, poor bacterial diversity of gut microbiota has been implicated in the development of recurrent CDI infection (rCDI) [2,5]. Unfortunately, antibiotics treatment for CDI, such as vancomycin and fidaxomicin, can affect the function and reduce the overall species diversity of gut microbiota, predisposing patients to rCDI and leading to a vicious cycle of recurrent disease [2]. A large body of evidence supports the role of faecal microbiota transplantation (FMT) in restoring colonization resistance to *C. difficile* [6–8], and such a therapeutic approach is recommended for patients with multiple CDI recurrences after failing antibiotics therapy by the European Society for Microbiology and Infectious Diseases as well as the American College of Gastroenterology [9,10]. As the term implies, faecal microbiota transplantation consists of transferring a faecal sample from a healthy donor into the gastrointestinal tract of a patient. A recent survey reported that approximately 2000 hospital-based FMT procedures were performed across European countries in 2019, with most referred to CDI clinical indication [11]. Despite the growing demand for FMT for patients with multiple recurrences of CDI, its incorporation into clinical practice remains a challenging task [11,12]. Indeed, no uniform perspective on FMT classification exists, and the regulatory authorities have developed different approaches to oversee the clinical FMT framework. The U.S. Food and Drug Administration (FDA) considers faecal microbiota a new biological drug, even though the introduction of enforcement discretion allows FMT use without an Investigational New Drug Application (IND) to treat *C. difficile* infection not responding to standard therapies [13]. In the U.K., FMT was initially regulated under the Human Tissue Authority, but it has been falling under the definition of a medicinal product and into the remit of the Medicines and Health care products Regulatory Agency since 2015 [14]. The U.K. change of perspective reflects the ongoing uncertainty surrounding the regulatory framework for faecal microbiota, considering that little is known about the active component and intrinsic mechanism of the action of FMT. The classification as a drug implies a strict monitoring of microbiota processing since the stool would be industrially manufactured in a batch-wise process to be placed on the market [15]. However, a stool is not a standardized mixture of bacteria, and the composition of a stool by itself is highly heterogeneous, donor-specific, and associated with significant day-to-day variability, even from a single individual [14,16]. Moreover, it is likely that a positive effect on FMT success rate in rCDI is given by the transfer of a complete faecal microbiome rather than specific bacterial strains [17]. Overall, high- microbial diversity and the balanced constitution of Bacteroidetes and Firmicutes of the donor stool correlate with improved FMT efficacy [18]. It is known that *C. difficile* colonization is associated with a marked decrease in Bacteroidetes and Firmicutes and a high increase in Proteobacteria [19]. Interestingly, FMT shifts the patient faecal microbiota profile to that of the healthy donor with relative reductions in Proteobacteria and relative increases in Bacteroidetes and Firmicutes [20]. Therefore, FMT reverses the dysbiotic state, restoring the normal composition of gut microbiota, and so it also has a significant impact on the host immune system and the metabolism of secondary bile acids, which can inhibit *C. difficile* germination and vegetative growth [19]. However, the underlying mechanism for FMT remains not fully understood, and further investigation is needed for the development of standardized microbiota replacement therapies.

In this context, the European Commission has left decision making in the hands of the individual Member States and left them free to decide on the most suitable framework at the national level, even though several European countries released no official determination on FMT regulation. Currently, some European Member States such as the Netherlands, Belgium, and Italy, have included faecal microbiota under the tissues and cells regulation, while in other countries, including France and Germany, stool has been classified as a drug [14]. However, it is worth mentioning the clear position of the United European Gastroenterology-funded working group on this issue, as it considers the stool a transplant product and demands that competent authorities supply a comprehensive regulatory framework to ensure FMT broad access and safety [21]. Accordingly, the Italian National Transplant Centre (CNT) has been leading the Italian National FMT Program for three years, addressed to all Italian FMT centres, with the aim of coordinating and standardizing the clinical framework for the application of FMT in rCDI.

2. Principles and Implementation of the Italian Regulatory Approach for FMT

The major challenges for the application of FMT as a treatment for rCDI are achieving well-defined safety and quality standards as well as ensuring FMT availability for patients. Many of the potential safety risks are linked to the donor selection and screening process, as an important safety alert about the transmission of multi-drug-resistant organisms through FMT has recently been released [22]. Therefore, stool samples need to be tested for antibiotic-resistant bacteria including methicillin-resistant Staphylococcus aureus (MRSA), vancomycin-resistant Enterococci (VRE), extended-spectrum β-lactamase-producing Enterobacteriaceae, and carbapenem-resistant Enterobacteriaceae/carbapenemase-producing Enterobacteriaceae. In Italy, all steps from donation to patient follow-up, including donor's selection and stool processing, must follow the stringent safety and quality requirements in compliance with Directives 2006/17/EC and 2006/86/EC implementing the European Union Tissues and Cells Directive (EUTCD) on the quality and safety of tissues and cells. In particular, Directive 2004/23/EC (EUTCD) lays down standards of quality and safety covering the donation, procurement, testing, processing, preservation, storage, and distribution of human tissues and cells [23]. In addition, specific Italian National guidance providing technical information on how to apply FMT in rCDI setting was issued, and the key characteristics have already been described [24]. As shown in Figure 1, the FMT process consists of sequential steps, from the patient selection to the follow-up evaluation, and it is based on a systematic and multidisciplinary approach requiring the involvement of an expert panel of microbiologists, gastroenterologists, and infectious disease specialists. In order to establish an FMT service, appropriate operational procedures must be in place.

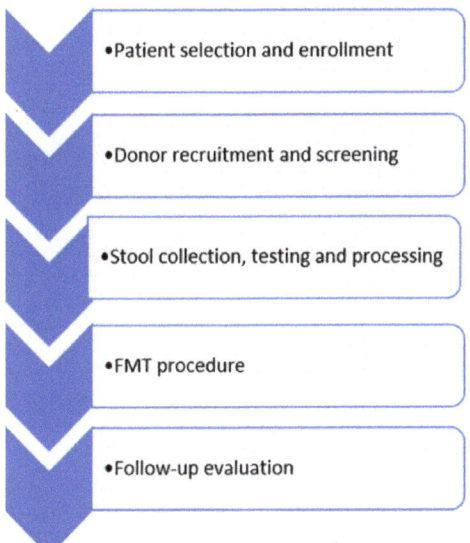

Figure 1. FMT process basic flow chart. The main sequential steps are represented.

Table 1 describes the measures required for FMT, as provided for the Italian National FMT Program and in accordance with EUTCD and the recommendations published by the European Directorate for the Quality of Medicines and HealthCare (EDQM) of the Council of Europe [25].

Table 1. Minimum requirements for FMT centres according to the Italian National FMT Program, EUTCD, and EDQM recommendations (4th edition).

EU Legislation	EDQM Guidance Principles	Italian National FMT Program Implementation Approaches
EC/23/2004 Art. 11;13;16;17;18 EC/86/2006 Art. 3;5;6EC/17/2006 Art. 2	Integrate FMT into a quality management system	- Use detailed written SOPs for each FMT activity (quality system in place). - Appoint a qualified responsible person and organizational chart which clearly defines roles and responsibilities in the FMT process. - Ensure continuous training and competency assessment of personnel involved. - Register the performance of all processing steps including the follow-up data. - Record any deviation, adverse events, and reactions. Notify the CNT of any serious adverse events and/or reactions. - Develop and use informed consents for both donors and patients according to National and International standards.

Table 1. Cont.

EU Legislation	EDQM Guidance Principles	Italian National FMT Program Implementation Approaches
EC/23/2004 Art. 12;13;14;15 EC/17/2006 Art. 3;4;5	Supply high-quality donor selection and testing	- Provide a standardized, three-step donor selection process, including a written questionnaire to assess medical history and lifestyle habits to exclude risk factors for infectious diseases, blood and stool testing for any potentially transmittable disease, and a further questionnaire and stool testing the day of donation. - Obtain and maintain the European (or equivalent) accreditation for microbiological testing. - Verify the blood and stool screening testing acceptability. - Develop formal procedures for minimizing the risk of cross-contamination for donating, including establishing a dedicated donor bathroom and utilizing sterile containers and utensils.
EC/23/2004 Art. 19;20;21;22;23;28 EC/86/2006 Art. 3;4	Guarantee the quality and safety of stool processing	- Identify a processing workspace within a Level 2 biosafety laboratory. - Adopt operating procedures for stool handling complying with European and National guidelines, in accordance with scientific and technical progress. - Validate and maintain the equipment and materials as well as any critical manipulation step influencing the quality and safety of the product. - Use single-use sterile consumables and reagents, when possible. - Specify expiry timescales for the stool storage, counting the microbial load of the fresh preparation compared to defrosted aliquots.
EC/23/2004 Art. 8; Art. 10;25 EC/86/2006 Art. 9;10	Ensure full traceability	- Develop an electronic central system of recording and labelling, ensuring full traceability from donor to recipient and vice versa. - Provide the following processing records: unique donor identification number, donor testing results, date and time of donation, identification of recipient, donation macroscopic features, consumable and reagent lot numbers and volumes used, operator name, date and time of stool manipulation, storage instructions, and expiry date. - For every critical activity, the materials, equipment, and personnel involved must be identified and documented. - Provide a formal written statement confirming the final FMT product compliance with quality and safety requirements prior to administration.

In particular, a quality system ensuring minimal risk for product, personnel, donor, and patient and maximal quality of the process shall be developed by the FMT centre, including an organizational chart with a clearly stated hierarchy of duties and responsibilities of the personnel involved. Personnel education and training need to be ensured and traced by specific procedures and records. Standard Operating Procedures (SOPs) for each step of the process shall be in place and periodically updated. According to Directive 2004/23/EC, a system shall be implemented with the aim to register and transmit to the Italian National Competent Authority (i.e., CNT) the information about serious adverse events and reactions influencing the quality and safety of FMT and attributable to the procurement, testing, processing, storage, distribution, and clinical application. The procurement of faecal microbiota shall be authorized only after informed consent of the donor once adequate information has been given. Likewise, consent approved by the local ethics committee shall be provided to the patient undergoing FMT. Donor recruitment and screening shall be carried out in compliance with the Italian National FMT program recommendations and in accordance with the European consensus guidelines [26]. Of note, the procurement procedures must preserve those properties of the stool material that are required for their ultimate clinical use and, at the same time, should be addressed to minimize the risk of microbiological contamination during stool collection and processing. Preferably, a dedicated bathroom should be used, or detailed instructions shall be provided to the donor in case of collection at home. In addition, the processing facility should provide sterile faecal containers in order to prevent contamination, and the stool preservation condition should be strictly monitored. The donor screening tests must be carried out by authorized and qualified laboratories, using EC-marked testing kits where appropriate, and be validated for the purpose in accordance with current scientific knowledge. Regardless of the findings, all results of the donor evaluation and testing procedures shall be documented. In order to guarantee the quality of stool handling, the laboratory is required to define critical parameters affecting the stool processing and the viability and composition of the microbial content. Moreover, a biosafety Level 2 processing facility is needed, and all personnel involved in processing activities must be trained and provided with protective clothing appropriate for the type of processing, wearing a sterile gown, sterile gloves, glasses, and a face shield or protective mask. Critical reagents and materials must meet documented requirements and specifications and, when applicable, should be single-use and disposable. The frozen faecal material should be stored in dedicated freezers under controlled storage conditions, subjected to appropriate monitoring, and provided with alerts for temperature. Maximum storage time shall be defined and validated by counting the microbial load of defrosted aliquots compared to the fresh preparation [27]. For each critical activity, the materials, equipment, and personnel involved must be identified and documented. The materials traceability shall be assured by recording data on materials and reagents (e.g., name of product and producer, lot, expiry date, and results of internal quality controls) used for the processing, and quality tests shall be successfully passed for the release of the final product. Overall, it is the responsibility of the processing laboratory to confirm final product compliance with the quality and safety requirements prior to distribution and administration. Finally, the implementation of the above-mentioned principles is a preliminary condition so that an FMT centre can be subjected to auditing by the CNT for the authorization purpose. Before applying for authorization, the FMT centre should review each step of the process to identify and improve all critical issues and procedures failing to comply with requirements of EU Directives/national law as well as the EDQM recommendations. Of note, the missing knowledge of the EU Directives requirements and the poor understanding on how to set out the SOPs often hamper and postpone the finalization of the accreditation process. More worryingly, a few centres are not fully aware that they have to report to the National Competent Authority for clinical FMT application. With the aim of supporting healthcare professionals at a practical level and promoting efficacious and safe clinical application, the CNT provides rules and organizational support to centres committed to developing a local clinical FMT framework in adherence to the European Tissue Act. Moreover, in order to foster continuous harmonization and to prevent fragmentation following different local approaches, the CNT promotes collaborative knowledge exchange through periodic virtual and face-to-face meetings as well as dissemination and training activities. However, it is worth noting that some differences remain regarding the organization of donor recruitment, the laboratory facilities and processing procedures. To monitor the overall functioning of the FMT centres network, the data of the centres' activities are collected in a dedicated database including quality and performance indicators such as the number of procedures performed according to Italian National FMT standards, transplant outcomes, any serious adverse events and/or reactions, as well as long-term follow-up evaluation. Currently, 57 patients (Female = 27, Male = 30; median age 70 years) have undergone FMT with faeces from 11 donors (Female = 8, Male = 3; median age 41 years). Overall, 68 transplants have been collected, as all patients were treated with at least one infusion, and 14 patients received multiple infusions. According to Ianiro G. et al. [28], our data show that sequential FMT is highly effective (success rate of 83% with single infusion versus 100% with sequential FMT). Notably, no serious adverse events and/or reactions were notified.

In order to gain insight into challenging issues, such as the FMT application in paediatric patients and in non-CDI clinical settings, a multidisciplinary network of experts in new potential indications for FMT is being established. Experts' participation in decision making will be strongly endorsed so that high-level evidence may be integrated more easily into clinical practice and translated into direct benefits for patients in terms of enhanced quality of care and safety. Meanwhile, to identify any patient safeguarding concerns, FMT in non-CDI indications must be conducted under a clinical trial to be submitted to the CNT for approval [24].

3. Conclusions

The FMT has been evaluated as a cost-effective strategy for the management of rCDI, with considerable cost savings mainly achieved by a significant reduction in the total days of hospital admission due to a faster recovery time [29]. Furthermore, emerging data support the intermediate to long-term safety profile of FMT for rCDI [30,31]. Interestingly, it has also been reported that FMT treatment could prevent as many as 32,000 CDI recurrences every year in the United States [32]. Therefore, the scale of FMT use may be increased to meet the significant need for patients with rCDI. Unfortunately, widespread access to this therapeutic option is hindered by regulatory frameworks' lack of uniformity, which is the primary barrier to embedding FMT into routine patient care. On one hand, faecal microbiota does not fall within the statutory scope of Directive 2004/23/EC on Tissue and Cells legislation because, although faeces are unquestionably substances of human origin, the human cells do not represent the active component [33]. On the other hand, the variability in gut microbial community composition and across stool samples does not meet the requirements of a batch-wise manufacturing process underlying the classification as a drug [15,34]. However, Member States' competent authorities agreed that FMT should be regulated by provisions equivalent to those existing for blood, tissue, and cells, because the FMT entails similar risks, including disease transmission [33]. For this reason, the Italian approach has been addressed to incorporate EUTCD and EDQM recommendations within hospital settings, supporting the development of FMT centres complying with high safety and quality standards. In order to provide ready-to-use screened faeces preparations and to facilitate patient access to the FMT treatment, specific transplant programs, including stool banks, will be set up. To this aim, detailed stool banking guidance is being developed at a national level, in accordance with European and International consensus reports [35,36]. Our model provides a FMT transplant framework including a stool bank responsible for the processing, storage, and distribution of faeces preparations to clinical centres, as well as additional infrastructures needed for donor recruitment, selection, testing, patient treatment, and follow-up. In terms of feasibility, all the facilities may be part of the same organization or placed in different hospitals, under the responsibility of a qualified director who coordinates the activities according to shared, approved, and validated protocols. Overall, the development of strictly regulated FMT transplant frameworks is pivotal for increasing the cost effectiveness and coordinating an FMT transplant service by standardized pathways. Improving the standardization of the procedures is crucial, as different regulatory frameworks of FMT across Europe have a negative impact on equitable, safe, and timely treatment. We agree with Keller J.J. et al. that FMT should be regarded as a transplant and covered by the EUTCD because donated faeces are not subjected to substantial modifications prior to administration [21]. Furthermore, as reported above, the EUTCD implementation ensures an extensive high-quality donor selection and testing as well as monitoring of the traceability and potential risk profile changes.

In conclusion, it has clearly emerged that there is a need for increased harmonization in FMT regulation among Member States. The achievement of a coordinated European approach, including establishing a custom regulatory solution, will contribute to the large-scale accredited use of FMT for patients with rCDI.

Author Contributions: Conceptualization, M.C.d.S., B.M. and L.L.; Analysis: F.V.; writing—original draft preparation, M.C.d.S.; writing—review and editing, M.C.d.S., B.M. and L.L.; supervision, M.C. All authors have read and agreed to the published version of the manuscript.

Funding: This communication received no external funding.

Conflicts of Interest: The authors declare no conflict of interest.

References

1. Sheitoyan-Pesant, C.; Abou Chakra, C.N.; Pépin, J.; Marcil-Héguy, A.; Nault, V.; Valiquette, L. Clinical and Healthcare Burden of Multiple Recurrences of Clostridium difficile Infection. *Clin. Infect. Dis.* **2016**, *62*, 574–580. [CrossRef] [PubMed]
2. Chilton, C.H.; Pickering, D.S.; Freeman, J. Microbiologic factors affecting Clostridium difficile recurrence. *Clin. Microbiol. Infect.* **2018**, *24*, 476–482. [CrossRef] [PubMed]
3. Olsen, M.A.; Yan, Y.; Reske, K.A.; Zilberberg, M.D.; Dubberke, E.R. Recurrent Clostridium difficile infection is associated with increased mortality. *Clin. Microbiol. Infect.* **2015**, *21*, 164–170. [CrossRef] [PubMed]
4. Singh, T.; Bedi, P.; Bumrah, K.; Singh, J.; Rai, M.; Seelam, S. Updates in Treatment of Recurrent *Clostridium difficile* Infection. *J. Clin. Med. Res.* **2019**, *11*, 465–471. [CrossRef]
5. Kelly, C.P. Can we identify patients at high risk of recurrent *Clostridium difficile* infection? *Clin. Microbiol. Infect.* **2012**, *18* (Suppl. 6), 21–27. [CrossRef]
6. Rokkas, T.; Gisbert, J.P.; Gasbarrini, A.; Hold, G.L.; Tilg, H.; Malfertheiner, P. A network meta-analysis of randomized controlled trials exploring the role of fecal microbiota transplantation in recurrent Clostridium Difficile Infection. *United Eur. Gastroenterol. J.* **2019**, *7*, 1051–1063. [CrossRef]
7. Hvas, C.L.; Jørgensen, S.M.D.; Jørgensen, S.P.; Storgaard, M.; Lemming, L.; Hansen, M.M.; Erikstrup, C.; Dahlerup, J.F. Fecal microbiota transplantation is superior to fidaxomicin for treatment of recurrent *Clostridium difficile* infection. *Gastroenterology* **2019**, *156*, 1324–1332. [CrossRef]
8. Kelly, C.R.; Khoruts, A.; Staley, C.; Sadowsky, M.J.; Abd, M.; Alani, M.; Bakow, B.; Curran, P.; McKenney, J.; Tisch, A.; et al. Effect of fecal microbiota transplantation on recurrence in multiply recurrent *Clostridium difficile* infection: A randomized trial. *Ann. Intern. Med.* **2016**, *165*, 609–616. [CrossRef]
9. Debast, S.B.; Bauer, M.P.; Kuijper, E.J.; on behalf of the Committee. European Society of Clinical Microbiology and Infectious Diseases: Update of the treatment guidance document for Clostridium difficile infection. *Clin. Microbiol. Infect.* **2014**, *20* (Suppl. 2), 1–26. [CrossRef]
10. McDonald, L.C.; Gerding, D.N.; Johnson, S.; Bakken, J.S.; Carroll, K.C.; Coffin, S.E.; Dubberke, E.R.; Garey, K.W.; Gould, C.V.; Kelly, C.; et al. Clinical Practice Guidelines for Clostridium difficile Infection in Adults and Children: 2017 Update by the Infectious Diseases Society of America (IDSA) and Society for Healthcare Epidemiology of America (SHEA). *Clin. Infect. Dis.* **2018**, *66*, e1–e48. [CrossRef]
11. Baunwall, S.M.D.; Terveer, E.M.; Dahlerup, J.F.; Erikstrup, C.; Arkkila, P.; Vehreschild, M.J.G.T.; Ianiro, G.; Gasbarrini, A.; Sokol, H.; Kump, P.K.; et al. The use of Faecal Microbiota Transplantation (FMT) in Europe: A Europe-wide survey. *Lancet Reg. Health Eur.* **2021**, *9*, 100181. [CrossRef] [PubMed]
12. Kelly, B.J.; Tebas, P. Clinical practice and infrastructure review of fecal microbiota transplantation for *Clostridium difficile* infection. *Chest* **2018**, *153*, 266–277. [CrossRef] [PubMed]
13. Enforcement Policy Regarding Investigational New Drug Requirements for Use of Fecal Microbiota for Transplantation to Treat Clostridium difficile Infection Not Responsive to Standard Therapies. Available online: https://www.fda.gov/downloads/BiologicsBloodVaccines/GuidanceComplianceRegulatoryInformation/Guidances/Vacines/UCM488223.pdf (accessed on 1 February 2022).
14. Merrick, B.; Allen, L.; Masirah, M.; Zain, N.; Forbes, B.; Shawcross, D.L.; Goldenberg, S.D. Regulation, risk and safety of Faecal Microbiota Transplant. *Infect. Prev. Pract.* **2020**, *2*, 100069. [CrossRef] [PubMed]
15. Mikkelsen, T.A.; McIlroy, J.R.; Mimiague, M.; Rouanet, A.; Sterkman, L. Towards an EU-wide suitable regulatory framework for faecally derived, industrially manufactured medicinal products. *United Eur. Gastroenterol. J.* **2020**, *8*, 351–352. [CrossRef]
16. Edelstein, C.A.; Kassam, Z.; Daw, J.; Smith, M.B.; Kelly, C.R. The regulation of fecal microbiota for transplantation: An international perspective for policy and public health. *Clin. Res. Regul. Aff.* **2015**, *32*, 99–107. [CrossRef]
17. Bibbò, S.; Settanni, C.R.; Porcari, S.; Bocchino, E.; Ianiro, G.; Cammarota, G.; Gasbarrini, A. Fecal Microbiota Transplantation: Screening and Selection to Choose the Optimal Donor. *J. Clin. Med.* **2020**, *9*, 1757. [CrossRef]
18. Ng, S.C.; Kamm, M.A.; Yeoh, Y.K.; Chan, P.K.S.; Zuo, T.; Tang, W.; Sood, A.; Andoh, A.; Ohmiya, N.; Zhou, Y.; et al. Scientific frontiers in faecal microbiota transplantation: Joint document of Asia-Pacific Association of Gastroenterology (APAGE) and Asia-Pacific Society for Digestive Endoscopy (APSDE). *Gut* **2020**, *69*, 83–91. [CrossRef]
19. Khoruts, A.; Sadowsky, M.J. Understanding the mechanisms of faecal microbiota transplantation. *Nat. Rev. Gastroenterol. Hepatol.* **2016**, *13*, 508–516. [CrossRef]
20. Weingarden, A.; González, A.; Vázquez-Baeza, Y.; Weiss, S.; Humphry, G.; Berg-Lyons, D.; Knights, D.; Unno, T.; Bobr, A.; Kang, J.; et al. Dynamic changes in short- and long-term bacterial composition following fecal microbiota transplantation for recurrent Clostridium difficile infection. *Microbiome* **2015**, *3*, 10. [CrossRef]

21. Keller, J.J.; Vehreschild, M.J.; Hvas, C.L.; Jørgensen, S.M.; Kupciskas, J.; Link, A.; Mulder, C.J.J.; Goldenberg, S.D.; Arasaradnam, R.; Sokol, H.; et al. Stool for fecal microbiota transplantation should be classified as a transplant product and not as a drug. *United Eur. Gastroenterol. J.* **2019**, *7*, 1408–1410. [CrossRef]
22. FDA. Fecal Microbiota for Transplantation: Safety Alert—Risk of Serious Adverse Events Likely Due to Transmission of Pathogenic Organisms. Available online: https://www.fda.gov/safety/medical-product-safety-information/fecal-microbiota-transplantation-safety-alert-risk-serious-adverse-events-likely-due-transmission (accessed on 3 February 2022).
23. European Parliament, Council of the European Union. Directive 2004/23/EC of the European Parliament and of the Council of 31 March 2004 on setting standards of quality and safety for the donation, procurement, testing, processing, preservation, storage and distribution of human tissues and cells. *Off. J. Eur. Union* **2004**, *L102*, 48–58.
24. de Stefano, M.C.; Mazzanti, B.; Vespasiano, F.; Cammarota, G.; Ianiro, G.; Masucci, L.; Sanguinetti, M.; Gasbarrini, A.; Lombardini, L.; Cardillo, M. The Italian National Faecal Microbiota Transplantation Program: A coordinated effort against *Clostridioides difficile* infection. *Ann. dell'Ist. Super. Sanita* **2021**, *57*, 239–243.
25. Council of Europe. European Directorate for the Quality of Medicines & HealthCare (EDQM). 4th Edition of the Guide to the Quality and Safety of Tissues and Cells for Human Application. Available online: https://www.edqm.eu/en/organs-tissues-and-cells-technical-guides (accessed on 3 February 2022).
26. Cammarota, G.; Ianiro, G.; Tilg, H.; Rajilić-Stojanović, M.; Kump, P.; Satokari, R.; Sokol, H.; Arkkila, P.; Pintus, C.; Hart, A.; et al. European consensus conference on faecal microbiota transplantation in clinical practice. *Gut* **2017**, *66*, 569–580. [CrossRef] [PubMed]
27. Quaranta, G.; Fancello, G.; Ianiro, G.; Graffeo, R.; Gasbarrini, A.; Cammarota, G.; Sanguinetti, M.; Masucci, L. Laboratory handling practice for faecal microbiota transplantation. *J. Appl. Microbiol.* **2020**, *128*, 893–898. [CrossRef]
28. Ianiro, G.; Maida, M.; Burisch, J.; Simonelli, C.; Hold, G.; Ventimiglia, M.; Gasbarrini, A.; Cammarota, G. Efficacy of different faecal microbiota transplantation protocols for *Clostridium difficile* infection: A systematic review and meta-analysis. *United Eur. Gastroenterol. J.* **2018**, *6*, 1232–1244. [CrossRef]
29. Dehlholm-Lambertsen, E.; Hall, B.K.; Jørgensen, S.M.D.; Jørgensen, C.W.; Jensen, M.E.; Larsen, S.; Jensen, J.S.; Lars, E.; Dahlerup, J.F.; Hvas, C.L. Cost savings following faecal microbiota transplantation for recurrent *Clostridium difficile* infection. *Ther. Adv. Gastroenterol.* **2019**, *12*, 1756284819843002. [CrossRef]
30. Saha, S.; Mara, K.; Pardi, D.S.; Khanna, S. Long-term safety of fecal microbiota transplantation for recurrent *Clostridioides difficile* infection. *Gastroenterology* **2021**, *160*, 1961–1969. [CrossRef]
31. Ooijevaar, R.E.; van Nood, E.; Goorhuis, A.; Terveer, E.M.; van Prehn, J.; Verspaget, H.W.; van Beurden, Y.H.; Dijkgraaf, M.G.W.; Keller, J.J. Ten-Year Follow-Up of Patients Treated With Fecal Microbiota Transplantation for Recurrent *Clostridioides Difficile* Infection from a Randomized Controlled Trial and Review of the Literature. *Microorganisms* **2021**, *9*, 548. [CrossRef]
32. Mamoon, L.; Olesen, S.W. Fecal Microbiota Transplants Annually and Their Positive Clinical Impact. *Clin. Transl. Gastroenterol.* **2020**, *1*, e00247. [CrossRef]
33. European Commission. Evaluation of the Union legislation on Blood, Tissues and Cells. 2019. Available online: https://ec.europa.eu/health/sites/health/files/blood_tissues_organs/docs/swd_2019_376_en.pdf (accessed on 3 February 2022).
34. Terveer, E.M.; van Beurden, Y.H.; Goorhuis, A.; Seegers, J.F.M.L.; Bauer, M.P.; van Nood, E.; Dijkgraaf, M.G.W.; Mulder, C.J.J.; Vandenbroucke-Grauls, C.M.J.E.; Verspaget, H.W.; et al. How to: Establish and run a stool bank. *Clin. Microbiol. Infect.* **2017**, *23*, 924–930. [CrossRef]
35. Cammarota, G.; Ianiro, G.; Kelly, C.R.; Mullish, B.H.; Allegretti, J.R.; Kassam, Z.; Putignani, L.; Fischer, M.; Keller, J.J.; Costello, S.P.; et al. International consensus conference on stool banking for faecal microbiota transplantation in clinical practice. *Gut* **2019**, *68*, 2111–2121. [CrossRef] [PubMed]
36. Keller, J.J.; Ooijevaar, R.E.; Hvas, C.L.; Terveer, E.M.; Lieberknecht, S.C.; Högenauer, C.; Arkkila, P.; Sokol, H.; Gridnyev, O.; Mégraud, F.; et al. A standardised model for stool banking for faecal microbiota transplantation: A consensus report from a multidisciplinary UEG working group. *United Eur. Gastroenterol. J.* **2021**, *9*, 229–247. [CrossRef] [PubMed]

MDPI AG
Grosspeteranlage 5
4052 Basel
Switzerland
Tel.: +41 61 683 77 34

Antibiotics Editorial Office
E-mail: antibiotics@mdpi.com
www.mdpi.com/journal/antibiotics

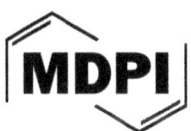

Disclaimer/Publisher's Note: The title and front matter of this reprint are at the discretion of the . The publisher is not responsible for their content or any associated concerns. The statements, opinions and data contained in all individual articles are solely those of the individual Editor and contributors and not of MDPI. MDPI disclaims responsibility for any injury to people or property resulting from any ideas, methods, instructions or products referred to in the content.